Stepping Hill Hospital

R30046

KT-448-158

Books are to be returned on or before
the last date below.

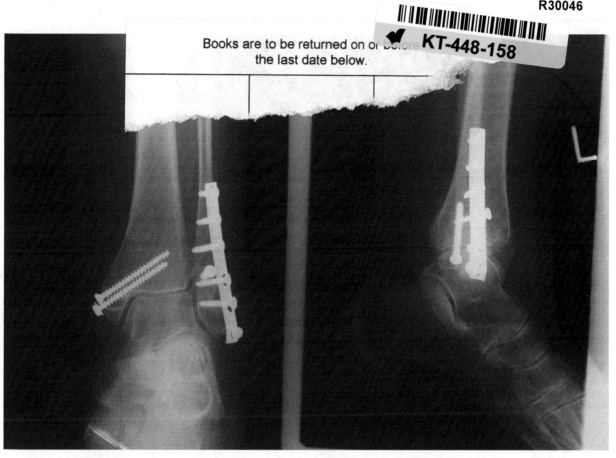

# Succeeding in the FRCS (T&O) Part 1 Exam

## Multiple choice revision questions in Trauma and Orthopaedics (T&O)

### Fahad G Attar & Talal Ibrahim

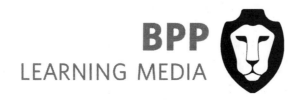

BPP
LEARNING MEDIA

610·76 ATT

**First edition October 2011**

ISBN 9781 4453 7954 8
e-ISBN 9781 4453 8574 7

**British Library Cataloguing-in-Publication Data**
A catalogue record for this book is available from the British Library

Published by
BPP Learning Media Ltd
BPP House, Aldine Place
London W12 8AA

www.bpp.com/health

Typeset by Replika Press Pvt Ltd, India
Printed in the United Kingdom

Your learning materials, published by BPP Learning Media Ltd, are printed on paper sourced from sustainable, managed forests.

All rights reserved. No part of this publication may be reproduced, stored in a retrieval system or transmitted in any form or by any means, electronic, mechanical, photocopying, recording or otherwise, without the prior written permission of BPP Learning Media.

The views expressed in this book are those of BPP Learning Media and not those of the NHS. BPP Learning Media are in no way associated with or endorsed by the NHS.

The contents of this book are intended as a guide and not professional advice. Although every effort has been made to ensure that the contents of this book are correct at the time of going to press, BPP Learning Media, the Editor and the Author make no warranty that the information in this book is accurate or complete and accept no liability for any loss or damage suffered by any person acting or refraining from acting as a result of the material in this book.

Every effort has been made to contact the copyright holders of any material reproduced within this publication. If any have been inadvertently overlooked, BPP Learning Media will be pleased to make the appropriate credits in any subsequent reprints or editions.

**A note about copyright**

Dear Customer

What does the little © mean and why does it matter?

Your market-leading BPP books, course materials and e-learning materials do not write and update themselves. People write them on their own behalf or as employees of an organisation that invests in this activity. Copyright law protects their livelihoods. It does so by creating rights over the use of the content.

Breach of copyright is a form of theft – as well as being a criminal offence in some jurisdictions, it is potentially a serious beach of professional ethics.

With current technology, things might seem a bit hazy but, basically, without the express permission of BPP Learning Media:

- Photocopying our materials is a breach of copyright
- Scanning, ripcasting or conversion of our digital materials into different file formats, uploading them to facebook or e-mailing them to your friends is a breach of copyright

You can, of course, sell your books, in the form in which you have bought them – once you have finished with them. (Is this fair to your fellow students? We update for a reason.)  But the e-products are sold on a single user license basis: we do not supply 'unlock' codes to people who have bought them secondhand.

And what about outside the UK? BPP Learning Media strives to make our materials available at prices students can afford by local printing arrangements, pricing policies and partnerships which are clearly listed on our website. A tiny minority ignore this and indulge in criminal activity by illegally photocopying our material or supporting organisations that do. If they act illegally and unethically in one area, can you really trust them?

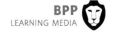

# Contents

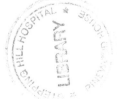

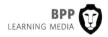

Contents

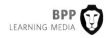

# About the Publisher

BPP Learning Media is dedicated to supporting aspiring professionals with top quality learning material. BPP Learning Media's commitment to success is shown by our record of quality, innovation and market leadership in paper-based and e-learning materials. BPP Learning Media's study materials are written by professionally-qualified specialists who know from personal experience the importance of top quality materials for success.

Every effort has been made to ensure the accuracy of the material contained within this guide. However it must be noted that medical treatments, drug dosages/formulations, equipment, procedures and best practice are currently evolving within the field of medicine.

Readers are therefore advised always to check the most up-to-date information relating to:

- The applicable drug manufacturer's product information and data sheets relating to recommended dose/formulation, administration and contraindications.
- The latest applicable local and national guidelines.
- The latest applicable local and national codes of conduct and safety protocols.

It is the responsibility of the practitioner, based on their own knowledge and expertise, to diagnose, treat and ensure the safety and best interests of the patient are maintained.

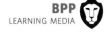

# Acknowledgements

We would like to thank our families for their support and understanding throughout the FRCS exam period and also for the late nights and loss of weekends during this project.

We are grateful to Assad Aziz Qureshi for his initiative and additional help through various stages in the overall culmination of this book.

We would also like to show our gratitude to all the consultants on our rotation who have been very supportive and helpful throughout our training period.

# Contributers

**Ibrar Majid**
SpR Trauma & Orthopaedics
Manchester

**Haroon A Mann**
SpR Trauma & Orthopaedics
London

**Assad Aziz Qureshi**
SpR Trauma & Orthopaedics
East Midlands

**Suhayl Tafazal**
SpR Trauma & Orthopaedics
East Midlands

**Gautam Tawari**
SpR Trauma & Orthopaedics
Wrightington

# Editors

**Fahad G. Attar, FRCS (Tr&Orth)**
Clinical Fellow in Arthroplasty and Lower Extremity Reconstruction Surgery
University Hospitals of Leicester NHS Trust
East Midland Rotation, Leicester

**Talal Ibrahim, MB BS (Hons.) MD FRCS (Tr&Orth)**
Clinical Lecturer in Orthopaedic Surgery
University of Leicester, Leicester
Clinical Fellow in Paediatric Orthopaedic Surgery
Great Ormond Street Hospital for Children, London

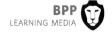

# Preface

While the orthopaedic literature is replete with works of outstanding calibre, our knowledge-base continues to grow with further developments worldwide in the field of Trauma & Orthopaedics. Amidst this backdrop of ever improving dissemination of knowledge, we introduce this latest addition to the succession of orthopaedic teaching materials. The inception of this project, can be traced back to our experiences and reflections while preparing for the written element of the FRCS (Orth) examination.

In devising this text, we have endeavoured to encompass the entire breadth of the FRCS (Orth) syllabus and we have intentionally not aimed for a level of abstraction greater than that which would be expected for the exam. We have attempted to provide comprehensive explanations for each question stem; suitably furnished with appropriate references based on recent review articles and current texts to pique the more discerning trainee's curiosity. As well as serving as a concise aide memoire and a means of identifying topics where further directed study is desirable for those sitting the exam, we hope that orthopaedic practitioners of all levels will benefit from the knowledge enshrined within these pages.

Multiple choice questions (MCQ) are a relatively recent inclusion to the FRCS (Orth) examination. The style allows for a vast scope of knowledge to be explored in a relatively short time and succinctly assesses reasoning and recall in equal measure. In preparation for the exam, we noted a distinct paucity in the available literature engendering a specific emphasis on this style of questioning set at a level suitable for the FRCS (Orth) exam. Only a few resources were available that matched astutely worded questions with a choice of several deliberately confusing answers. The pleasure in answering such questions for the enthusiastic orthopaedic trainee is analagous to that of completing a harsh Sudoku. As nature abhors a vacuum and with the solemn intention of filling this void, we stepped into the abyss and hence the inception of this book!

Guided by our ambition, this book is the product of our love and dedication to the scientific and, at times, sublime art which is Orthopaedics. We cannot hold ourselves above scrutiny and it is our intention that this book will be successively revised and contributed to by the readership to better meet the needs of the modern curriculum. Change is inexorable and we look forward from this humble beginning to the future of a continually growing and improving MCQ collection.

**Fahad Attar**
**Clinical Fellow in Arthroplasty and Lower Extremity Reconstruction Surgery**
**East Midlands Deanery**

**Talal Ibrahim**
**Clinical Lecturer in Orthopaedic Surgery**
**East Midlands Deanery**

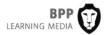

BPP
LEARNING MEDIA

# Foreword by Mr Tim Green

Assessments, tests and examinations have long been a part of medical training. These days, in response to the advice of educationalists, and for the future of our speciality, we must be certain that any system designed to select candidates must be clear, reproducible and fair. In the case of a final or exit type exam, these criteria are particularly important as they directly affect a candidate's future career.

Having sat the Intercollegiate Examination myself and now been an examiner for several years, I have been fortunate to see it from both sides of the table. What is most impressive is the effort expended to make sure that every exam is of the highest quality. Obvious efforts are made to expose the candidates to as wide a variety of cases and examiners in the clinical section, but less clear is the work that goes on behind the scenes to ensure a fair written exam.

Multiple choice questions on the face of it seem easy to write and to answer. Sadly, as we all know, reality brings inconsistency and lack of precision. The Intercollegiate Board subject all questions to panels of examiners before and after exams, constantly polishing and refining the wording and the subject until it can be shown to be reliable. Any that repeatedly fail to demonstrate success in picking out the best candidates will be dropped.

I know that the authors of this book have set themselves similar standards in writing this book of questions based on the broad spread of Orthopaedics. Hours of work have been spent researching, writing, validating and testing. They now represent a realistic example of the sort of questions seen in the Intercollegiate exam, and as such provide an ideal revision aid for the trainee approaching this final professional hurdle.

Tim Green
Consultant Orthopaedic Surgeon
Intercollegiate Examiner
MB ChB FRCS Ed. (Orth.)

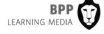

BPP
LEARNING MEDIA

# Foreword by Mr Chris Kershaw

The trouble with relying on experience as a guide to learning is that the final exam often comes first and only afterwards comes the lesson. The FRCS (Trauma & Orthopaedics) exam is set so that learning is demonstrated to be in place before the lessons become too harsh. Knowledge, judgement and skill are all requirements of a competent surgeon. Any way in which the knowledge can be revised and reinforced can only be a help, and this book seeks to aid stressed orthopaedic trainees in the run up to the all important test. As a wise consultant told me, 'Knowledge is like clay; the more that is thrown at you, the more will stick.' Hopefully this clay will stick.

I am admiring of anybody who can see a task such as this through to completion. Even writing Christmas cards exhaust me and something of this magnitude is impressive. George Orwell commented 'Writing a book is a horrible, exhausting struggle, like a long bout of some painful illness. One would never undertake such a thing if one were not driven on by something which one can neither resist nor understand.' I suppose the 'thing' here is the desire to help those who follow them through the crucible of the FRCS (Trauma & Orthopaedics), and that is a very creditable motive.

I am sure that those who use this book will find it helpful in the final months before the exam. Orthopaedic surgery is a dynamic subject and this book will hopefully continue to help learners of all types, evolving as orthopaedic surgery evolves.

**Chris Kershaw MB ChB FRCS**
**Consultant Orthopaedic Surgeon (University Hospitals of Leicester)**
**FRCS (Tr & Orth) Examiner**
**Retired Training Programme Director for South Trent**

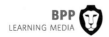

BPP
LEARNING MEDIA

# Basic Sciences

## Question Bank

Asad A Qureshi & Talal
Ibrahim

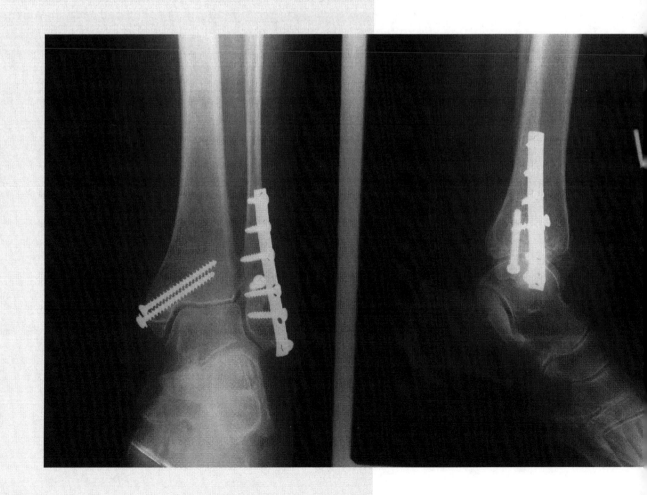

1.  Which of the following is **false** regarding the structure of human bone?
    A.  Contains osteoblasts which secrete osteoid through Howship's lacunae
    B.  Can be thought of as a composite material on many levels
    C.  Contains Volkman's canals connecting different Haversian systems
    D.  Contains BMPs which are members of the TGFβ family
    E.  Contains hydroxyapatite deposited in small crystals

2.  Achondroplasia gives rise to defects in which region of the growth plate?
    A.  Reserve zone
    B.  Zone of proliferation
    C.  Zone of maturation
    D.  Zone of degeneration
    E.  Zone of provisional calcification

3.  Which of the following is **false** regarding osteoclasts?
    A   They are multinuclear cells that are derived from the monocyte cell line
    B.  Microscopic ruffling of the cell border in contact with bone markedly increases the surface area for acidification and subsequent resorption
    C.  Attach to bone surfaces occurs via integrins
    D.  Apoptosis typically occurs after 10–14 days of activity
    E.  Express parathyroid hormone (PTH) receptors

4.  A patient is taken to theatre for repair of a median nerve injury after a screwdriver is inadvertently driven into his wrist. At surgery the findings are that of a crush injury with the epineurium disrupted but the architecture of individual fascicles and surrounding perineurium preserved. How would you classify this peripheral nerve injury?
    A.  First degree
    B.  Second degree
    C.  Third degree
    D.  Fourth degree
    E.  Fifth degree

5.  What is the expected order of recovery in nerve fibre sensory modalities after injury?
    A.  Pain, temperature, touch, proprioception
    B.  Temperature, pain, touch, proprioception
    C.  Proprioception, touch, temperature, pain
    D.  Touch, proprioception, temperature, pain
    E.  Slow simultaneous recovery of all modalities

6.  When articular cartilage is stained, a tidemark is seen separating which two regions in cross-section?
    A.  The calcified zone and the subchondral bone
    B.  The middle circular zone and the deep zone
    C.  The deep zone and the calcified zone
    D.  The superficial zone and the middle zone
    E.  The transition points in collagen fibre orientation

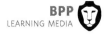
BPP
LEARNING MEDIA

7.  Regarding the menisci, which of the following statements is **false**?
    A.  The lateral meniscus is more mobile than the medial
    B.  The medial meniscus acts as a secondary restraint for anterior translation of the tibia when the ACL is sectioned
    C.  The majority of collagen fibres are arranged circumferentially
    D.  Collagen type II is the most abundant collagen type
    E.  Ninety percent of joint forces are transmitted through the menisci in knee flexion.

8.  Comparing cortical bone with cancellous bone, which of the following statements is **false**.
    A.  Cortical bone demonstrates more isotropicity than cancellous bone
    B.  Cortical bone has a greater metabolic cost than cancellous bone
    C.  Cortical bone is denser with a greater modulus of elasticity
    D.  Material properties are less dependent on porosity and more dependent on direction of applied force
    E.  Cortical bone remodels at a slower rate

9.  Regarding the structure of articular cartilage, which of the following is **false**?
    A.  Water content is greatest in the superficial zone
    B.  Aggrecan content is greatest in the deep zone
    C.  Collagen type IX crosslinks parallel longitudinal collagen chains forming a loose mesh in the superficial zone
    D.  Collagen type XI acts as a template for collagen fibril growth to occur
    E.  Proteoglycan content decreases with a period of joint immobilisation

10. Which of the following is an inhibitor of normal bone calcification?
    A.  Interleukin – 1 (IL1)
    B.  Interleukin – 6 (IL6)
    C.  Citrate
    D.  Bone sialoprotein
    E.  PDGF

11. Which of the following statements regarding action potential generation and propagation is **false**?
    A.  The cellular resting membrane potential is produced by the action of ion channels and transporters and is typically around −70mV
    B.  Action potentials are generated by the inward flow of sodium (Na) ions through voltage gated channels driven by the electrochemical gradient
    C.  The amplitude of an action potential is proportional to the stimulus strength
    D.  Action potentials are regenerated at each node of Ranvier in myelinated axons
    E.  A period exists during the action potential when the cell is completely refractory to further stimulation

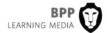

12. A motor unit is defined as:
    A. The region of the motor homonculus where activity is demonstrated during functional imaging while performing an isolated contraction of a specific muscle
    B. The nerve fibres and innervated muscle in the efferent limb of a reflex arc
    C. A skeletal muscle under voluntary control innervated by a single nerve
    D. An α motor neuron and all the skeletal muscle fibres that its axon supplies
    E. The motor end plate and the skeletal muscle fibre where it terminates

13. Which of the following statements is **false** regarding the structure of skeletal muscle?
    A. The basic unit of a myofibril is the sarcomere
    B. Individual sarcomeres are separated by H bands
    C. Filaments within the I band are principally composed of actin
    D. The A band is formed by the overlap of thick and thin filaments
    E. Thick filaments are found centrally within the sarcomere

14. Which of the following statements regarding the structure of cartilage is **false**?
    A. The perichondrium covers the outer surface of intra-articular mature hyaline cartilage
    B. Most cartilage is devoid of blood vessels
    C. Nutrition occurs through flow of water and metabolites through the porous permeable structure of the matrix
    D. The thickest layer of cartilage in the human body lines the articular surface of the patella
    E. Fibrocartilage is composed of alternating layers of hyaline cartilage matrix and layers of closely packed collagen fibres orientated in the direction of stresses

15. Which of the following is **false** regarding osteoblasts?
    A. Synthesise extracellular matrix known as osteoid which is mineralised with hydroxyapatite to form bone
    B. Produce collagen types I, III and V
    C. Produce osteocalcin which is though to recruit octeoclasts to resorb bone
    D. Express vitamin D receptors
    E. Are excitable cells

16. According to the Sillence classification of Osteogenesis Imperfecta which type has an autosomal recessive pattern of inheritance typically associated with blue sclera and severe deformities in utero?
    A. Type I
    B. Type II
    C. Type III
    D. Type IV
    E. Type V

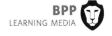
BPP
LEARNING MEDIA

17. What is the inheritance pattern of Duchenne muscular dystrophy?
    A. Autosonal dominant
    B. Autosomal recessive
    C. X-linked dominant
    D. X-linked recessive
    E. Sporadic

18. What is the inheritance pattern of Osteogenesis Imperfecta type IV according to the Sillence classification?
    A. Autosomal dominant
    B. Autosomal recessive
    C. X-linked dominant
    D. X-linked recessive
    E. Sporadic

19. Which of the following statements regarding hereditary sensorimotor neuropathy is **false**?
    A. The overall incidence is 1 in 2500
    B. The disease is commonly classified based on the results of motor nerve conduction velocities
    C. The type II disorder is characterised by thickened nerves on biopsy with reduced motor conduction velocities
    D. The type I disorder has an autosomal dominant pattern of inheritance
    E. The commonest gene defect in type I is found on chromosome 17

20. Which of the statements regarding the embryological development of the skeletal system is **false**?
    A. The somites are formed from segmentation of the paraxial mesoderm
    B. Bone is continually remodelled in utero by the action of osteoblasts alone
    C. Formation of the somites occurs around the third week in utero with each somite differentiating into two parts
    D. Most flat bones develop by inttramembranous ossification
    E. BMPs are throught to regulate some aspects of skeletal development

21. Regarding enchondral ossification, which of the statements is **false**?
    A. Cartilage first appears in embryos in the second trimester
    B. Lengthening of long bones occurs at the diaphyseal-epiphyseal junction
    C. Secondary centres of ossification arise in the first few years of life
    D The perichondrium develops into the periosteum and is responsible for circumferential growth of long bones
    E. With growth, bone resorption occurs on the endosteal surface

22. Regarding limb development, which of the following statements is **false**?
    A. The lower limb buds develop before the upper limb buds
    B. The limb buds first appear at 3 months
    C. Apoptosis is crucial to normal limb development
    D. The entirety of the limb bud develops from mesodermal tissue
    E. During development, the limb buds rotate on their longitudinal axes in different directions

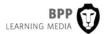

23. At what stage of embryological development does the neural tube form?
    A. 1$^{st}$ week
    B. 2$^{nd}$ week
    C. 4$^{th}$ week
    D. 8$^{th}$ week
    E. 12$^{th}$ week

24. Which of the following statements regarding limb bud formation is **false**?
    A. Limb bud formation is initiated at around 28 days
    B. HOX genes control FGF expression which determines whether limb is forelimb or hindlimb
    C. The apical ectodermal ridge produces FGF which maintains further growth
    D. The zone of polarising activity is found on the anterior aspect of the limb bud and establishes the anteroposterior axis
    E. Mutations in gene p63 often lead to cleft limb deformations

25. The G$_1$ phase in the cell cycle usually lasts a length of time equal to:
    A. 15 minutes
    B. 1 hour
    C. 6–12 hours
    D. 12–24 hours
    E. 48 hours

26. Which of the following statements regarding bone morphogenetic proteins (BMPs) is **false**?
    A. They are members of the TGFβ superfamily
    B. They are dimeric disulphide bonded proteins
    C. They utilise SMAD signalling pathways
    D. Overexpression has been associated with fibrodysplasia ossificans progressiva
    E. Clinical trials have shown no benefit from exogenous application in the healing of long bone nonunions

27. Which of the following statements regarding Ehlers-Danlos syndrome (EDS) is **false**?
    A. Ehlers Danlos syndromes are a heterogenous group of disorders characterised by laxity and weakness of the dermis, ligaments and blood vessels
    B. Type I is characterised by lax joints and hyperextensible skin and usually inherited in an autosomal recessive pattern
    C. Type II is more severe than type I
    D. Type IV is associated with fatal ruptures of large vessels in midlife
    E. Types I and II result from a mutation in the gene coding for type V collagen

28. Osteoporosis is defined by the World Health Organization criteria as:
    A. Z score < −2.5
    B. Z score < −1
    C. T score > 2.5
    D. T score < −1 but > −2.5
    E. T score < −2.5

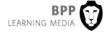

29. The average dietary requirement of calcium for an adult man is:
   A. 50mg/day
   B. 100mg/day
   C. 250mg/day
   D. 750mg/day
   E. 1500mg/day

30. Which of the following is **false** regarding vitamin D metabolism?
   A. Vitamin D is hydroxylated to the 25-(OH)-vitamin D3 in the liver
   B. Vitamin D metabolism is impaired by phenytoin
   C. 1, 25-dihydroxycholecalciferol is the most sensitive marker for total body vitamin D3 stores
   D. Conversion to the active form occurs in response to increased levels of PTH
   E. Hydroxylation of vitamin D at the first position occurs in the distal convoluted tubules

31. Which of the following is not a feature of primary hyperparathyroidism?
   A. Hypercalcaemia
   B. Hyperphosphatemia
   C. Pathological fractures
   D. Renal tract calculi
   E. Loss of lamina dura around the teeth

32. Which of the following is not a radiological feature of Paget's disease?
   A. Loss of corticomedullary differentiation
   B. Cortical expansion
   C. Femoral bowing
   D. Abnormal trabeculation
   E. Looser zones

33. Which of the following is **false** regarding Paget's disease?
   A. Associated with osteosarcoma
   B. Rarely presents below the age of 50 years
   C. Commonly affects the pelvis
   D. Rarely found in Asian ethnicity individuals
   E. Disease activity is inversely related to urine hydroxyproline levels

34. Which of the following is **not** a feature of gout?
   A. Periarticular erosions
   B. Synovitis and inflammation of overlying soft tissues
   C. Deposition of monosodium urate crystals which are strongly negatively bifringent under polarised light
   D. Intra-articular calcification
   E. Ankle joint involvement

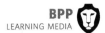

35. Which of the following is **true** regarding the fatigue endurance limit?
    A. Can be calculated for most non-ferrous alloys
    B. Is the stress level at which failure occurs at a set number of cycles
    C. Is the number of cycles at which failure occurs at a particular stress level
    D. Is the largest value of fluctuating stress that will not cause failure for a 1,000,000 cycles
    E. Is the largest value of fluctuating stress that will not cause failure for an infinite number of cycles

36. Which of the following is **false** regarding the fluid film lubrication?
    A. The minimum thickness of fluid has to exceed the surface roughness of the bearing surfaces
    B. Lubricant can act as both a squeeze film and exhibit hydrodynamic lubrication
    C. Is more likely with a large head size and high velocity in hard on hard bearings
    D. Friction depends on the properties of the both the bearing surfaces and the lubricant
    E. Is important in human diarthrodial joints

37. Which of the following is **false** regarding polyethylene wear in prosthetic hip joints?
    A. Can be measured from explanted joints using a shadowgraph technique
    B. Is always underestimated when measured radiographically
    C. Is dependent on scratch profile
    D. When determined using a joint simulator, should have a single loading cycle per gait cycle
    E. Typically occurs superolaterally

38. Which of the following is **false** regarding polythylene manufacture for tibial inserts in total knee arthroplasty?
    A. Utilises the Ziegler process
    B. Ram extrusion produces a finished product with superior wear properties compared to heat pressing
    C. White band subsurface oxidation is associated with an increased wear rate
    D. Polyethylene can be rigidly cross linked using peroxide chemistry
    E. Polyethylene should be irradiated in an inert environment

39. With respect to the bone cement interface in cemented hip replacement, which of the following is **false**?
    A. Presence of active bleeding can reduce the shear strength of the interface by up to 20%
    B. Ten 5mm keyholes provide better torsional resistance in comparison to three 10mm holes
    C. A zone of bone death occurs around the cement mantle
    D. Bone turnover is dictated by the mechanical environment around the implant
    E. Pressurised lavage leads to improved bone-cement shear strength compared with brushing and washing

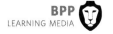

40. Wear is equal to:
    A. Coefficient of friction × Polar moment of area
    B. Coefficient of friction × Sliding distance
    C. Load × Polar moment of area
    D. Load × Sliding distance
    E. Load × Coefficient of friction × Sliding distance

41. Which of the following statements regarding fatigue of materials is **false**?
    A. Largest cause of failure in metals
    B. Failure occurs in response to dynamic and fluctuating stresses
    C. It usually occurs insidiously and catastrophically
    D. Extensive plastic deformation is evident at time of fracture
    E. The fracture surface is perpendicular to the direction of applied stress

42. Which of the following is not an effective means of reducing corrosion in metals?
    A. Ceramic outer coating
    B. Partially coating metal to be protected in a more electropositive metal
    C. Minimising articulations between components
    D. Impressed current cathode
    E. Reduce fluctuating stresses

43. Passivity in metals occurs as a result of which of the following?
    A. The formation of a thin adherent oxide layer on the surface
    B. The coupling of a more electropositive metal with the metal to be protected
    C. The coupling of a more electronegative metal with the metal to be protected
    D. The net accumulation of dislocations at the grain boundary interfaces
    E. The ductile brittle transition which occurs as the temperature is reduced

44. Out of the following benign bone tumours, which arises within the epiphysis?
    A. Giant cell tumour
    B. Chondroblastoma
    C. Osteoblastoma
    D. Osteochondroma
    E. Enchondroma

45. A patient has a high grade osteosarcoma in the proximal tibia with plain radiographs revealing ossification in the surrounding tissues but no further lesions on a bone scan. How would you grade this tumour according to the Enneking classification?
    A. IA
    B. IB
    C. IIA
    D. IIB
    E. III

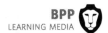

46. What is the characteristic signal intensity of soft tissue sarcomas on MRI?
    A. T1 high T2 low
    B. T1 high T2 high
    C. T1 low T2 low
    D. T1 low  T2 high
    E. T1 low T2 low with signal drop out on gradient echo sequences


47. A patient presents with severe pain in their proximal humerus and plain radiographs reveal a lytic lesion in the proximal humerus encompassing both cortices. According to Mirels' classification the score is:
    A. 4
    B. 7
    C. 10
    D. 12
    E. 16


48. A Mirels' score of 8 is associated with a:
    A. 5% risk of fracture
    B. 15% risk of fracture
    C. 33% risk of fracture
    D. 50% risk of fracture


49. A 15-year-old boy is seen in clinic due to a painful lump near his knee. Plain radiographs reveal a well defined expansile lesion contained within the epiphysis of the distal femur with cortical thinning but no pathological fracture. How would you stage this lesion according to the Musculoskeletal Tumor Society?
    A. Stage 1a
    B. Stage 1b
    C. Stage 2a
    D. Stage I
    E. Stage II


50. In which joint is pigmented villonodular synovitis most commonly found?
    A. Ankle
    B. Knee
    C. Hip
    D. Elbow
    E. Shoulder


51. The most common location of parosteal osteosarcoma is:
    A. Anterior cortex proximal tibia
    B. Posterior cortex proximal tibia
    C. Anterior cortex distal femur
    D. Posterior cortex distal femur
    E. Femoral calcar

BPP
LEARNING MEDIA

52. Which of the following is not recommended when biopsying musculoskeletal tumours?
    A. Biopsy can be performed before investigations complete
    B. Biopsy should be performed in a specialist centre
    C. Tourniquets can be used
    D. The approach should minimise the number of compartments entered
    E. Drains should be placed in the line of the incision

53. The most common location for a unicameral bone cyst is:
    A. Proximal femur
    B. Distal femur
    C. Proximal tibia
    D. Proximal humerus
    E. Spine

54. The most sensitive imaging modality for detecting malignant transformation of osteochondromas is:
    A. Plain radiographs
    B. Ultrasound
    C. CT scan
    D. MRI
    E. Bone scan

55. Which of the following statements regarding osteoid osteoma is **false**?
    A. May occur in cortical, cancellous bone or subperiosteally
    B. They are more common in males
    C. Characteristically produce nocturnal pain relieved by salicylates
    D. Greater than 2 cm radiolucent nidus surrounded by reactive sclerotic bone
    E. Commonly treated by CT guided radiofrequency ablation

56. Regarding free body diagrams, which of the following is **false**?
    A. Sketch of body under consideration
    B. Assumes all skeletal links rigid
    C. Friction in joints is taken into account
    D. Usually more than one free body diagram can be drawn for a particular situation
    E. The line of action of muscles passes along the centre of the cross sectional area.

57. Regarding strain, which of the following is **false**?
    A. Is linearly related to stress only along the elastic portion of the stress-strain curve
    B. Can be expressed as a percentage
    C. Defined as the deformation per unit length of element subjected to load
    D. Can be calculated from the stress, and Young's modulus, using the Poisson's ratio
    E. Strain in the elastic portion of the curve is recoverable and occurs due to the resistance to interatomic seperation

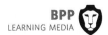

58. With respect to the below stress-strain diagram, which of the following is true?

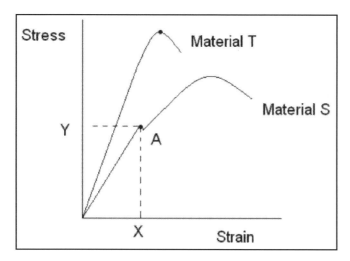

    A. Material S is stiffer than Material T
    B. Material S is more ductile than Material T
    C. A approximates the ultimate tensile strength of Material S
    D. The stiffness of Material S can be defined by X/Y
    E. The stress strain curve of Material S up to point A represents the plastic portion of the curve

59. Which of the following experiments best demonstrates the creep phenomenon?
    A. A viscoelastic material is subjected to stress to impose a level of strain which is kept constant over time
    B. A viscoelastic material is subjected to a stress which is maintained at a constant level over time
    C. A ferrous alloy is subjected to a repeated fluctuating stress level whose amplitude is 2.5 times less than the ultimate tensile stress
    D. A ferrous alloy is subjected to stress to impose a level of strain which is kept constant over time
    E. A ceramic material is subjected to a stress which is maintained at a constant level over time

60. Which of the following fracture patterns is created by a bending moment applied to a long bone while the bone is loaded along its longitudinal axis?
    A. Buckle fracture
    B. Pilon fracture
    C. Spiral fracture
    D. Transverse fracture with butterfly fragment
    E. Short oblique fracture

BPP
LEARNING MEDIA

61. Which of the following statements regarding the study of forces acting on a stationary body is **false**?
    A. Forces cannot be characterised by magnitude alone
    B. External forces are the forces of one body on another
    C. The centre of gravity of a body is the point in the body about which all parts balance each other exactly and in the human body approximates to just anterior to the third lumbar segment
    D. The magnitude of a moment is equal to the magnitude of the applied force multiplied by the perpendicular distance between its line of action and the axis of rotation
    E. A couple is two forces with same magnitudes and parallel lines of action but the opposite sense

62. Which of the following statements regarding metallic structure is **false**?
    A. The stiffness of a metal is a function of its resistance to interatomic separation
    B. Thermal and electrical conductivity arises as a result of a mobile electron cloud composed of valence electrons
    C. The crystalline structure of metals can be described in terms of the unit cell
    D. Two types of unit cell crystalline structure exist
    E. Polymorphism describes how some metals can have more than one crystalline structure

63. Which of the following statements regarding plastic deformation in metals is **false**?
    A. Plastic deformation is typically observed when the stress-strain curve deviates from proportionality
    B. The strength of a metal is defined as its resistance to plastic deformation
    C. The toughness of a metal is its ability to absorb energy up to the point of failure
    D. The ductility of a metal is independent of impurities
    E. Plastic deformation can occur as a result of the movement of dislocations through the crystalline lattice

64. Which of the below mechanisms is **not** associated with an increase in the strength of a metal?
    A. Grain size reduction
    B. Introduction of impurities into the crystal lattice
    C. Formation of precipitates within metallic structure
    D. Cold working
    E. Testing material in different directions

65. Which of the following is **false** regarding fracture in ductile materials?
    A. There is high energy absorption and plastic deformation at the point of fracture
    B. Cracks usually extend slowly
    C. Cracks resist further extension unless there is an increase in the applied stress
    D. Characteristically occurs in ceramics
    E. Fractures usually have a cup and cone appearence

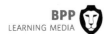

66. With respect to the ankle joint sagittal plane kinetics and kinematics during the 'heel off' to 'toe off' phase of the gait cycle:
    A. There is plantarflexion from 10° dorsiflexion to 30° plantarflexion and the ground reaction force is posterior to the joint
    B. There is plantarflexion from 10° dorsiflexion to 30° plantarflexion and the reaction force is anterior to the joint
    C. There is plantarflexion from 20° dorsiflexion to 60° plantarflexion and the ground reaction force is anterior to the joint
    D. There is plantarflexion from 20° dorsiflexion to 60° plantarflexion and the ground reaction force is posterior to the joint
    E. There is plantarflexion from 10° dorsiflexion to 60° plantarflexion and the ground reaction force passes from posterior to anterior to the joint

67. Which of the following is an intrinsic characteristic of a material?
    A. Ductility
    B. Stiffness
    C. Strength
    D. Toughness
    E. Fatigue resistance

68. What is the Young's modulus of polymethylmethacrylate (PMMA)?
    A. 0.5 Gpa
    B. 2 Gpa
    C. 10 Gpa
    D. 50 Gpa
    E. 100 Gpa

69. Which of the following is **false** regarding P values?
    A. Are a type of inferential statistic
    B. Do not always demonstrate clinically significant differences despite demonstrating statistical significance
    C. Are arbitrarily deemed as statistically significant when less than 0.05
    D. Are a probability statement of rejecting the null hypothesis
    E. Provide information on magnitude and direction of measured clinical effect or difference

70. Which of the following is **false** regarding the power of a study?
    A. Can be calculated for both numerical and categorical data
    B. Commonly gives rise to a type I error
    C. Requires the use of a nomogram which assumes independent groups with normal distributions
    D. Demonstrates that a much larger sample is required if the measured clinical effect or difference is very small
    E. Requires determination of the smallest true clinical or experimental difference that we consider as valuable

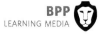

71. Which of the following defines the sensitivity of a diagnostic test?
    A. Proportion of patients with the condition correctly identified by the test
    B. Proportion of patients without the condition correctly diagnosed as not having the condition
    C. Proportion of patients with a positive test result who are correctly diagnosed as having the condition
    D. Proportion of patients with a negative test result who are correctly diagnosed as not having the condition
    E. Proportion of patients with a positive test result

72. Which of the following best describes the difference between an ordinal and nominal variable?
    A. Ordinal variables are continuous whereas nominal variables are discrete
    B. Ordinal variables are discrete whereas nominal variables are continuous
    C. Ordinal variables are numerical whereas nominal variables are categorical
    D. Nominal variables are categorical variables which can be ranked in a specific order whereas ordinal variables cannot be ordered in such a way
    E. Ordinal variables are categorical variables which can be ranked in a specific order whereas nominal variables cannot be ordered in such a way

73. A research question comparing outcomes from patients with fixed and rotational bearing total knee replacements utilises a matched case control study design. What would be the level of evidence of the findings of such a study?
    A. Level 1a
    B. Level 1b
    C. Level 1c
    D. Level 2
    E. Level 3

74. A study is being designed on the following research question 'Does postoperative use of drug A reduce the risk of venous thromboembolism (VTE) as measured on ultrasound at 6 weeks post surgery in comparison to postoperative use of drug B?' The null hypothesis of this study is:
    A. The incidence of VTE is less with drug A compared with drug B
    B. The incidence of VTE is greater with drug A compared with drug B
    C. The incidence of VTE with use of drug A is equal to that with use of drug B
    D. The incidence of VTE is less with drug A compared with drug B and is statistically significant
    E. The incidence of VTE is less with drug A compared with drug B but this difference is not statistically significant

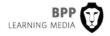

75. A study is designed to determine the relationship between 2 variables in hip fracture patients – age at the time of fracture and bone mineral density on DEXA scanning. The data is collected for both variables and the plotted distributions demonstrate the data to be skewed for both variables. The most appropriate statistical test to demonstrate correlation between the two variables is:
   A. Pearson correlation co-efficient
   B. Spearman Rho test
   C. Mann-Whitney test
   D. Student's T test
   E. Chi squared test

76. The 95% confidence interval of a data set is derived from the following calculation:
   A. mean $+/-$ (1.96 × standard deviation)
   B. mean $+/-$ (1.96 × standard error of the mean)
   C. mean $+/-$ (2.49 × standard deviation)
   D. mean $+/-$ (2.49 × standard error of the mean)
   E. mean $+/- \sqrt{}$sample variance

77. Which of the following statements is **false** regarding the age related structural changes in ground substance in hyaline cartilage?
   A. Chondroitin 6 sulphate levels increase
   B. Chondroitin 4 sulphate levels increase
   C. Keratin sulphate levels increase
   D. Net aggrecan levels decrease
   E. Hydration may initially increase but in the long term decrease

78. What is the main structural change in hyaline cartilage that is observed when a joint is immobilised?
   A. Sulphation pattern of proteoglycans changes
   B. Decrease in proteoglycan content
   C. Reorientation of collagen fibrils
   D. Decrease in collagen type II
   E. Chondrocyte apoptosis

79. Parathyroid hormone exerts which of the following effects on serum biochemistry?
   A. Increased serum calcium, increased serum phosphate
   B. Increased serum calcium, decreased serum phosphate
   C. Decreased serum calcium, increased serum phosphate
   D. Decreased serum calcium, decreased serum phosphate
   E. Increased serum calcium, serum phosphate unchanged

80. Which of the following statements regarding the structure and function of collagen molecules is **false**?
   A. Type I collagen is the most abundant collagen in bone
   B. The highest collagen content in articular cartilage is in the superficial zone
   C. Type XI collagen assists in collagen growth by acting as a template for the growth and orientation of collagen type II fibrils
   D. Type V collagen binds type II collagen fibres in the superficial zone
   E. Type III collagen is commonly found in the vessel walls of medium and large sized arteries

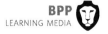

# Basic Sciences

## Answers

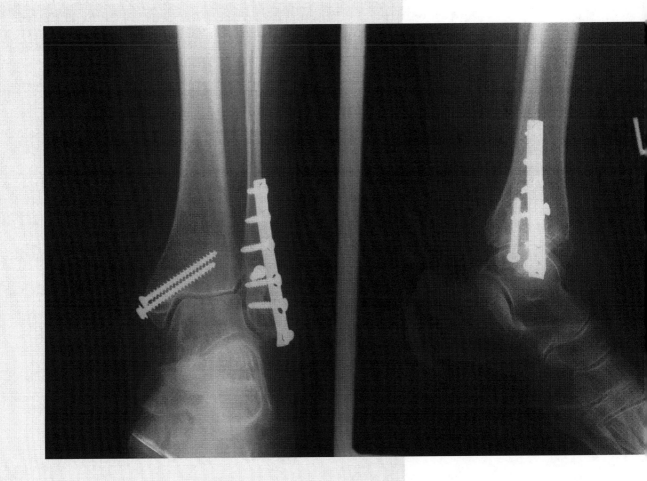

1. **A**

   Osteoblasts secrete osteoid containing type I collagen at the mineralisation front. Bone resorption is undertaken by osteoclasts within depressions within bone known as Howship's lacunae.

   Ref:
   Buckwalter, J; Einhorn, T and Simon, S. (2nd ed.) (2000) *Orthopaedic Basic Science: Biology and Biomechanics of the Musculoskeletal System*, American Academy of Orthopaedic Surgeons, Rosemont.

2. **B**

   It is worthwhile remembering the more common conditions which affect the different regions of the growth plate:

   | | |
   |---|---|
   | Reserve | Lysosomal storage diseases (eg Gauchers) |
   | Proliferation | Achondroplasia |
   | Hypertrophic | rickets, Mucopolysaccharidoses, Enchondromas, SUFE |

   Ref:
   Miller, M. (5th ed.) (2008) *Review of Orthopaedics*, Saunders, Philadelphia.

3. **E**

   Osteoclastic resorption of bone occurs in response to PTH. However, PTH receptors are only found on osteoblasts. The presumed signalling mechanism is that activated osteoblasts release pro-inflammatory cytokines which activate osteoclastic activity. This is an example of a site directing coupling mechanism between both cell types' opposing activities with respect to bone. Another is that residues from enzymatic secretion from osteoclasts may serve to attract osteoblasts to areas of resorption.

   Ref:
   Buckwalter, J; Einhorn, T and Simon, S. (2nd ed.) (2000) *Orthopaedic Basic Science: Biology and Biomechanics of the Musculoskeletal System*, American Academy of Orthopaedic Surgeons, Rosemont.

4. **D**

   | | |
   |---|---|
   | First | Neuropraxia, nerve structure intact, full recovery expected |
   | Second | Axontemesis, axons disrupted but endoneurial sheath continuity preserved, recovery is likely once neurons regroup down their respective conduits after distal Wallarian degeneration has occurred. |
   | Third | Neurotmesis, Axonal degeneration and loss of endoneurial tube connectivity; individual fascicles preserved ie perineurium intact, recovery variable |
   | Fourth | Neurotmesis, Nerve trunk continuity preserved but fascicles disrupted, recovery variable |
   | Fifth | Neurotmesis, Complete loss of nerve trunk continuity |

   Ref:
   Buckwalter, J; Einhorn, T and Simon, S. (2nd ed.) (2000) *Orthopaedic Basic Science: Biology and Biomechanics of the Musculoskeletal System*, American Academy of Orthopaedic Surgeons, Rosemont.

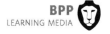

5.  **A**

    The order of recovery is pain, temperature, touch and finally proprioception. Motor recovery in mixed sensory and motor nerve injury usually occurs last which can be remembered by the observation of patients with sciatica whose painful symptoms have resolved but are left with a residual foot drop.

    Ref:
    Canale T. (10th ed.) (2003) *Campbell's Operative Orthopaedics*, Elsevier, St Louis.

6.  **C**

    The tidemark is a histological staining artefact which marks the calcification front separating calcified and uncalcified cartilage. It tends to migrate towards the surface with ageing and can be duplicated in arthritic degeneration of the cartilage.

    Ref:
    Ramachandran, M. (2007) *Basic Orthopaedic Sciences: The Stanmore Guide*, Hodder Arnold, London.

7.  **D**

    The important functions of the menisci are:

    1.  Load transmission and improving articular congruity
    2.  Shock absorption
    3.  Contributing to joint lubrication
    4.  Aiding stability
    5.  Articular cartilage nutrition
    6.  Most of the collagen is type I

    Ref:
    Ramachandran, M. (2007) *Basic Orthhopaedic Sciences: The Stanmore Guide*, Hodder Arnold, London.

8.  **A**

    Cortical bone is denser, less isotropic and incurs a greater metabolic cost than trabecular or cancellous bone. It also remodels at a slower rate with a reduced rate of turnover.

    Ref:
    Nordin, M and Frankel, V. (3rd ed.) (2001) *Basic biomechanics of the musculoskeletal system*, Lippincott Williams and Wilkins, Philadelphia.

9.  **E**

    It is useful to remember the various constituents of articular cartilage and their distribution. Water – mainly concentrated near articular surface (80%) and decreases with increasing depth (65% deep zone). Movement is essential for nourishment of cartilage and circulation of mobile free cat-ions.

    Chondrocytes – differentiate from mesenchymal cells and cluster in groups of two or more cells in a structure called a chondron. Responsible for generation and turnover of matrix.

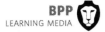

Collagen – mainly type II (90%) but other types are also found. Type IX is mainly found in the surface and links parallel collagen fibres to form an outer mesh which counteracts shear forces and aids in porosity. Type VI forms a 3D meshwork in the peri-cellular region and may aid in cell-matrix interactions. Type XI is found in the core of fibres and is thought to act as a template and regulate the diameter of growing fibres. Type X is present in the calcified layer and its expression is also increased in osteoarthritis. Type I cartilage is not normally found unless injury has occurred and healing by fibrocartilage has taken place.

Proteoglycans – large protein polysaccharide molecules which are concentrated in the deeper zones, less so in the superficial zone. Proteoglycan content decreases dramatically in the first two weeks following joint immobilisation.

Glycoproteins – these are dispersed throughout the matrix and assist in cell-matrix interactions as well as cell adhesion and lubrication mechanisms.

Enzymes – turnover of matrix contents is regulated by opposing enzyme systems such as matrix metalloproteinases eg aggrecanase and tissue induced inhibitors (TIMP).

Ref:
Nordin, M and Frankel, V. (3rd ed.) (2001) *Basic biomechanics of the musculoskeletal system*, Lippincott Williams and Wilkins, Philadelphia.


10. **C**
Physiologic bone calcification is regulated by many different matrix proteins.

Promoters – type I collagen, bone sialoprotein, matrix vesicles, phosphoproteins, proteolipids and biglycan.

Inhibitors – large proteoglycans, pyrophosphate, ATP and citrate.

Ref:
Buckwalter, J; Einhorn, T and Simon, S. (2nd ed.) (2000) *Orthopaedic Basic Science: Biology and Biomechanics of the Musculoskeletal System*, American Academy of Orthopaedic Surgeons, Rosemont.


11. **C**
The resting membrane potential of a cell is determined by the net effect of electrochemical gradients of various ions across the plasma membrane that exist due to the presence of ATP dependent ion transporters. The typical resting membrane potential of most cells, including neurons, is around −70mV. An action potential (spike) is generated when an excitable cell is stimulated by depolarisation above a threshold membrane potential. The action potential is a characteristic response in that it is an 'all or nothing phenomenon' ie the stimulus either produces an action potential if high enough or doesn't. The other important characteristics are that this depolarising spike has a constant amplitude irrespective of stimulus strength. Similarly, it is propagated without detriment along the length of the nerve fibre. To better understand this phenomenon we must consider the underlying electrochemical processes.

The action potential is a result of sudden transient changes in the plasma membrane conductance of Na and K ions. A depolarising stimulus above the threshold value activates

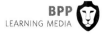

a critical number of voltage gated Na channels causing a rapid influx of this ion into the cell causing a crescendo effect in terms of further depolarisation and activating more Na channels. However, this effect is short lived as a secondary gate function of the Na channels leads to a propensity for closure with further depolarisation thus terminating the influx. The Na channels are then unable to open until repolarisation has been achieved. This accounts for the insensitivity to further stimuli during the action potential known as the absolute refractory period. The move towards repolarisation is aided by the opening of voltage gated K channels which are similarly opened by the depolarisation but cause an opposing shift of current towards repolarisation. These K channels remain active even when repolarisation is achieved accounting for the after hyperpolarisation that is seen at the end of an action potential.

In myelinated axons, conduction velocities are faster for several reasons. First, myelin increases the membrane resistance ensuring that less of the conducting signal is lost through the membrane and that the amplitude is maintained. The thickened myelin layers also act to create greater separation of the internal and external cellular environments which decreases the capacitance of the cell membrane allowing more rapid depolarisation. Additionally, the voltage gated Na channels are preferentially concentrated at gaps in the myelin sheath known as the nodes of Ranvier. Therefore transmembrane currents only occur at these regions and the action potential is regenerated only at these points rather than continuously along the length of the fibre. This action potential 'leaping' behaviour speeds up conduction vastly and is known as salutatory conduction (saltare – Latin for 'leap').

Ref:
Koeppen, B and Stanton, B. (6$^{th}$ ed.) (2008) *Berne and Levy Physiology*, Mosby, Philadelphia.

12. **D**
Skeletal muscles are innervated by large diameter neurons called $\alpha$ motor neurons. These are situated in the ventral horn of the spinal cord as well as the cranial nerve nuclei. A motor unit is a single $\alpha$ motor neuron and all the skeletal muscle fibres its axon supplies. The number of muscle fibres supplied differs depending on muscle size and function. Typically large lower limb muscles have very large motor units where hundreds of muscle fibres are innervated by a single motor unit. In small motor units, only a few fibres are innervated and this allows for very fine control such as in the ocular muscles.

Ref:
Koeppen, B and Stanton, B. (6$^{th}$ ed.) (2008) *Berne and Levy Physiology*, Mosby, Philadelphia.

13. **B**
Each skeletal muscle fibre is composed of bundles of myofibrils. Each myofibril in turn is composed of multiple sarcomeres connected end to end. Striations appear in skeletal muscle as a result of the repeating arrangement of thick and thin filaments within the myofibrils. A sarcomere is delineated by two dark lines called Z lines and is in essence the basic repeating unit of skeletal muscle. On either side of the Z line is an A band which is lighter and corresponds to thin filaments predominantly made up of actin filaments. The area between the two I bands is known as the A band which contains thick filaments made up of myosin. In the centre of the sarcomere is a dark M line. This is flanked by a light

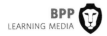

region known as the H band. This part of the A band is lighter because it only contains thick filaments whereas the remainder of the A band is darker due to the overlap of both thick and thin filaments.

Ref:
Koeppen, B and Stanton, B. (6<sup>th</sup> ed.) (2008) *Berne and Levy Physiology*, Mosby, Philadelphia.

14.  **A**
Most mature cartilage masses have a surrounding layer known as the perichondrium which is made up of collagen fibres and spindle shaped cells resembling fibroblasts. These have the potential of transforming into chondroblasts and producing cartilage matrix by a process of appositional growth. Interstitial growth whereby remaining chondroblasts divide and increase synthetic activity is more limited. Most mature hyaline cartilage in joints does not have a perichondrium and consequently does not regenerate after injury.

Most of cartilage is devoid of a blood supply relying on diffusion of water and metabolites into its porous structure from the surrounding synovial fluid. This does limit the thickness of achievable viable cartilage. Larger cartilage masses eg costal cartilages are able to retain viable tissue at their core due to small channels which convey blood vessels to these regions.

Hyaline, fibro- and elastic cartilage differ in the number and type of collagen fibres. In fibrocartilage the matrix is periodically interspersed with dense layers of collagen fibres whereas in elastic cartilage, elastin fibres are commonly found.

Ref:
Wheater, P; Heath, J and Young, B. (4<sup>th</sup> ed.) (2000) *Wheater's functional histology: A text and color atlas*, Churchill Livingstone, Edinburgh.

15.  **E**
Although osteoblasts respond to many different stimuli, including proposed piezo-electric impulses between fully differentiated osteocytes dictating bone formation and resorption, they are in themselves not excitable cells i.e. unable to propagate action potentials. Examples of excitable cells include neurons, smooth muscle cells and pacemaker cells within the heart.

Ref:
Miller, M. (5<sup>th</sup> ed.) (2008) *Review of Orthopaedics*, Saunders, Philadelphia.

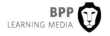

16. **B**

The Sillence classification defines 4 subtypes of Osteogenesis Imperfecta (OI) based on genetic, clinical and radiographic features.

| Type | Inheritance | Sclera | Features |
|------|-------------|--------|----------|
| I | Autosomal dominant | Blue | Most common type Mild–moderate severity |
| II | Autosomal dominant/ Autosomal recessive | Blue | Almost always die in utero |
| III | Autosomal dominant/ Autosomal recessive | Normal | Moderate to severe Dentnogenesis imperfecta |
| IV | Autosomal dominant | Normal | Mild to moderate |

Ref:
Sillence DO. (1988) Osteogenesis imperfecta nosology and genetics. *Ann NY Acad Sci,* 543: 1–15.

17. **D**

Duchenne muscular dystrophy (DMD), first described by Guillaume Duchenne in 1861, is the most severe form of muscular dystrophy. It is inherited in an x-linked recessive pattern with an incidence of 1 in 20,000. Presentation is at the age of 3–5 years with progressive muscle weakness causing an awkward gait, difficulty in rising from the floor (Gower sign) and calf pseudohypertrophy due to replacement with fibrous tissue. The condition is universally progressive with death at a mean age of 18 years. Consequently, new cases principally arise from mutation rather than passage of genes to the next generation.

Ref:
Turnpenny, P and Ellard, S. (12th ed.) (2005) *Emery's elements of medical genetics,* Elsevier, Philadelphia.

18. **A**

(refer to answer to question 16)

Ref:
Sillence DO. (1988) Osteogenesis imperfecta nosology and genetics. *Ann NY Acad Sci,* 543: 1–15.

19. **C**

Hereditary sensory motor neuropathy (HSMN) is the most common inherited neuropathy with a incidence of around 1 in 2500. The condition is also referred to as Charcot-Marie Tooth disease and Peroneal muscular atrophy. There are many different types and subtypes of the disease described. The disorder is classified on the basis of motor nerve conduction velocities. Type I is an autosomal dominant disorder with reduced conduction velocities and thickened 'hypertrophic' nerves which can occasionally be palpable. In the type II disorder, defecits arise as a result of axon loss and thus conduction velocities are unaffected. HSMN can arise in an autosomal dominant, autosomal recessive or x-linked inheritance

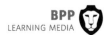

pattern although autosomal dominant forms are the most common. Over 70% of cases of type I are associated with a defect in chromosome 17 causing a duplication effect of the PMP-22 gene.

Ref:
Turnpenny, P and Ellard, S. (12<sup>th</sup> ed.) (2005) *Emery's elements of medical genetics*, Elsevier, Philadelphia.

**20. B**

During embryological development, the mesoderm lateral to the developing neural tube forms two dorsolateral longitudinal columns of mesoderm known as the paraxial mesoderm. These begin to segment around the third week of life into blocks of mesodermal tissue known as somites. Each somite itself further differentiates into a ventromedial sclerotome (later forms the vertebrae and ribs) and a dorsolateral dermatome (gives rise to fibroblasts and myoblasts). Bones first arise within this mesenchymal tissue as condensations of cells. This important point marks the onset of selective gene activity after which cell differentiation is seen. Bone is continuously remodelled in-utero by the action of both osteoblasts and osteoclasts. Most flat bones develop within preformed membranous sheets by a process of ossification appropriately referred to as intramembranous ossification. Conversely, long bones develop by a process of endochondral ossification whereby the mesenchymal elements are transformed into a cartilage bone model. Many cytokines have been implicated in the regulation of bone and cartilage formation with BMPs 5 and 7 thought to play important roles.

Ref:
Moore, K, and Persaud, T. (8<sup>th</sup> ed.) (2007) *The Developing Human: Clinically Orientated Embryology*, Elsevier, Philadelphia.

**21. A**

Mesenchyme condenses to form chondrification centres in regions where cartilage is to develop. Differentiation of the mesenchymal cells into chondroblasts occurs and cartilage first starts to appear in the embryo at 5 weeks. In long bones, the primary centre of ossification is in the diaphysis and the process of ossification occurs throughout much of the embryonic period such that most of the diaphyses are largely ossified at birth. Due to the location of the ossification centre, growth occurs at the diaphyseal-epiphyseal junction. Secondary ossification centres appear in the epiphyses of most long bones after birth (birth appropriately marking the distinction between primary and secondary). Bones grow circumferentially by the deposition of bone by the periosteum formed from the perichondrium. A medullary cavity is maintained relative to the diameter of the bone by the action of osteoclasts resorbing bone on the endosteal surface as the bone widens.

Ref:
Moore, K, and Persaud, T. (8<sup>th</sup> ed.) (2007) *The Developing Human: Clinically Orientated Embryology*, Elsevier, Philadelphia.

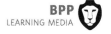

22.   **C**
The limb buds develop from the ventrolateral body wall as small projections in the 4th week of life. Development of the upper limb buds preceeds that of the lower limb buds by a few days. Both mesodermal and ectodermal tissues contribute to their development. There is a substantial change in the orientation of the limb buds during growth. Initially they are pointing caudally but later project ventrally (7th week). This is followed by rotation along the longitudinal axis in different directions. The upper limbs rotate laterally by 90 degrees and the lower limbs medially by slightly less. This is best remembered by appreciating that our elbows point backwards and our knees point forwards. Longitudinal limb growth occurs by proliferation of the mesenchymal elements. However, apoptosis is a necessity to form the clefts between digits (8th week) and its absence at this stage gives rise to syndactyly.

Ref:
Moore, K, and Persaud, T. (8th ed.) (2007) *The Developing Human: Clinically Orientated Embryology*, Elsevier, Philadelphia.

23.   **C**
The spinal cord develops from the ectoderm. Dorsal thickening of this tissue forms the neural plate during the third week of life. Subsequent infolding of the neural plate occurs forming a groove and two folds which eventually meet to form the neural tube in the 4th week. The neural tube susequently develops into the brain and spinal cord

Ref:
Moore, K, and Persaud, T. (8th ed.) (2007) *The Developing Human: Clinically Orientated Embryology*, Elsevier, Philadelphia.

24.   **D**
Limb bud formation usually commences around 28 days in response to the action of members of the FGF family under the control of HOX genes which determine limb type and number. These fibroblast growth factors continue to be important throughout most of limb development. The apical ectodermal ridge is a thickened part of ectoderm at the tip of the developing limb bud which is responsible for ensuring further growth and determining the proximo-distal axis. The p63 gene is crucial to maintaining this structure and defects in this gene commonly give rise to cleft limb type deformities. The zone of polarising activity is found on the posterior aspect of the limb bud and signals through Sonic Hedgehog and many other molecules to establish the anteroposterior axis. Development at the distal end of the limb is governed by the activation of HOX genes in the undifferentiated mesenchymal cells beneath the apical ectodermal ridge. Selective expression of genes in this region known as the progress zone dictate local cell proliferation and differentiation.

Ref:
Moore, K, and Persaud, T. (8th ed.) (2007) *The Developing Human: Clinically Orientated Embryology*, Elsevier, Philadelphia.

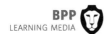

**25.  C**

The cell cycle is divided into 4 active phases

| | | | |
|---|---|---|---|
| $G_0$ | Resting phase | | Phase exists outside of cell cycle (inactive) |
| $G_1$ | Growth phase (1) | 6–12 hours | Active RNA and protein synthesis |
| S | Synthesis phase | 6–8 hours | DNA replication<br>Cells can be identified by labelling with bromodeoxyuridine |
| $G_2$ | Growth phase (2) | 3–4 hours | Active RNA and protein synthesis |
| M | Mitosis | 1 hour | Chromosomes segregate via activity of mitotic spindle<br>Cell divides |

Ref:

Buckwalter, J; Einhorn, T and Simon, S. ($2^{nd}$ ed.) (2000) *Orthopaedic Basic Science: Biology and Biomechanics of the Musculoskeletal System*, American Academy of Orthopaedic Surgeons, Rosemont.

**26.  E**

The role of BMPs in osseous repair has been demonstrated in several animal models. A prospective randomised controlled trial has demonstrated a role for BMP 7 in the treatment of tibial nonunions. A smilar rate of union was seen in the other arm of the study treated with bone autograft although there was an incidence of donor site morbidity in this group. Other studies have also demonstrated a role for BMP 7 in spinal fusion.

Ref:

White AP, Vaccaro AR, Hall JA, Whang PG, Friel BC, McKee MD. (2007) Clinical applications of BMP-7/OP-1 in fractures, nonunions and spinal fusion. *Int Orthop*, 31: 735–41.

**27.  B**

There are at least 9 clinical and genetic types described of this broad range of disorders. EDS types I and II both result from a mutation in the gene coding for collagen type V and are usually inherited in an autosomal dominant manner. This collagen molecule has an important role in the formation of collagen I fibrils and typically EDS types I and II have lax joints and hyperextensible skin. EDS type II has a similar presentation to type I but is a milder form of the disease. EDS IV is caused by a mutation in the gene coding for type III collagen – an important constituent of blood vessels (accounts for 50% of the collagen found here). The disorder is associated with the rupture of large and medium sized arteries which can occur as early as the second decade of life.

Ref:

Buckwalter J, Einhorn T, Simon S. ($2^{nd}$ ed.) (2000) *Orthopaedic Basic Science : Biology and Biomechanics of the Musculoskeletal System*, American Academy of Orthopaedic Surgeons, Rosemont.

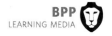

28.   **E**

The World Health Organisation definition of osteoporosis is a T score less than 2.5. The T score is derived from bone densitometry readings which are matched for sex and race and compared with the peak bone mass of young normal adults. In contrast the Z score is matched for sex, race and age and gives an indication as to whether there is an aetiology other than age related bone loss.

Ref:

Ramachandran, M. (2007) *Basic Orthhopaedic Sciences: The Stanmore Guide*, Hodder Arnold, London.

29.   **D**

The dietary requirement of calcium differs according to age and physiological status:

| | |
|---|---|
| Child | 600mg/day |
| Adolescent | 1300mg/day |
| Adult man/woman | 750mg/day |
| Lactating women | 2000mg/day |
| Postmenopausal women | 1500mg/day |
| Healing long bone fracture | 1500mg/day |

Ref:

Miller, M. (5th ed.) (2008) *Review of Orthopaedics*, Saunders, Philadelphia.

30.   **C**

Serum 25(OH) Vitamin D3 levels are the best indication of body stores of Vitamin D3.

Ref:

Buckwalter, J; Einhorn, T and Simon, S. (2nd ed.) (2000) *Orthopaedic Basic Science: Biology and Biomechanics of the Musculoskeletal System*, American Academy of Orthopaedic Surgeons, Rosemont.

31.   **B**

Primary hyperparathyroidism leads to an increase in serum calcium and a decrease in serum phosphate because of increased renal excretion. Osteoclastic activity also increases and characteristic bone changes which may be seen include osteopenia, brown tumours, chondrocalcinosis and loss of lamina dura around the teeth.

Ref:

Miller, M. (5th ed.) (2008) *Review of Orthopaedics*, Saunders, Philadelphia.

32.   **E**

Looser zones are characteristically seen in rickets and are associated with pathological fractures. The typical appearance is that of fracture on the compression side of the bone.

Ref:

Ramachandran, M. (2007) *Basic Orthhopaedic Sciences: The Stanmore Guide*, Hodder Arnold, London.

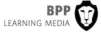

**33.**   **E**

Paget's disease occurs due to abnormal bone remodelling. It is rare below the age of 40 years and exhibits a strong geographical prevalence in both the UK and US. Abnormal osteoblastic and osteoclastic activity leads to the formation of disorganised bone with an increased propensity to fracture. The characteristic radiographic signs are cortical expansion, abnormal trabeculation and loss of corticomedullary differentiation. Activity of the disease process can be monitored by collagen degradation products such as urine hydroxyproline. There is an associated risk of sarcomatous change within the diseased bone which is one of the reasons for the late peak seen in osteosarcoma.

Ref:
Ramachandran, M. (2007) *Basic Orthhopaedic Sciences: The Stanmore Guide*, Hodder Arnold, London.

**34.**   **D**

Pseudogout is caused by calcium dehydrate pyrophosphate crystals being deposited in joints and can lead to intra-articular calcification seen on radiograph.

Ref:
Miller, M. (5th ed.) (2008) *Review of Orthopaedics*, Saunders, Philadelphia.

**35.**   **E**

Fatigue is a form of failure occurring in structures subjected to dynamic and fluctuating stresses and is the most common cause of failure in metals. The S-N curve was devised by Wohler in the 19th century during the experimental determination of fatigue properties of various materials using rotating bending tests. In these tests, a specimen is subjected to repetitive stress cycles to the point of failure. This procedure is repeated on specimens of the same material with a different maximum stress amplitude each time. A curve can be plotted of the maximum stress amplitude against the logarithm of the number of cycles to failure. For most ferrous alloys the curve plateaus to a level of stress below which failure will not occur for an infinite number of cycles, typically 35–60% of the ultimate tensile strength of the material. This largest value of fluctuating stress that will not cause failure for an infinte number of cycles is defined as the fatigue limit. S-N curves for most non-ferrous alloys do not plateau and demonstrate failure through fatigue no matter how low the stress level.

For these materials, fatigue can be quantified in two ways:

Fatigue strength – stress level at which failure occurs for a set number of cycles

Fatigue life – number of cycles at which failure occurs for a particular stress

Ref:
Callister, W. (7th ed.) (2006) *Materials science and engineering: an introduction*, John Wiley, New York.

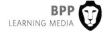

**36.    D**

In the fluid film model of lubrication, a film of fluid separates the surfaces so that asperities from neither surface are in contact. The fluid film thickness thus has to exceed the surface roughness of the bearing surfaces. The friction is determined solely by the viscous properties of the fluid and is independent of the physical or chemical properties of the bearing surfaces. This is thought to be an important mechanism of lubrication in human synovial joints.

Ref:

Nordin, M and Frankel, V. (3rd ed.) (2001) *Basic biomechanics of the musculoskeletal system*, Lippincott Williams and Wilkins, Philadelphia.

**37    D**

Wear can be measured either directly from explanted joints using a shadowgrapgh technique or co-ordinate measuring system; or indirectly using sequential radiographs. Other means of assessment are joint wear simulators. However, these do not replicate invivo loading conditions and should be taken as an underestimate of true wear. In addition, the load bearing cycle of the hip demonstrates two peaks – one at heel strike and one at load transfer to the other leg. Therefore, during the gait cycle, we need to consider two cycles of hip loading/unloading rather than just one.

Ref:

Buckwalter, J; Einhorn, T and Simon, S.(2nd ed.) (2000) *Orthopaedic Basic Science: Biology and Biomechanics of the Musculoskeletal System*, American Academy of Orthopaedic Surgeons, Rosemont.

**38.    B**

When considering the properties of a finished polyethylene implant, four aspects require attention:

- The nature of the starting product
- The method of manufacture
- The method of sterilisation
- The storage conditions

All of these factors affect the mechanical properties of the produced poyethylene. In ram extrusion, the starting product in the form of a powder is fed into a hopper and is pushed through a heated die by a hydraulic ram to give you polyethylene bar stock which is subsequently machined to give you the finished product. The result is cheap with inferior wear characteristics (typically 0.1mm/year wear rate). Direct compression moulding and heat pressing are manufacture methods whereby the polyethylene is heated and compressed to give the final product which, though expensive to produce, confers better wear characteristics (0.05mm/year wear rate).

Ref:

Buckwalter, J; Einhorn, T and Simon, S. (2nd ed.) (2000) *Orthopaedic Basic Science: Biology and Biomechanics of the Musculoskeletal System*, American Academy of Orthopaedic Surgeons, Rosemont.

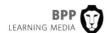

**39. B**

When an implant is cemented into bone, the mechanical and thermal trauma creates a zone of bone death around the implant which is replaced by a thin glycoprotein interface conversion film[1]. Pressurised lavage has been shown to be superior to washing and brushing with respect to shear strength of the bone cement interface and active bleeding can reduce the shear strength of this interface by up to 20%[2]. Three 10mm keyholes provide better trosional resistance to twelve 5mm keyholes with respect to macrolocking of cemented acetabular implants[3].

Ref:
1. Buckwalter, J; Einhorn, T and Simon, S.(2nd ed.) (2000) *Orthopaedic Basic Science: Biology and Biomechanics of the Musculoskeletal System*, American Academy of Orthopaedic Surgeons, Rosemont.
2. Majkowski, R; Bannister, G and Miles, A. (1994) The effect of bleeding on the cement-bone interface: an experimental study. *ClinOrthop*, 299: 293–297.
3. Reading, A; Miles, A and Bannister, G. (2002) Keyholes in acetabular preparation. *J Bone Joint Surg (Br)*, 85(S1): 57.

**40. D**

Wear is directly related to both load and sliding distance and with this in mind, Charnley designed his low frictional torque arthroplasty with a small head on the basis that this should produce reduced wear.

Ref:
Nordin, M and Frankel, V. (3rd ed.) (2001) *Basic biomechanics of the musculoskeletal system*, Lippincott Williams and Wilkins, Philadelphia.

**41. D**

Fatigue usually occurs in response to cyclical loading with stress levels much lower than the ultimate tensile strength of the material. Cracks develop at the site of imperfections or other regions of high stress concentration and propagate with each loading cycle until a critical size is reached at which point rapid propagation and final failure occur. Consequently, there is very little if any plastic deformation at the time of failure.

Ref:
Callister, W. (7th ed.) (2006) *Materials science and engineering: an introduction*, John Wiley, New York.

**42. B**

Corrosion occurs in metals by several different mechanisms:

(a) Uniform attack eg generalised rusting
(b) Galvanic corrosion – occurs when two metals electrochemically dissimilar are connected in solution. The more electronegative of the two acts as an anode and is destroyed electrochemically ie corrodes. This situation can be beneficial in that more electronegative metals can be used as scarificial anodes or by enforcing a cathode status on the metal to be protected by an external supply of electrons from an applied current
(c) Crevice corrosion – solution in crevice stagnates and oxygen is locally depleted leading to enhanced corrosion eg between modular components, between screw threads

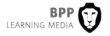

(d) Pitting corrosion – similar to crevice corrosion but highly localised attack with gravity aiding the formation of pits with high levels of solute concentration and oxygen depletion at the base

(e) Erosion corrosion – corrosive attack intensified due to mechanical wear from fluid motion

(f) Fretting corrosion – corrosion enhanced by mechanical wear from moving parts

(g) Fatigue enhnced corrosion – combination of fatigue in a corrosive environment

Ref:
Callister, W. (7<sup>th</sup> ed.) (2006) *Materials science and engineering: an introduction*, John Wiley, New York.

**43.** **A**

Passivity is the phenomenon by which normally active metals or alloys lose all reactivity and become inert depending on their environmental conditions. This occurs due to the formation of a thin highly adherent oxide film on the surface which acts as a protective barrier. Stainless steel exhibits this where the chromium content forms this protective oxide layer. With respect to corrosion resistance it offers an additional benefit over a standard protective coating such as paint in that if it is scratched the exposed metal is oxidised and the layer reforms.

Ref:
Callister, W. (7<sup>th</sup> ed.) (2006) *Materials science and engineering: an introduction*, John Wiley, New York.

**44.** **B**

Two benign bone tumours can be found in the epiphysis-chondroblastomas and giant cell tumours. Whereas the giant cell tumour commonly arises on the metaphyseal side of the physis and crosses over into the epiphysis, the chondroblastoma almost exclusively arises from the epiphysis.

Ref:
Ramachandran, M. (2007) *Basic Orthhopaedic Sciences: The Stanmore Guide*, Hodder Arnold, London.

**45.** **D**

The Enneking classification of tumour grading is:

| Stage | Grade | Site | Metastases |
|---|---|---|---|
| IA | G1 (low) | T1 (intracompartmental) | M0 (none) |
| IB | G1 (low) | T2 (extracompartmental) | M0 (none) |
| IIA | G2 (high) | T1 (intracompartmental) | M0 (none) |
| IIB | G2 (high) | T2 (extracompartmental) | M0 (none) |
| III | Any | Any | M1 (present) |

Ref:
Buckwalter, J; Einhorn, T and Simon, S.(2<sup>nd</sup> ed.) (2000) *Orthopaedic Basic Science: Biology and Biomechanics of the Musculoskeletal System*, American Academy of Orthopaedic Surgeons, Rosemont.

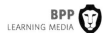

**46.** **D**

On MRI scans, soft tissue sarcomas have a characteristic appearence of high signal intensity on T2 weighted images and low signal intensity on T1 weighted images.

|  | T1 | T2 |
|---|---|---|
| Fat | high | intermediate |
| Muscle | intermediate | intermediate |
| Cortical bone | low | low |
| Normal marrow | high | intermediate |
| Pigmented villonodular synovitis | very low | very low |
| Soft tissue sarcomas | low | high |

Ref:
Buckwalter, J; Einhorn, T and Simon, S.(2<sup>nd</sup> ed.) (2000) *Orthopaedic Basic Science: Biology and Biomechanics of the Musculoskeletal System*, American Academy of Orthopaedic Surgeons, Rosemont.

**47.** **C**

Mirels developed a scoring system to predicte fractures of long bone. In his system, there are four categories each rated on a scale of 1–3 points reflecting severity. The categories are:

- Site – upper limb, lower limb, peritrochanter
- Pain – mild, moderate, severe
- Lesion – blastic, mixed, lytic
- Size – <1/3, 1/3–2/3, >2/3

From his series he concluded that a score of 8 out of 12 was associated with a 15% risk of fracture. However, a score of 9 increased this risk to 33% and he argued that this should be used as an indication of prophylactic fixation.

Ref:
Mirels H. Metastatic disease in long bones. (1989) *Clin Orthop Rel Res*, 249: 256–264.

**48.** **B**

See answer to question 47.

Ref:
Mirels H. Metastatic disease in long bones. (1989) *Clin Orthop Rel Res*, 249: 256–264.

**49.** **E**

Benign tumours are staged as follows:

- Stage 1 – Latent. Intracapsular, asymptomatic and usually incidental findings. On radiographs, well defined margin with no cortical destruction or expansion.
- Stage 2 – Active. Intracapsular but actively growing and can cause symptoms or pathological fracture. Radiographs show well defined margins but there may be cortical thinning or expansion.

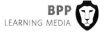

- Stage 3 – Aggressive. Extracapsular with frequent spread beyond bones into surrounding soft tissues and the possibility of metastases.

Ref:
Buckwalter J, Einhorn T, Simon S. (2nd ed.) (2000) *Orthopaedic Basic Science : Biology and Biomechanics of the Musculoskeletal System*, American Academy of Orthopaedic Surgeons, Rosemont.

**50. B**

Pigmented villonodular synovitis most commonly occurs in the joints of the lower limb. The knee is most common followed by the hip and shoulder. The lesion has been reported in other joints less frequently.

Ref:

Buckwalter, J; Einhorn, T and Simon, S. (2nd ed.) (2000) *Orthopaedic Basic Science: Biology and Biomechanics of the Musculoskeletal System*, American Academy of Orthopaedic Surgeons, Rosemont.

**51. D**

Parosteal osteosarcoma usually presents as a lobulated ossific mass on the posterior aspect of the distal femur. The lesion usually has a medullary cavity continuous with that of the host bone as demonstrated on computed tomography.

Ref:
Canale, T. (10th ed.) (2003) *Campbell's Operative Orthopaedics*, Elsevier, St Louis.

**52. A**

Mankin (1982) conducted a study looking at the complications of biopsy of musculoskeletal tumours and based on his results provided the following recommendations:

(a) Biopsy should be performed after investigations are complete
(b) Biopsy should be performed in a specialist centre by a surgeon who is familiar with incisions of limb salvage and flaps and who will perform the definitive resection
(c) A tourniquet is allowed but compressive exanguination is deleterious
(d) Transverse incisions should be avoided as they are difficult to excise
(e) As few compartments as possible should be violated during the biopsy and the tract should be marked
(f) If a hole is to be made in a bone, it should be filled with a cement plug to minimise the risk of pathological fracture and seeding
(g) A frozen section should be sent for histology as if the tumour is found to be benign, definitive resection and curettage can be performed
(h) Haemostasis should be meticulous as any blood clot will fill up with tumour cells
(i) Any drains should be placed in the line of the incision so that the tract can be excised later

Ref:
Canale, T. (10th ed.) (2003) *Campbell's Operative Orthopaedics*, Elsevier, St Louis.

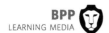

**53.  D**

Unicameral bone cysts usually arise in the first two decades of life and are most commonly found in the proximal humerus. The next most common site is the proximal femur. They usually appear on radiographs as cystic lesions with septa which expand the bone but do not elicit a periosteal reaction. Occasionally a shard of cortical bone is seen at the base of the lesion (fallen leaf sign). They are usually asymptomatic until pathological fracture occurs and healing of the fracture usually obliterates the cyst.

Ref:
Ramachandran, M. (2007) *Basic Orthhopaedic Sciences: The Stanmore Guide*, Hodder Arnold, London.

**54.  D**

Malignant transformation of osteochondromas is quite rare but should be suspected when a longstanding lesion becomes painful and enlarged. An increase in the thickness of the cartilaginous cap beyond 1cm is an indication for surgical resection.

Ref:
Ramachandran, M. (2007) *Basic Orthhopaedic Sciences: The Stanmore Guide*, Hodder Arnold, London.

**55.  D**

Osteoid osteomas can frequently be missed on plain films as their diameter is less than 1 cm and usually require fine cut CT. Osteoblastomas may resemble osteoid osteomas but are chiefly differentiated on the basis of size with osteoblastomas having a diameter greater than 1.5 cm.

Ref:
 Canale, T. (10th ed.) (2003) *Campbell's operative orthopaedics*, Elsevier, St Louis.

**56.  C**

A free body diagram is a sketch of a body under consideration which is isolated from all other bodies and shows all external forces acting on it. In terms of orthopaedic biomechanics these forces include the results of muscle action, gravity and supports eg walking sticks. Usually more than one free body diagram can be drawn for a particular situation, the choice usually dictated by the information available. However, there are certain assumptions and exclusions to this type of analysis:

- Skeletal links are assumed to be rigid.
- Joints are considered to act as frictionless hinges.
- Muscles act only in tension with a line of action along the centre of the cross sectional area.
- All body weight passes through an exact centre of body mass.
- Internal forces are usually excluded from the analysis.

Ref:
Nordin, M and Frankel, V. (3rd ed.) (2001) *Basic biomechanics of the musculoskeletal system*, Lippincott Williams and Wilkins, Philadelphia.

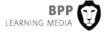

57.  **D**
     Strain ('E) is defined as the change in length of a material as a fraction of the original length at a point in time. It is given by the equation:

     'E $= l_i - l_o/l_o$  $l_i$ instantaneous length

     $\qquad\qquad\qquad$ $l_o$ original length before load applied

     It is dimensionless but can be expressed as a percentage by multiplying by 100. Stress and strain are linearly related to each other on the elastic portion of the stress strain curve by the equation Stress = Strain × Young's modulus

     It can be seen that when stress is plotted against strain, the gradient of the linear part of the curve is equivalent to Young's modulus or the stiffness of the material. The imposed stress which causes the resultant deformation or strain is recoverable once the stress is removed. This resistance to elastic deformation relates to the material's resistance to interatomic seperation. Thus materials which have a greater number of interatomic bonds are stiffer, more resistant to deformation, and produce far less strain under an imposed stress.

     Poisson's ratio describes the changes in dimensions which occur as a result of a uniaxial applied stress. For example, when a metal bar is stressed in tension, the resultant deformation or strain leads to changes in both the length and width of the metal bar. Poisson's ratio is simply the ratio of change in the longitudinal dimension with respect to the change in the transverse dimension.

     Ref:
     Callister, W. (7th ed.) (2006) *Materials science and engineering: an introduction*, John Wiley, New York.

58.  **B**
     The stress-strain curve is devised by imposing an increasing load or stress on a structure or material and measuring the extent of deformation or strain up to the point of failure. In most testing situations, a tensile stress is applied. Young's modulus which defines the stiffness of a material is given by the steepness of the gradient of the elastic portion of the stress strain curve. It can be seen that Material S is stiffer than T. Ductility is a measure of the extent of plastic deformation at the time of fracture. A material which demonstrates greater strain under an applied load is more ductile. At the same stress level, Material S demonstrates more strain and therefore more deformation than T and is therefore more ductile.

     At some point on the linear portion (elastic deformation) of the stress-strain curve, the curve deviates from proportionality as in point A for Material S. This is the yield point of the Material and thereafter as the imposed stress increases the material demonstrates plastic deformation ie non-reversible deformation. The small peak which occurs at this point in the curve for metals corresponds to a reduction in stress due to this initial plastic deformation.

     The highest point on the stress-strain curve marked for material T is the ultimate tensile strength of this material which corresponds to the maximum stress that can be sustained by the material under the conditions of the test performed.

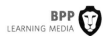

Ref:
Callister, W. (7<sup>th</sup> ed.) (2006) *Materials science and engineering: an introduction*, John Wiley, New York.

**59.  B**

Creep is defined as the viscoelastic property of certain materials whereby if a stress is imposed and held at a constant level over time, the material exhibits deformation. The opposing phenomenon that is seen when strain is kept constant over time rather than the stress level is stress relaxation whereby the stress within the material decreases over time as it is held in this state of persistent deformation.

Ref:
Nordin, M and Frankel, V. (3<sup>rd</sup> ed.) (2001) *Basic biomechanics of the musculoskeletal system*, Lippincott Williams and Wilkins, Philadelphia.

**60.  D**

Applications of certain force profiles have a tendency to be associated with certain fracture patterns. This understanding of relationships between the force profile in terms of point of application, sense (direction) and magnitude; and the resultant bone injury is invaluable in closed reduction techniques. From a forensic perspective it also allows insight into third party accounts of mechanisms of injury in pediatric trauma.

Buckle and greenstick fractures are commonly observed in paediatric bone which is more flexible and has a thicker periosteum restricting displacement of the fragments. Pilon fractures are observed in certain joints where a pure axial load drives the harder of the two bones into the expanded end of the softer one frequently causing fractures in multiple planes. Characteristic sites include the distal tibia and base of phalanx. Spiral fracture results from the application of a torsional force to long bone whereas pure bending usually gives rise to a transverse fracture. Combined longitudinal compression with bending leads to failure that begins first on the side under tension. The crack that develops here propagates along the planes of maximum shear stress as a result of the combined force profile. This creates the characteristic wedge or butterfly fragment seen at the fracture site.

Ref:
Buckwalter, J; Einhorn, T and Simon, S. (2<sup>nd</sup> ed.) (2000) *Orthopaedic Basic Science: Biology and Biomechanics of the Musculoskeletal System*, American Academy of Orthopaedic Surgeons, Rosemont.

**61.  C**

Forces can be defined as the action of one body with another and are vectors. Fundamentally, they can not be described by magnitude alone as they also have a point of application and direction (or sense). In most biomechanical analysis we mainly consider external forces of bodies rather than the internal forces between constituent molecules. The centre of the gravity in the human body is most consistently mapped just anterior to the vertebral body of S2. A couple is an important biomechanical concept because the resultant force is zero yet movement in the form of rotation occurs. An example is the action of the serratus anterior and trapezius muscles rotating the scapula.

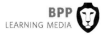

Ref:
Buckwalter, J; Einhorn, T and Simon, S. (2nd ed.) (2000) *Orthopaedic Basic Science: Biology and Biomechanics of the Musculoskeletal System*, American Academy of Orthopaedic Surgeons, Rosemont.

**62.    D**

The stiffness of a material relates to the gradient of the stress-strain curve in its elastic portion. In essence, the steepness of the gradient dictates how much deformation occurs for a particular level of imposed strain. Therefore, the steeper the gradient, the greater the resistance to elastic deformation. As elastic deformation is completely reversible once the stress is removed this resistance translates to the resistance to interatomic separation as it is these bonds which are stretched. In metallic bonding, each atom gives up 1–3 surplus valence electrons which form a mobile electron sea which shields the positive cores of nuclei and remaining valence electrons from each other. This sea of electrons can also be likened to a cloud which drifts throughout the entire metal giving rise to some metals' excellent thermal and electrical conductivity.

Most crystalline structures such as metals and many ceramics can be described in terms of the unit cell. This is the smallest repeating unit that can be used to describe the whole structure. In metals, close packing of atoms is necessary to maximise the shielding provided by the electron cloud and three three types of structure exist:

(a)    Face centred cubic eg Al, Au, Ag
(b)    Body centred cubic eg Fe, Cr
(c)    Hexagonal close packed eg Mg, Zn

Polymorphism is the phenomenon whereby some metals and non-metals have more than one crystalline structure. The type of structure that exists is dictated by the prevailing conditions. Iron has a body centred cubic structure at room temperature but at 900 degrees this transforms into a face centred cubic configuration along with a change in physical properties such as volume and density.

Ref:
Callister, W. (7th ed.) (2006) *Materials science and engineering: an introduction*, John Wiley, New York.

**63.    D**

As the applied stress increases, a certain point is reached where stress is no longer proportional to strain. This is known as the yield point and signals the onset of plastic deformation. Plastic deformation differes from elastic deformation in that permanent change results which is not immediately reversible on unloading. The strength of a material is dictated by its resistance to plastic deformation much in the way that the stiffness of a material is dictated by its resistance to elastic deformation. Ductility is a measure of the extent of plastic deformation at the time of fracture. Toughness is the ability of a material to absorb energy up to the point of fracture and depends on specimen geometry and load application. Strength, ductility and toughness are all sensitive to the presence of impurities, heat treatments and prior deformation because all of these effect plastic deformation. Elastic deformation which is recoverable occurs as a result of interatomic bonds being stretched. There are several possible mechanisms by which plastic deformation can occur in metals which relate to defects in the crystalline structure. These defects are known as

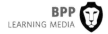

dislocations and occur as a result of planes of atoms being misaligned due to missing atoms. These disruptions in the crystal lattice structure are mobile and plastic deformation principally arises as a result of movement in a multitude of dislocations along different planes. This can be rudimentarily compared to mechanisms of plastic deformation in biological structures whereby tendons elongate under prolonged stress due to interfibrillar sliding.

Ref:
Callister, W. (7th ed.) (2006) *Materials science and engineering: an introduction*, John Wiley, New York.

64.  **A**
Strength is the resistance to plastic deformation. Plastic deformation occurs as a result of defects in the crystal lattice, known as dislocations, moving through the structure by a process known as slip. Therefore, anything that restricts the movement of these dislocations will increase the strength of the metal. These include:

a.  Grain size reduction – most crystalline structures are polycrystalline. The individual crystals that make up the structure are made up of different lattice orientations. Disloctions are only able to move along predetermined crystallographic planes and can therefore not jump from crystal to crystal. These grain boundaries between crystals therefore act to restrict the movement of dislocations. Grain size reduction leads to an increase in the number of grain boundaries and so increases the strength of the metal.

b.  Solid solution hardening – the presence of foreign atoms within a metal distorts the crystal lattice which restricts the movement of dislocations and therefore increases the strength. This was first noted to occur by a process of age hardening whereby a metal left over time became stronger due to the formation of precipitates throughout the structure which acted to limit the movement of dislocations.

c.  Strain hardening / cold working – progressive plastic deformation leads to preferentially aligned dislocations being used up. The hard to move dislocations left in the lattice require more force to move and cause plastic deformation thus strengthening the material. The problem here is that as the strength of the material goes up, the ductility decreases because after a while all the dislocations can move no further and there is a build-up of stresses at the grain boundaries. Eventually, the material becomes very brittle and fractures.

Metals, due to their polycrystalline structure, may be thought of as isotropic in that they have similar properties regardless of the direction of measurement. Therefore, if a cube of metal was turned on its side and tested again in tension, the results would be no different. This is in contrast to biological materials which tend to be highly anisotropic eg cortical bone.

Ref:
Callister, W. (7th ed.) (2006) *Materials science and engineering: an introduction*, John Wiley, New York.

65.  **D**
Ductile materials usually absorb a lot of energy and deform significantly before fracture. Cracks that are formed are usually stable in contrast to brittle materials where the cracks

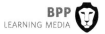

are unstable and spread rapidly with little or no plastic deformation. In brittle materials, the crack propagation continues spontaneously without an increase in the applied stress and usually propagates at the speed of sound. Ceramics usually fracture in this way and the fractured surface is usually flat and featureless with occasionally noticeable characterstic chevron markings radiating out from the site of the defect. Conversely, fracture usually occurs in ductile materials due to the coalescement of microvoids which propagate along the lines of maximal shear stress giving rise to a cup and cone appearence of the fractured specimen.

Ref:
Callister, W. (7th ed.) (2006) *Materials science and engineering: an introduction*, John Wiley, New York.

**66. B**

During 'heel off' to 'toe off', the ankle plantarflexes from 10 degrees dorsiflexion to 30 degrees plantarflexion. The Ground Reaction Force acts anterior to the joint which produces a dorsiflexion movement. However, the calf plantarflexors act to oppose this movement.

Ref:
Whittle, M. (3rd ed.) (2001) *Gait analysis: an introduction*, Elsevier, Oxford.

**67. B**

Strength, ductility, toughness all relate to structures or materials stressed to beyond their elastic limits such that plastic deformation occurs. Failure through fatigue relates to the number, size and geometry of defects within a material as well as the mechanism of crack propagation which the structure or material permits. It can be seen that all of these can be influenced by the extent of prior deformation, presence of impurities and effects of heat treatment. In contrast, stiffness is a measure of resistance to elastic deformation which in itself relates to resistance to interatomic separation. Stiffness is therefore independent of all such factors which can alter the mechanics of plastic deformation and is a intrinsic characteristic of a material.

Ref:
Callister, W. (7th ed.) (2006) *Materials science and engineering: an introduction*, John Wiley, New York.

**68. B**

It is useful to remember the material properties of materials commonly utilised in orthopaedics.

| Material | Young's modulus |
| --- | --- |
| Steel | 20 GPa |
| Titanium | 110 GPa |
| PMMA | 2 GPa |
| Cortical bone | 17 GPa |
| Trabecular | 100 MPa |

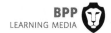

Ref:

Buckwalter, J; Einhorn, T and Simon, S.(2nd ed.) (2000) *Orthopaedic Basic Science : Biology and Biomechanics of the Musculoskeletal System*, American Academy of Orthopaedic Surgeons, Rosemont.

**69.  E**

P values like confidence intervals are examples of inferential statistics. As it is very difficult to conduct studies on entire populations, such statistical analyses are used to infer findings from a discrete sample to an entire population and determine the likelihood that any differences could have occurred by chance. The P value corresponds to the probability of obtaining the observed difference or one more extreme when the null hypothesis is true. It is in essence a probability statement that the statistical observation in a study is due to chance alone. By convention a cut off value of 5% (p <0.05) is deemed as statistically significant. However, P values should never be viewed in isolation. For example, a P value may be less than 0.05 and deemed statistically significant. However, the actual measured difference to which this P value corresponds may not be clinically significant eg a difference in length of hospital stay from 8 to 9 days. This can be the case in studies with very large numbers. Conversely a drug may be three times more effective than its rival but as the P value for the observed difference is 0.16, this difference may be dismissed. For this reason, confidence intervals are preferable as they provide the reader with information on the direction and magnitude of effect or difference.

Ref:

Buckwalter, J; Einhorn, T and Simon, S. (2nd ed.) (2000) *Orthopaedic Basic Science : Biology and Biomechanics of the Musculoskeletal System*, American Academy of Orthopaedic Surgeons, Rosemont.

**70.  B**

A type I error is when the null hypothesis is rejected when it is in fact true ie you think there is a difference when there isn't one. This relates to **false** positives and the questionable nature of the specificity of the test which has given these significant results. A type II error is when the null hypothesis has been accepted when in fact it is **false**. This means that a difference does exist but the sample size may have been too small to detect it. This relates to the power of a study.

The power of a test is the probability that a study of a given size would register as statistically significant a real difference of a given magnitude. To perform a power caculation requires determination of the smallest true clinical or experimental difference that would be considered as valuable ie if it exists you can say there is a benefit and if it does not exist there is no benefit. If this value is very small a much larger sample size is required.

Having calculated the standardised difference from the above value and the standard deviation of the primary variable for both groups, a nomogram can be used to calculate the sample size or power. The use of a nomogram assumes two independent groups with roughly equal sample sizes and normal distributions.

Ref:

Buckwalter, J; Einhorn, T and Simon, S. (2nd ed.) (2000) *Orthopaedic Basic Science: Biology and Biomechanics of the Musculoskeletal System*, American Academy of Orthopaedic Surgeons, Rosemont.

BPP LEARNING MEDIA

71.   **A**

The sensitivity of a test is the proportion of positives that are correctly identified by the test as positive. The specificity of a test is the proportion of negatives that are correctly identified by the test as negative. This contrasts with the positive and negative predictive values. The positive predictive value is the number of patients with a positive test result who are correctly diagnosed as positive. The negative predictive value is the number of patients with a negative test result who are correctly diagnosed as negative.

Ref:
Buckwalter, J; Einhorn, T and Simon, S.(2nd ed.) (2000) *Orthopaedic Basic Science: Biology and Biomechanics of the Musculoskeletal System*, American Academy of Orthopaedic Surgeons, Rosemont.

72.   **D**

Variables that can be measured on a scale are defined as numerical variables. Two types exist:

1.   Continuous variables – on this scale measurements can be directly quantified at any point on a given range eg visual analogue scale for pain
2.   Discrete – these reflect counts where in between values don't exist and are therefore usually a whole number eg number of births

Variables that are entirely qualitative whereby no quantitative distinction can be made between individual values are known as categorical variables. Two types exist:

1.   Ordinal – individual values can be ranked although no precise relationship exists between ranks eg grading pain as mild, moderate, severe
2.   Nominal – 'in name only.' Such variables can not be ranked eg gender, blood group

Ref:
Buckwalter, J; Einhorn, T and Simon, S. (2nd ed.) (2000) *Orthopaedic Basic Science: Biology and Biomechanics of the Musculoskeletal System*, American Academy of Orthopaedic Surgeons, Rosemont.

73.   **E**

The current levels of evidence as defined by the Oxford Centre for Evidence-based Medicine for experimental study designs looking at therapeutic intervention are

1a   Systematic review (with homogeneity) of RCTs
1b   Individual RCT (with narrow confidence interval)
1c   'All or none' case series. Two scenarios
     –   all patients died before treatment became available, but some now survive on it
     –   some patients died before treatment became available but none now die on it
2a   Systematic review (with homogeneity) of cohort studies
2b   Individual cohort study (including low quality RCT eg <80% follow up)
2c   'Outcomes' research; ecological studies
3a   Systematic review (with homogeneity) of case-control studies
3b   Individual case control study

Ref:
Centre for Evidence-based Medicine (www.cebm.net)

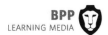

74. **C**

The research question outlined that the incidence of VTE is less with drug A than drug B is the research hypothesis. Hypothesis testing works on the basis that proving that a difference exists does not disprove the possibility of there being no difference. Consequently, research sets out to disprove the hypothesis that no difference exists. This hypothesis is known as the null hypothesis. Thus, for our present study, the appropriate null hypothesis is that the incidence of VTE with drug A is equal to that of drug B. The alternate hypothesis is that a difference in VTE incidence does exist between the two treatments. Choice of statistical tests employed and at what level we set significance allow us to appropriately accept or reject the null hypothesis but in themselves are not the basis of the null hypothesis.

Ref:

Buckwalter, J; Einhorn, T and Simon, S. (2nd ed.) (2000) *Orthopaedic Basic Science: Biology and Biomechanics of the Musculoskeletal System*, American Academy of Orthopaedic Surgeons, Rosemont.

75. **B**

An important consideration in appropriate use of statistical tests is whether the data sets assume a normal distribution. A histogram should always be plotted to assess skewness and kurtosis. When data is skewed the mean is not found in the centre of the distribution (demonstrated graphically by the curve not being symmetrical about the mean). Kurtosis of a variable implies that the tail ends of the distribution do not taper off in the classic bell shaped normal distribution in that there are either too many or too few numbers of cases in the tail end(s) of the distribution. Data sets that deviate from the normal distribution in either or both of these ways are known as non-parametric data and consequently parametric (normal distribution) tests can not be appropriately used. The options in this instance are to apply a transformation function such as logarithms to transform the data set to resemble a normal distribution or to use non-parametric designed tests that do not hold the same assumptions regarding skewness about the mean. Below are given examples of equivalent non-parametric tests:

| Parametric | Non-parametric |
| --- | --- |
| Pearson correlation co-efficient | Spearman Rho test |
| Student's T test | Mann-Whitney |
| Paired T test | Wilcoxon signed rank |
| One way analysis of variance | Kruskal-Wallis |
| Two way analysis of variance | Friedman |

Ref:

Buckwalter, J; Einhorn, T and Simon, S. (2nd ed.) (2000) *Orthopaedic Basic Science: Biology and Biomechanics of the Musculoskeletal System*, American Academy of Orthopaedic Surgeons, Rosemont.

76. **B**

The standard deviation and confidence intervals are methods of expressing the dispersion of a data set. The standard deviation is the square root of the variance of a sample ie the average of the distance of each point from the mean. The confidence interval is a range within the data set that we can be confident includes the true population value. It encompasses two features:

BPP
LEARNING MEDIA

(1) a point estimate of the true value (the mean)
(2) variation in the sample (the standard error)

The 95% confidence interval is derived from the following formula:

mean +/− (1.96 × standard error of the mean)

The 99% confidence interval is derived from the following formuala:

mean +/− (2.49 × standard error of the mean)

The 95% confidence interval does not mean that there is a 95% chance that this range contains the true population mean. It actually means that there is a 95% probability that the limits calculated from a random sample will contain the true population value ie take 100 similar sized samples from the population and derive 95% confidence intervals then 95 of these constructed confidence intervals would enclose the true population value.

Ref:
Buckwalter, J; Einhorn, T and Simon, S. (2nd ed.) (2000) *Orthopaedic Basic Science: Biology and Biomechanics of the Musculoskeletal System*, American Academy of Orthopaedic Surgeons, Rosemont.

77. **B**
There are several important structural changes which occur in cartilage with ageing. There are qualitative and quantitative differences in proteoglycan and collagen content as well as changes in hydration of the porous permeable matrix. The changes which occur in the proteoglycan content are:

(a) Chondroitin 4 sulphate levels decrease
(b) Chondroitin 6 sulphate levels increase
(c) Keratin sulphate: chondroitin sulphate ratio increases
(d) Aggrecan levels decrease

Ref:
Buckwalter, J; Einhorn, T and Simon, S. (2nd ed.) (2000) *Orthopaedic Basic Science: Biology and Biomechanics of the Musculoskeletal System*, American Academy of Orthopaedic Surgeons, Rosemont.

78. **B**
Immobilisation has several effects on bone, tendons and cartilage. The most profound change is a marked reduction in proteoglycan content which decreases the hydration of the cartilage porous permeable matrix structure. Consequently, there is a greater capacity for deformation. The potentially deleterious effects this may have on integrity of the matrix are minimised by the fact that the collagen content does not change. Therefore, the bulk restrictive properties of the matrix and its structural integrity are preserved until the joint is once again loaded and proteoglycan and hydration levels can be restored.

Ref:
Buckwalter, J; Einhorn, T and Simon, S. (2nd ed.) (2000) *Orthopaedic Basic Science: Biology and Biomechanics of the Musculoskeletal System*, American Academy of Orthopaedic Surgeons, Rosemont.

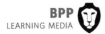
BPP
LEARNING MEDIA

79. **B**

Parathyroid hormone acts to increase serum calcium and decrease serum phosphate. The active form of vitamin D increases serum levels of both calcium and phosphate.

Ref:

Buckwalter, J; Einhorn, T and Simon, S. (2nd ed.) (2000) *Orthopaedic Basic Science: Biology and Biomechanics of the Musculoskeletal System*, American Academy of Orthopaedic Surgeons, Rosemont.

80. **D**

There are several different types of collagen and it is worthwhile remembering where they are commonly found and what their functions are.

| | |
|---|---|
| Type I | Commonly found in bone |
| Type II | Most predominant type of collagen found in articular cartilage. Collagen content is highest in the superficial zone. |
| Type III | Found in the periosteum where it enhances the migration of osteoprogenitor cells and capillary ingrowth. Accounts for up to 50% of collagen found in vessel walls of medium and large sized arteries |
| Type V, XI | Act as templates regulating the diameter and orientation of collagen fibrils |
| Type IX | Commonly found in the superficial zone of articular cartilage where it stabilises the collagen fibrous network improving the wear resistance and enhances the bulk restrictive properties of the porous permeable matrix |

Ref:

Buckwalter, J; Einhorn, T and Simon, S. (2nd ed.) (2000) *Orthopaedic Basic Science: Biology and Biomechanics of the Musculoskeletal System*, American Academy of Orthopaedic Surgeons, Rosemont.

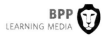

# Trauma

## Question Bank

Gautam Tawari & Fahad
G Attar

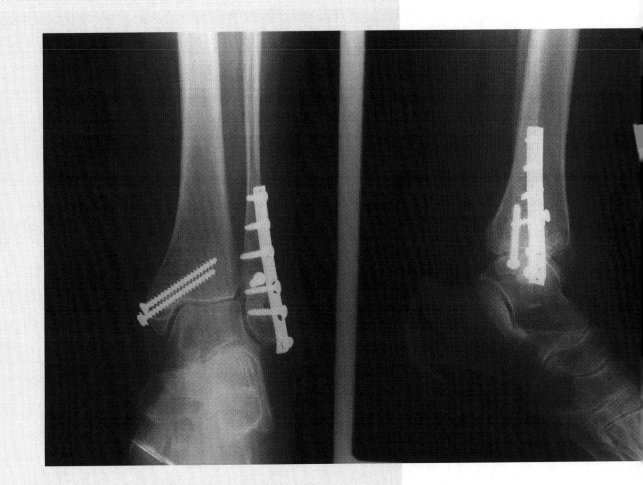

Trauma

1. Following a distal radius fracture, ligaments useful in restoring palmar tilt during fracture reduction with the help of ligamentotaxis include all of the below except:
   A. Radioscapholunate ligament
   B. Radioscaphoid ligament
   C. Radiocapitate ligament
   D. Volar radiotriquetral ligament
   E. Radial collateral ligament

2. The following classification for distal radius fracture is based on the mechanism of injury:
   A. Frykman's classification
   B. Melone's classification
   C. Rayhack's classification
   D. Fernandez's classification
   E. AO/ASIF classification

3. The following statement indicates towards an unstable distal radius fracture pattern requiring internal or external fixation:
   A. Articular depression of 1mm
   B. Radial shortening of 8mm
   C. Dorsal tilt of 15 degrees
   D. None of the above
   E. All of the above

4. Which of the below is the definitive method to confirm the diagnosis of Avascular Necrosis of scaphoid?
   A. Clinical examination
   B. Plain radiographs
   C. CT scan
   D. MRI scan
   E. Surgical biopsy

5. The following statements are **true** for the scaphocapitate syndrome except
   A. This is a combined scaphoid and capitate fracture resulting from extreme dorsiflexion of the wrist
   B. Results from a direct blow to the radial styloid
   C. The proximal pole of the capitate may rotate by up to 180 degrees
   D. Treatment includes internal fixation of both scaphoid and capitates
   E. It is associated with AVN of scaphoid.

6. The pattern for ligamentous failure in progressive perilunar disruption is:
   A. Capitolunate tear, scapholunate tear, lunotriquetral tear, dorsal radiolunate tear
   B. Scapholunate tear, lunotriquetral tear, capitolunate tear, dorsal radiolunate tear
   C. Scapholunate tear, capitolunate tear, lunotriquetral tear, dorsal radiolunate tear
   D. Capitolunate tear, lunotriquetral tear, scapholunate tear, dorsal radiolunate tear
   E. Lunotriquetral tear, capitolunate tear, scapholunate tear, dorsal radiolunate tear

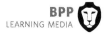

7.  All of the following are included as the radiological features of a DISI in the wrist, except:
    A.  Widening of the scapholunate interval of >3 mm on PA view
    B.  A scapholunate angle of 30 degrees on lateral view
    C.  Evidence of scaphoid fracture
    D.  Presence of 'cortical ring' sign
    E.  A capitolunate angle of 15 degrees

8.  Isolated disruption of intrinsic ligaments between the same row of carpal bones results in carpal instability pattern commonly described as one of the following:
    A.  Carpal Instability Dissociative (CID)
    B.  Carpal instability Non-Dissociative (CIND)
    C.  Carpal Instability Complex (CIC)
    D.  Carpal Instability Adaptive (CIA)
    E.  Midcarpal Instability (MCI)

9.  The treatment for Class 1A TFCC tear include:
    A.  Arthroscopic repair of the TFCC
    B.  Arthroscopic debridement of TFCC
    C.  Open repair of the TFCC
    D.  Reattachment of the avulsed TFCC
    E.  Splint and rest

10. To prevent bowstringing deformity of the finger, the following pulleys should be preserved:
    A.  A1, A3
    B.  A2, A4
    C.  A1, A2
    D.  A3, A4
    E.  A3, A5

11. Passive mobilisation provides with a greater tensile strength, fewer adhesions and improved excursion when applied to the following healing phase of the flexor tendons:
    A.  Inflammatory phase
    B.  Fibroblastic phase
    C.  Remodeling phase
    D.  None of the above
    E.  All of the above

12. Primary repair of the flexor tendons in the following zone have a good prognosis and result:
    A.  Zone I, zone III
    B.  Zone II, zone III
    C.  Zone III, zone IV
    D.  Zone IV, zone II
    E.  Zone III, zone V

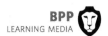

13. A 'Stener's' lesion of the thumb is associated with the following:
    A. Rupture of ulna collateral ligament with interposition of abductor pollicis aponeurosis
    B. Rupture of ulna collateral ligament with interposition of extensor pollicis aponeurosis
    C. Rupture of ulnar collateral ligament with interposition of the flexor pollicis aponeurosis
    D. Rupture of ulnar collateral ligament with interposition of the adductor pollicis aponeurosis
    E. Rupture of ulnar collateral ligament with interposition of volar plate

14. Extensor tendon laceration leading to Boutonniere's deformity typically occurs at the following zone:
    A. Zone 1
    B. Zone 2
    C. Zone 3
    D. Zone 4
    E. Zone 5

15. The following statement is **true** regarding the epidemiology of spinal cord injury (SCI):
    A. The incidence is significantly higher in females as compared to males
    B. The mean age for both genders at the time of injury is 30 years
    C. Motor vehicle accidents are the second most common cause of the injury
    D. Occurrence of SCI in context of sports is 2%–5%
    E. Falls is the predominant cause of SCI in younger age group

16. In case of occlusion of the radicular artery, which area of the spinal cord is most prone to ischaemia?
    A. Cervical cord
    B. Thoracic cord
    C. Lumbar cord
    D. Sacral cord
    E. All segments are equally affected

17. The central cord syndrome is best characterised by which of the following statements?
    A. Disproportionately greater loss of motor power in the lower extremity
    B. Bladder dysfunction (generally overflow incontinence)
    C. Sensory loss below the lesion
    D. All of the above
    E. None of the above

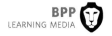

18. The pattern of recovery following the central cord syndrome is best described by the following statement (in the order of its recovery):
    A. Motor power of upper extremity, motor power of hands, motor power of lower extremity, bladder function
    B. Motor power of hands, motor power of upper extremity, bladder function, motor power of lower extremity
    C. Motor power of lower extremity, motor power of upper extremity, bladder function, motor power of the hands
    D. Motor power of lower extremity, bladder function, motor power of upper extremity, motor power of hand
    E. Motor power of upper extremity, motor power of lower extremity, bladder function, motor power of hands

19. The following statements are **true** to both conus medularis and cauda equina syndrome except:
    A. This is an incomplete SCI syndrome
    B. This can be caused by burst fractures of the vertebrae or an acute disc prolapse
    C. This is associated with radicular pain and leg weakness
    D. This is associated with sphincter disturbances
    E. This is associated with areflexic bladder

20. In atlanto-axial rotatory subluxation, a transverse ligament insufficiency with a 5 mm of anterior displacement of atlas is described as the following type:
    A. Type I
    B. Type II
    C. Type III
    D. Type IV
    E. Type V

21. Which of the following mechanism of injury is commonly associated with central cord syndrome in elderly patients with spondylosis of cervical spine?
    A. Compressive flexion injury
    B. Compressive extension injury
    C. Distractive extension injury
    D. Distractive flexion injury
    E. Lateral flexion injury

22. The most common type of compression fracture of the thoraco-lumbar spine usually involves:
    A. Both the endplates
    B. Superior endplate
    C. Inferior endplate
    D. Central body failure with intact endplates
    E. Central body failure with involvement of both endplates

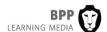

23. 'Chance fracture' of the thoraco-lumbar spine occur following which type of injury?
    A. Transitional injury
    B. Flexion distraction injury
    C. Flexion compression injury
    D. Compression injury
    E. Flexion injury

24. Atlanto-occipital dissociation injuries are always considered as unstable. The most commonest pattern seen based on the Traynelis classification is:
    A. Anterior displacement of the occiput on the C-spine.
    B. Posterior displacement of the occiput on the C-spine
    C. Vertical displacement of the occiput on the C-spine
    D. Oblique displacement of the occiput on the C-spine
    E. Lateral displacement of the occiput on the C-spine

25. An unstable C1 fracture is:
    A. Posterior arch fractures
    B. Anterior arch fractures
    C. Transverse process fracture
    D. Simple lateral mass fractures
    E. All of the above

26. Patients sustaining a spinal fracture at C2 level following blunt trauma has the following statistical risk for another spinal fracture:
    A. 10%
    B. 20%
    C. 30%
    D. 40%
    E. 50%

27. The most common complication following halo jacket treatment is:
    A. Pin tract infection
    B. Pin tract loosening
    C. Severe pain
    D. Loss of reduction
    E. Pressure sores

28. All of the following are **true** with regards to the 'PINCER' fracture of the vertebrae, except:
    A. Associated with implosion of the disc through the vertebral body
    B. Caused by excessive axial loading of the vertebra resulting in failure of endplate
    C. Mid-body separation of the vertebra in sagittal plane
    D. Associated with poor prognosis for healing compared to compressive fractures
    E. There is a combined disc and vertebral body injury

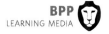

29.  In compression fractures of the thoraco-lumbar vertebrae, the following parameter indicates some element of a posterior ligamentous injury
     A.  Loss of >10% of anterior column height
     B.  Loss of >20% of anterior column height
     C.  Loss of >30% of anterior column height
     D.  Kyphosis of >10 degrees
     E.  Kyphosis of >30 degrees

30.  In a burst fracture of the thoraco-lumbar vertebra, all of the following indicate a need for operative intervention except:
     A.  Progression of >30 degrees of kyphosis
     B.  Presence of neurological deficit
     C.  Presence of bony retropulsion with intact posterior ligament complex
     D.  Presence of painful instability
     E.  >50% loss of anterior column height

31.  The following injury has the highest specificity for 'child abuse':
     A.  Spinous process avulsion fracture
     B.  Long bone fracture
     C.  Multiple fractures
     D.  Fractures in various stage of healing
     E.  Epiphyseal separation

32.  The following statements are **true** regarding the epidemiology of fractures in children, except:
     A.  Boys sustain more fractures than girls
     B.  Distal radius is the most common anatomic site for fractures
     C.  Right-sided fractures are more common than left
     D.  Physeal fractures account for common pattern just before skeletal maturity
     E.  Open fractures are relatively uncommon

33.  All of the following are **true** with consideration for the technique in treatment of physeal fractures, except:
     A.  Internal fixation should not cross the physis
     B.  Stable articular congruity should be achieved by compression screw
     C.  Compression screw across epiphyseal fragment should be parallel to physis
     D.  Smallest pin feasible should be used when crossing the physis
     E.  Manipulation should be undertaken until anatomical reduction is achieved

34.  The following statement is **false** regarding partial arrest of physis:
     A.  Peripheral bar is the commonest form
     B.  Arrest affecting more than 25% has poor prognosis
     C.  Post traumatic partial arrest has better prognosis than Blount's disease
     D.  Conversion of partial arrest to complete arrest prevents further angulation
     E.  Bar resection should be considered if > 2 years of growth remains

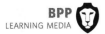

35. The most commonest complication following a distal femoral physeal fracture is:
    A. Angular deformity
    B. Leg length discrepancy
    C. Physeal bar
    D. Neurovascular injury
    E. Extensive contracture of the knee

36. The following meniscal tears can be managed non-operatively in children, except:
    A. Tear of 2mm in the outer 30% of the meniscus
    B. Tear of 5mm in the outer 30% of meniscus
    C. Tear of 8mm in the outer 30% of meniscus
    D. Radial tear of 5mm
    E. Stable partial tears

37. The following are **true** regarding compartment syndrome of the leg in children, except:
    A. Poorly controlled pain is the earliest sign
    B. Splitting of the cast and the underlying padding reduces pressure by 50%
    C. Two incision four compartment fasciotomy achieves full decompression
    D. Decompression with partial fibulectomy is a good alternative method
    E. All of the above are true

38. The following parameters are unacceptable for conservative treatment of closed diaphyseal fractures of the tibia in children:
    A. At least 50% apposition of the fragments
    B. Up to 10 degrees of anterior angulation
    C. Up to 5 degrees of valgus or varus deformity
    D. Up to 2cm of shortening
    E. Up to 5 degrees of posterior angulation

39. A bucket handle metaphyseal fracture of the proximal tibia is diagnostic of:
    A. High energy injury
    B. Bicycle spoke injury
    C. Child abuse
    D. Congenital pseudoarthrosis of tibia
    E. Stress fracture

40. Tillaux and Triplane injuries are related to the pattern of closure of the distal tibial physis. This pattern correctly described as (earliest to latest)
    A. Medial, central, lateral physeal closure
    B. Lateral, central, medial physeal closure
    C. Central, medial, lateral physeal closure
    D. Central, lateral, medial physeal closure
    E. Medial, lateral, central physeal closure

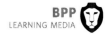

41. Triplane and tillaux fractures are respectively classified according to the Salter-Harris classification as:
    A. Type II, Type IV
    B. Type III, Type IV
    C. Type II, Type III
    D. Type IV, Type II
    E. Type III, Type II

42. The following statement is **false** for a talar fracture in children:
    A. Usually occurs due to forced dorsiflexion of foot in some eversion or inversion
    B. Undisplaced fractures are treated with non weight bearing cast for 6 weeks
    C. Avascular necrosis occurs during the first 6 months following the injury and presence of 'Hawkins' sign is its indicator
    D. Closed reduction can be accepted with up to 5mm of displacement; more displacement requires open reduction and fixation
    E. This most commonly involves the talar neck

43. The antibiotic choice for treatment of metatarsal osteochondritis following a punctured wound of the foot from a nail through the sole of a sneaker in a child is
    A. Benzyl penicillin
    B. Amoxicillin
    C. Flucloxacillin
    D. Temocillin
    E. Piperacillin

44. The following fracture is associated with the loss of radiological radio-capitellar relationship of the elbow:
    A. Fracture of lateral condyle
    B. Supracondylar fracture
    C. Transphyseal humeral fracture
    D. Kilfoyle Type I fracture
    E. All of the above

45. The neurological injury of ulnar nerve is most commonly seen with the following displacement of supracondylar fracture of elbow:
    A. Posteromedial displacement
    B. Posterolateral displacement
    C. Extension angulation displacement
    D. Flexion angulation displacement
    E. None of the above

46. The most stable percutaneous bicortical pinning construct for treatment of supracondylar fracture of the elbow is:
    A. Two parallel lateral pins
    B. Two lateral pins crossing near the fracture
    C. One lateral pin and one medial pin
    D. Two medial pins
    E. Two divergent lateral pins

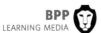

47. The following statements is **not true** regarding the medial epicondylar fracture of elbow:
    A. 50 % of these injuries are associated with elbow dislocation, reduced spontaneously
    B. No association with growth disorder around the elbow
    C. Commonly present with haemarthrosis
    D. Peak age of injury is 11–12 years
    E. Open reduction and fixation is recommended for displacement > 5 mm & rotation of 90 degrees

48. The following statement is **true** regarding the Milch type I fracture of the lateral condyle of the elbow:
    A. The fracture extends to the apex of the trochlear notch
    B. This is a Salter-Harris Type II fracture
    C. The elbow joint is considered stable
    D. Treatment is operative
    E. Malunion commonly results in a cubitus valgus deformity

49. An injury to the nutrient vessel supplying the lateral condyle of elbow during operative treatment leads to avascular necrosis. The location of this vessel is
    A. Anterolateral
    B. Posterolateral
    C. Anteromedial
    D. Posteromedial
    E. Anterior

50. The following displacement based on Wilkin's classification for an olecranon fracture is associated with posterior interosseous nerve injury
    A. Type A
    B. Type B – valgus
    C. Type B – varus
    D. Type C
    E. Type D

51. Based on Bado's classification of Monteggia fracture, a type II injury is described as:
    A. Presence of ulna fracture and radial head is dislocated anterior
    B. Presence of ulna fracture and radial head is dislocated laterally
    C. Presence of ulna fracture and radial head is dislocated posterior
    D. Presence of ulna fracture and radial shaft fracture and anterior dislocation
    E. Presence of ulna fracture and radial neck fracture and anterior dislocation

52. Avulsion fracture around the pelvis in children is most commonly seen at:
    A. Ischium
    B. Anterior superior iliac spine
    C. Anterior inferior iliac spine
    D. Iliac apophysis
    E. Lesser trochanter

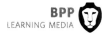

53. The following is recognised as the 'most dangerous' pelvic fracture in children:
    A. Sacro-iliac joint fracture
    B. Straddle fracture
    C. Ischial body fracture
    D. Duverney fracture
    E. Fracture of pubis

54. Which of the following is the most sensitive test in revealing an occult femoral neck fracture:
    A. Physical examination
    B. Antero-posterior and lateral hip radiographs
    C. Magnetic resonance imaging scan
    D. Bone scan
    E. None of the above

55. While using cannulated screws for fixation of an undisplaced fracture of the neck of femur in young patients, care should be taken for the screws to be placed in the following positions:
    A. Superior, anterior, posterior
    B. Anterior, posterior, inferior
    C. Central, anterior, posterior
    D. Central, superior, inferior
    E. Central, anterior, superior

56. A contraindication for treatment of undisplaced femoral neck fracture with the use of cannulated screws is:
    A. Parkinsonism disease
    B. Severe dementia
    C. Chronic renal failure
    D. Paget's disease
    E. Rheumatoid disease

57. The following are related to femoral fracture fixation in patients with multiple injuries, except:
    A. Lower incidence of fat embolism following early stabalisation
    B. Decrease hospital and intensive stay following early stabalisation
    C. Lower incidence of ARDS following early stabilisation
    D. Clinical benefits of early stabilisation were seen in patients with lower Injury Severity Score (ISS)
    E. Reduced healthcare costs were seen in patients with early stabilisation

58. All of the following statements are **true** regarding intramedullary nail breakage in femoral shaft fractures, except:
    A. Use of larger diameter nail reduces breakage
    B. Limitation of weight bearing until 50% femoral stiffness regained reduces breakage
    C. Use of titanium nails reduces breakage
    D. Fracture within 5cm of the proximal distal locking screw is associated with breakage
    E. Use of locked nails increases stiffness compared to unlock nails

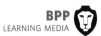

59. While using the piriform fossa as an entry point for a cephalomedulary femoral nail, the following displacement at the piriform fossa entry point should be avoided:
    A. Anterior displacement of > 6mm
    B. Medial displacement of > 6mm
    C. Lateral displacement of > 6mm
    D. Posterior displacement of > 6mm
    E. All of the above.

60. The most common deformity following closed treatment of femoral shaft fractures is:
    A. Rotational deformity
    B. Angular deformity
    C. Shortening of the leg
    D. Lengthening of the leg
    E. All of the above

61. The following type of knee dislocation based on the joint position classification, is irreducible by closed reduction:
    A. Posterior
    B. Anteromedial
    C. Posterolateral
    D. Anterolateral
    E. Posteromedial

62. Limb loss following a popliteal artery injury after a knee dislocation is imminent if re-vascularisation is not performed within:
    A. 1–2 hours
    B. 2–4 hours
    C. 4–6 hours
    D. 6–8 hours
    E. 8–10 hours

63. In a KD-IIIM type knee dislocation, the following statement is **true** regarding ligamentous reconstruction:
    A. Posterolateral approach is used, peroneal nerve is isolated before exploring the joint
    B. Posterior cruciate ligament is reconstructed along with medial collateral ligament
    C. Anterior cruciate ligament is reconstructed along with lateral collateral ligament
    D. Anterior cruciate ligament is reconstructed to allow stability
    E. In a combined anterior and posterior ligament reconstruction, the anterior cruciate ligament is tensioned first following the posterior cruciate ligament.

64. The most common proximal tibio-fibular dislocation is:
    A. Superior
    B. Posteromedial
    C. Posterolateral
    D. Anterolateral
    E. Posterior

BPP
LEARNING MEDIA

65. A 'lateral capsular sign' is seen in which type of fracture dislocation of knee:
   A. Type I
   B. Type II
   C. Type III
   D. Type IV
   E. Type V

66. The following feature is associated with dislocation of patella
   A. Genu varus
   B. Patellofemoral sulcus angle of 140 degrees
   C. Q angle of 15 degrees
   D. 10 mm lateralisation of tibial tubercle
   E. Merchant's congruence angle of −6 degrees

67. The medial patello-femoral ligament (MPFL) is a part of which layer around the knee
   A. First
   B. Second
   C. Third
   D. Fourth
   E. Fifth

68. Meniscal injury following a tibial plateau fracture is seen in the following percentage of cases:
   A. 15%
   B. 30%
   C. 50%
   D. 65%
   E. 80%

69. Which Schatzker Type tibial plateau fracture is associated with peripheral lateral meniscal tear with possibility of incarceration of the meniscus:
   A. Type I
   B. Type II
   C. Type III
   D. Type V
   E. Type VI

70. A high percentage of malunion and nonunion is seen in Schatzker Type VI fractures of the tibial plateau when treated with the following modality:
   A. Double plates
   B. Single plates
   C. Single plate with a contra-lateral external fixator
   D. 'Hybrid' external fixator
   E. All of the above

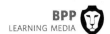

71.  A tibial shaft fracture with extensive muscle contusion and deep contaminated skin abrasion is classified into the following grade according to Tscherne soft tissue injury classification:
     A.  Grade 0
     B.  Grade 1
     C.  Grade 2
     D.  Grade 3
     E.  Grade 4

72.  The following angulation following tibial shaft fracture warrants a re-manipulation:
     A.  > 10 degrees angulation in sagittal plane, > 5 degrees angulation in coronal plane
     B.  > 5 degrees angulation in sagittal plane, > 10 degrees angulation in coronal plane
     C.  > 10 degrees in sagittal plane, > 10 degrees in coronal plane
     D.  All of the above
     E.  None of the above

73.  The following are absolute indications for operative treatment of a tibial shaft fracture, except:
     A.  Compartment syndrome
     B.  Significantly comminuted fracture
     C.  Multiple injuries
     D.  Vascular injury
     E.  Open fracture

74.  All of the following are important statements regarding stiffness of the construct following use of an external fixator in tibial shaft fractures, except:
     A.  Stiffness increases with contact of the fracture ends
     B.  Stiffness is directly proportional to the fourth power of the radius of the half pins
     C.  Stiffness is inversely proportional to the square of the distance between the bar and the bone
     D.  Stiffness increases by increasing the number of half pins
     E.  Use of lag screw with an external fixator increases the risk of nonunion and re-fracture

75.  When performing a fasciotomy, using two incision technique for the leg, a lateral incision is used to decompress the following compartments:
     A.  Superficial posterior and deep posterior compartments
     B.  Superficial posterior and anterior compartments
     C.  Anterior and lateral compartments
     D.  Deep posterior and lateral compartments
     E.  Superficial posterior and lateral compartment

76.  A pilon fracture with extensive posterior articular comminution occurs due to:
     A.  Axial loading with ankle in dorsiflexion
     B.  Axial loading with ankle in plantar flexion
     C.  Axial loading with ankle in neutral position
     D.  Shear force
     E.  Combined axial loading and rotation

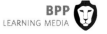

77. The following statement is **true** regarding comminuted tibial plafond fracture:
    A. Low energy injury leads to smaller articular fragment fracture
    B. High energy injury leads to large articular fragment fracture
    C. High energy injuries are best treated by open reduction and fixation
    D. Low energy injuries consistently require external fixator
    E. Use of interfragmentary diaphyseal screw is associated with increased risk of re-fracture

78. A Weber 'B' type fracture corresponds to the following Lauge Hansen mechanism of injury:
    A. Supination – adduction injury
    B. Supination – external rotation injury
    C. Pronation – external rotation injury
    D. Pronation – abduction injury
    E. Supination – abduction injury

79. The National Acute Spinal Cord Injury Study III concluded:
    A. No statistical difference between the three groups receiving bolus dose of methyl prednisolone within 3–8 hours
    B. Significant statistical improvement in the neurological recovery of the patients treated within 3–8 hours with a bolus dose methyl prednisolone followed by a 24 hour infusion of methyl prednisolone
    C. Significant statistical improvement in the neurological recovery of the patients treated within 3–8 hours with a bolus dose methyl prednisolone followed by a 48 hour infusion of methyl prednisolone
    D. Significant statistical improvement in the neurological recovery of the patients treated within 3–8 hours with a bolus dose methyl prednisolone followed by a 6 hour infusion of tirilazad mesylate for 48 hours
    E. Significant statistical improvement in the neurological recovery of the patients treated within 3 hours with a bolus dose methyl prednisolone

80. What type of loading procedure produces a fracture with a butterfly fragment?
    A. Torsion
    B. Torsion and tension
    C. Compression and shear
    D. Compression and bending
    E. Shear

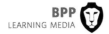

BPP
LEARNING MEDIA

# Trauma

## Answers

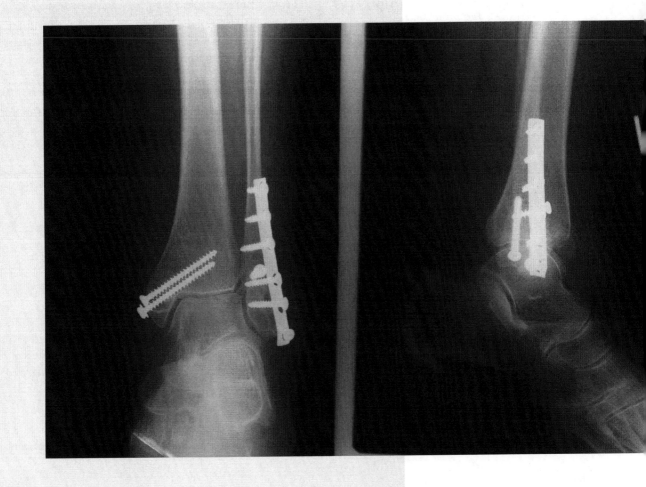

1.  **B**

    The volar extrinsic ligaments of the wrist are more vertical and stronger than the weaker and 'Z' shape oriented dorsal ligaments. The dorsal ligaments are also less well defined and hence are not very effective at restoring palmar tilt with ligamentotaxis during fracture reduction.

    The volar extrinsic wrist ligaments include:

    1.  Radioscapholunate ligament
    2.  Radial collateral ligament
    3.  Radiocapitate ligament
    4.  Volar radiotriquetral ligament

    The dorsal extrinsic wrist ligament includes:

    1.  Radioscaphoid ligament
    2.  Dorsal radiotriquetral ligament.

    Ref:
    Bartosh RA, Saldana MJ. Intra-articular distal radius fracture: A cadaveric study to determine if ligamentotaxis restores radiopalmar tilt. *J Hand Surg* 15A: 18–21, 1990.

2.  **D**

    Description of the distal radius fractures of the wrist has been commonly based on the eponyms like Colles' fractures, Smith's fracture, Barton's fracture and so on, which are an imprecise mode of description of fractures. The modern classification systems for distal radius fractures are more specific and orient towards the treatment of these fractures.

    These include:

    1.  Frykman's classification – based on fracture pattern
    2.  Melone's classification – based on the orientation of the four main intra-articular fragments
    3.  Rayhack's classification – based on the stability of the fracture pattern
    4.  Fernandez's classification – based on the mechanism of injury
    5.  AO/ASIF classification – based on the fracture pattern and involvement of articular surface

    Ref:
    Fernandez DL. Fractures of the distal radius: operative treatment. *Instr Course Lect.* 1993, 42; 73–88.

3.  **B**

    The treatment of distal radius fractures is determined by considering the stability of the fracture. As a general rule the stable fractures can be treated by closed reduction and plaster immobilisation while unstable fractures require either an internal or an external fixation. The following factors are the hallmarks of an unstable fracture:

    1.  Articular depression more than 2mm
    2.  Radial shortening of more than 5 mm

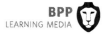

3.  Dorsal tilt of more than 20 degrees
4.  Metaphyseal comminution involving both the volar and the dorsal cortices.

Certain eponym's patterns are known to be unstable and are invariably treated with fixation. These include Barton's and Chauffeur's fractures. (These fractures have displaced articular margins.)

Ref:
1.  Knirk J, Jupiter J. Intraarticular fractures of distal end of radius in young adults. *JBJS* 1986, 68(5): 647–659.
2.  Porter M, Stockley I. Fractures of distal radius. *Clin. Orthopaed Rel Res* 1987; 220: 241–252.
3.  McQueen MM, Hajducka C, Court-Brown C. Redisplayed Unstable fractures of the distal radius: a randomised prospective study of bridging versus non-bridging external fixator. *JBJS* 1996; 78(3): 404–409.

4.  **E**

    Evaluation of avascular necrosis of the scaphoid can be performed by plain radiographs that show radio dense proximal scaphoid fragment. MRI scan is both sensitive and specific for the diagnosis of AVN and is performed in the absence of radiographic features in plain films. But the most definitive test for the diagnosis of AVN of the scaphoid is a surgical biopsy with the absence of punctate bleeding surface seen during open reduction.

    Ref:
    Green DP. The effect of avascular necrosis on Russe bone grafting for scaphoid nonunion. *J Hand Surg* 1985; 10-A: 597–605.

5.  **E**

    Scaphocapitate syndrome includes combined fractures of scaphoid and capitate bones. These fractures result from extreme dorsiflexion of the wrist or a direct blow to the radial styloid. This represents a serious injury to the wrist and can result in the rotation of the proximal pole of the capitate by 180 degrees. The diagnosis for this syndrome is difficult and this can be missed as the fragments have a tendency to remain collinear. Complication of AVN of capitate, principally the proximal pole, due to disruption of the blood supply may occur. Treatment is open reduction internal fixation of both scaphoid and capitate bones.

    Ref:
    Vance RM, Gelberman RH, Evans EF. Scaphocapitate fractures. *JBJS* 1980; 62-A: 271–276.

6.  **C**

    Description: the perilunar disruption has been described in four stages of progressive ligamentous failure.
    1st stage – scapholunate ligamentous tear leading to scapholunate dissociation
    2nd stage – capitolunate ligamentous tear
    3rd stage – lunotriquetral ligamentous tear leading to perilunate dissociation
    4th stage – dorsal radiolunate ligament tear leading to lunate dislocation.

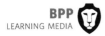

Ref:
Mayfield JK, Kilcoyne RK, Johnson RP. Carpal dislocation: pathomechanics and progressive perilunate instability. *J Hand Surg* 1980; 5: 226–241.

7.   **B**

Scapholunate dissociation can occur due to fracture of scaphoid or scapholunate ligament tear. This leads to DISI instability in the wrist. Lunate gets separated from the scaphoid and rotates dorsally due to lunotriquetral ligament and scaphoid rotates into flexion. This is radiologically seen as increase in the scapholunate angle > 60 degrees when measured on the lateral view (normal angle 30–60 degrees). Widening of scapholunate space of >3mm on PA view or evidence of scaphoid fracture. Triangular appearance of lunate and 'cortical ring' sign of scaphoid and a capitolunate angle of up to 15 degrees.

Ref:
Cautilli GP, Wehbe MA. Scapholunate distance and cortical ring sign. *J Hand Surg* 1991; 16-A: 501–503.

8.   **A**

Carpal Instability Dissociative refers to intrinsic ligament disruption that occurs between the same rows of the carpal bones. These include: scapholunate and lunotriquetral dissociations. The Carpal Instability Non-Dissociative refers to extrinsic ligament disruption that connects the proximal and distal carpal rows. Disruption of these ligaments leads to a midcarpal instability. Carpal instability complex is a combination of dissociative and non-dissociative types and includes perilunate dislocations. Carpal instability adaptive refers to instability due to an adaptive response to a prior malalignment. This includes midcarpal instability due to malunited distal radius fracture.

Ref:
Cooney WP, Dobyns JH, Linscheid RL. Arthroscopy of the wrist: Anatomy and classification of carpal instability. *Arthroscopy* 1990; 6: 133–140.

9.   **B**

Traumatic TFCC tears can be classified into four groups:
Class 1A – central tears treated with arthroscopic debridement of the tear, as this is an avascular area

Class 1B – complete tears with dislocation of DRUJ, treated with suture repair of the TFCC or ORIF ulnar styloid if present

Class 1C – located distally with disruption of Ulnolunate ligament, lunotriquetral ligament or both. Treated with open or arthroscopic repair along with anatomical reduction of the lunate fossa fracture

Class 1D – avulsion of TFCC from its radial attachment of sigmoid notch. Treated with open or arthroscopic repair and immobilisation for 6–8 weeks

Ref:
Melone CP Jr, Nathan R. Traumatic disruptions of triangular fibrocartilage complex, pathoanatomy. *Clin Orthop Rel Res* 1992; 275: 65–73.

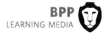

**10. B**

The annular pulley provides mechanical stability and the cruciate pulley permits flexibility. To prevent bowstringing deformity of the finger it is imperative to preserve the A2 pulley at the proximal phalanx and the A4 pulley at the middle phalanx. The A1, A3 and A5 pulleys arise from the palmar plates of the MCPJ, PIPJ and DIPJ respectively.

Ref:
Strickland JW. Flexor tendon injuries. *Hand Clin* 1985; 1(1).

**11. B**

The healing process following a flexor tendon injury undergoes the following phases:

The inflammatory phase – first 3–5 days, strength of the repair is imparted by the sutures entirely. The fibroblastic phase – 5–21 days, collagen is produced and the strength of the repair increases rapidly as the granulation tissue bridges the defect. Controlled passive mobilisation in this phase leads to a greater tensile strength, fewer adhesions ad improved excursion. Remodelling phase – after 21 days, allows complete maturation and reversion of fibroblasts to tenocytes by 112 days.

Ref:
Strickland JW. Flexor tendon injuries. *Hand Clin* 1985; 1(1).

**12. E**

The primary surgical repair of the flexor tendon is indicated for all flexor tendon laceration including zone 2. It is most difficult to get a good result following repair of flexor zone at zone 2. However a good prognosis and result is obtained after primary repair in zone 3 because of absence of fibro-osseous pulley in this zone. Zone 1 is distal to FDS insertion, rupture of the insertion of the flexor tendon in this zone should be treated with a re-insertion with a pull button technique through the bone. Zone 4 is at the carpal tunnel and is associated with median nerve injury, zone 5 is in the forearm and a repair generally has a good prognosis.

Ref:
Strickland JW. Flexor tendon injuries. *Hand Clin* 1985; 1(1).

**13. D**

A Stener's lesion is characterised with rupture of ulnar collateral ligament with interposition of the adductor pollicis aponeurosis. This does not heal with conservative management and requires a surgical treatment.

Ref:
Harammati N, Hiller N, Dowdie J, *et al.* MRI of Stener Lesion. *Skelet Radiolo.* 1995; 24: 515–518.

**14. C**

The extensor tendon laceration has been classified according to zones into 1 to 9. The zones 1, 3, 5 are at the DIP, PIP and MCP joints. Disruption of the central slip of the extensor tendon at the PIPJ leads to the volar migration of the lateral bands leading to a

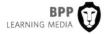

Boutonnière's deformity. There is a loss of the extension of the PIPJ with a compensatory hyperextension of the DIPJ.

Ref:
Schneider LH. Extensor tendon Injuries. *Hand Clin* 1995, 11(3).

15.  **B**
The incidence of spinal cord injury (SCI) is discrete and varies in geographic regions within a specific time frame, this is however estimated to be around 40 per million per year. The incidence of SCI is higher in males than females. The mean age for both genders at the time of injury is around 30 years. The peak age of incidence is 20–24 years for males and 25–29 years for females. Motor vehicle accident is the most frequent cause (50%), the second most frequent cause (20%) is falls (accidental or suicidal). Approximately 10–20% of the cases occur in the context of sports or recreational activities. Fall from a standing height is the most common cause for older patients (age > 65 years).

Ref:
Burney RE, Maio RF, Maynard F, *et al.* Incidence, characteristics and outcome of spinal cord injury at trauma centers in North America. *Arch Surg* 1993; 128(5): 596–599.

16.  **B**
The thoracic cord has the greatest distance between each of its supplying radicular arteries compared to the lumbar and sacral cord. The cervical cord has equal bilateral supply form the radicular arteries. Hence the thoracic cord is the most prone to ischaemia following occlusion of the radicular artery.

Ref:
Carpenter MB: *Coretext of neuroanatomy*. Baltimore, 1991. Williams & Wilkins.

17.  **C**
The central cord syndrome is characterised by disproportionate loss of motor power between the upper and lower extremities; however the loss is greater in the upper extremity than the lower. There is a sensory loss below the lesion and presence of bladder dysfunction usually in the form of urinary retention. The mechanism of injury in the central cord syndrome consists of hyperextension of the cervical spine. The syndrome has good prognosis compared to the other syndromes of incomplete SCI.

Ref:
Brodkey JS, Miller CF Jr, Harmody RM. The syndrome of acute central cervical spinal cord injury revisited. *Surg Neurol* 1980; 14: 251–257.

18.  **D**
The recovery from central cord syndrome generally follows a pattern. The recovery pattern is as follows: first, motor power of lower extremity; second, recovery of bladder function; third, motor recovery of upper extremity. Hands and finger movements are the last to recover and may not recover fully. Cases of spontaneous recovery following the anterior cord syndrome have been reported.

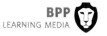

Ref:

Ditunno JF Jr, Stover SL, Freed MM. Motor recovery of the upper extremities in traumatic quadriplegia: A multicentre study. *Arch Phys Med Rehab*. 1992; 73: 431–436.

19. **C**

The conus medullaris syndrome is caused by compression of the tapering distal end of the cord. The syndrome is characterised by lower motor neuron deficit leading to flaccid paralysis of the lower extremity, bladder areflexia, variable sensory deficits. The upper motor neuron findings are seen in the chronic phase. The cauda equina syndrome is caused by compression of the lumbar and sacral roots beyond the termination of the cord. Compression can be caused by fractures or acute disc prolapse. The clinical picture consists of perianal anaesthesia, sphincter dysfunction, bladder areflexia, normal leg strength and absence of radicular pain. The prognosis in general is better than other SCI's. Treatment is urgent surgical decompression.

Ref:

Singh K, Vaccaro AR. Thoracic and lumbar trauma. In: Bono CM, Garfin SR eds. *Orthopaedic surgery essential: Spine*. Philadelphia: Lippincott Williams & Wilkins. 2004: 45–57.

20. **B**

Atlantoaxial rotatory subluxation is being classified by Fielding into 4 types. The condition is difficult to diagnose and is usually related to vehicular trauma. The condition is associated with fracture of the lateral mass. The types are:

1.  Type I – most common, fixed rotation deformity without disruption of transverse ligament
2.  Type II – transverse ligament insufficiency with 3–5 mm anterior displacement of atlas
3.  Type III – associated with > 5mm anterior displacement
4.  Type IV – associated with posterior displacement of atlas and rotatory subluxation. Least common.

Ref:

Fielding JW, Hawkins RJ. Atlanto-axial Rotatory Fixation (fixed rotatory subluxation of Atlanto-axial joint). *JBJS Am* 1977; 59: 37–44.

21. **C**

Distraction extension injuries cause failure of the anterior longitudinal ligament or result in a transverse vertebral body fracture. These injuries are less common and difficult to diagnose as it can be primarily a soft tissue injury and spontaneous reduction can occur following neutralisation in the head position. In spondylosis cervical spine of the elderly patients, these injuries commonly cause a central cord syndrome. Vertical compression injuries result in burst fractures. Distraction flexion injuries result in rupture of the PLL. Lateral flexion injuries result in fracture of the neural arches due to asymmetric compression.

Ref:

Allen BL Jr, Ferguson RL, Lehmann TR, *et al*. A mechanistic classification of closed, indirect fractures and dislocations of lower cervical spine. *Spine* 1982; 7: 1–27.

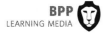

**22.**   **B**

Compression fracture of the thoracolumbar spine involves the anterior column and results from flexion force to the spine. The compression fracture is classified by Denis into four types:

1.   Type A – fracture involving both the endplates
2.   Type B – fracture involving the superior endplate (most common)
3.   Type C – fracture involving the inferior endplate
4.   Type D – fracture involving the vertebral body and both the endplates.

Ref:
Denis F. The three-column spine and its significance in the classification of acute thoracolumbar spine injuries. *Spine* 1983; 8: 817–831.

**23.**   **B**

The seat belt injuries or 'chance fractures' occurs due to a flexion-distraction injury to the spine. A flexion force leads to a distraction failure of all the three vertebral columns. It can occur through the soft tissue or may contain bony fragments. It has a high association with intra-abdominal injuries and presence of seat belt ecchymosis should raise suspicion. Bony chance injuries heal better than soft tissue chance injuries. Soft tissue chance injury can result in chronic instability symptoms.

Ref:
Gertzbein SD, Court-Brown CM. Flexion distraction injuries of the lumbar spine: mechanism of injury and classification. *Clin Orthop* 1988; 227: 52–60.

**24.**   **D**

Atlanto-occipital dissociations are considered as unstable injuries. Traynelis classified these injuries into four types based on the displacement of the occiput on the C-spine.

1.   Type I – anterior displacement of the occiput
2.   Type II – vertical Displacement of the occiput
3.   Type III – posterior displacement of the occiput
4.   Type IV – oblique displacement of the occiput. This is the commonest type and occurs in 85% of the cases.

Ref:
Traynelis VC, Marano GD, Dunker RO, *et al.* Traumatic Atlanto-occipital dislocation. Case report. *J Neurosurg* 1986; 65: 863–870.

**25.**   **B**

The C1 ring fractures are described based on their position and number of fragments. The stability of the fracture is depended on its position and pattern

The stable C1 fractures include posterior arch fracture, transverse process fracture and simple lateral mass fracture.

The unstable C1 Fractures include anterior arch fractures, comminuted lateral mass fracture and Jefferson's fracture.

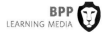

Ref:
Levine AM, Edwards CC. Fracture of atlas. *JBJS Am*.1991; 73: 680–691.

26. **E**

With a history of blunt trauma to the cervical spine, a fracture of any of the cervical spine vertebra is associated with a 10–30% chance of finding another spinal fracture. This figure increases to 50% with a fracture of C2. Hence in the presence of C2 fracture due to blunt trauma, the whole spine should be carefully examined to exclude another fracture.

Ref:
Reid DC, Henderson R, Saboe L, Miller JDR. Etiology of missed spine fractures. *J Trauma*.1987; 27: 980–986.

27. **D**

A halo jacket uses at least four pins tightened on an adult skull with 6–8 in/lbs to allow a stable skull fixation and immobilisation of the fracture. Children require six to eight pins with 2–6 in/lbs tightening. The complication following the use of a halo jacket include: loss of reduction (most common), pin tract infection, pins loosening, severe pain, pressure sores. Injury to supra-orbital nerve and dural pin penetration are rare. Pulmonary complications and aspiration have been associated with halo vest in elderly patients.

Ref:
Anderson PA, Budorick TE, Easton Kb, *et al*. Failure of halo vest to prevent in vivo motion in patients with injured cervical spine. *Spine* 1991; 16: S501–505.

28. **C**

Axial compression injury of the vertebral column ranges from a simple compression fracture (pure axial load) to significant burst fracture (axial load in flexion). A pincer fracture is a special type of fracture of the vertebral body and is a part of this spectrum caused by excessive axial loading, which results in the failure of the endplates. This is associated with implosion of the disc through the vertebral body after a mid body separation of the vertebra in coronal plane. As there is interposition of disc material healing is slow and prognosis poor.

Ref:
Eismont FJ, Grafin SR, Abitbol JJ. Thoracic and upper lumbar spine injuries, in Browner BD, Jupiter JB, Levine AM, Trafton PG. *Skeletal Trauma: Fracture, dislocation, ligamentous injuries*. Vol 1, 1992. Philadelphia, WB Saunders.

29. **E**

Compression fracture by definition results in failure of the anterior column, with intact middle column. However involvement of the posterior ligamentous complex renders the fracture unstable and is an indication for further investigation and stabilisation. These fractures are unsuitable for treatment with TLSO. The presence of following parameters in a compression fracture indicates involvement of the posterior ligamentous complex:

a.    > 50% loss of the height of the anterior column
b.    >30 degrees of kyphosis

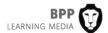

Ref:
Willen J, Anderson J, Toomako K, *et al.* The natural history of burst fracture at the Thoraco lumbar junction. *J Spinal Disord.* 1990; 3: 39–46.

**30.    C**

Following a burst fracture of the thoracolumbar vertebra, operative intervention is required in the presence of: progressive kyphosis of > 30 degrees, loss of >50% anterior column height, presence of neurological deficit and presence of painful instability. However presence of bony retropulsion, with no neurological deficit and intact posterior ligament complex is treated conservatively. Presence of retropulsive fragments is not an indication for surgery and favourable results with conservative treatment can be achieved in the absence of posterior ligament complex injury.

Ref:
Mohanty SP, Venkatram N. Does neurological recovery in the thoracolumbar and lumbar burst fractures depend on the extent of canal compromise? *Spinal Cord* 2002; 40: 295–299.

**31.    A**

Skeletal injuries following child abuse can be categorised based on their specificity to diagnose this condition into high, moderate and low specificity. The injuries highly specific for child abuse include: posterior rib fractures, sternal fractures, scapular fractures and spinal process avulsion fracture. Long bone fractures, though commonly seen have a low specificity. Multiple fractures with varying ages on the injury are of moderate specificity.

Ref:
1.   Kocher MS, Kasser JR. Orthopaedic aspects of child abuse. *J Am Acad Orthop Surg.* 2000; 16: 121–123.
2.   Campbell RM Jr, Schrader T. Child abuse. In Rockwood & Wilkins. *Fracture in Children.* 6th ed. (2006) Philadelphia. Lippincott Williams & Wilkins.

**32.    C**

The epidemiology of fractures in children has been described to show a linear increase in the annual incidence of fractures with age. Boys sustain more fractures than girls (2.7:1) and the peak age is 12 years with a decline until the age of 16 years. Left sided fractures are more common than right sided (1.3:1) and is consistently related to the number of hours of sunshine. Open fractures are uncommon in children and constitute 2.9% of all fractures. The commonest long bone to fracture is radius with a relative frequency of 45.1% and physeal injuries are most common before skeletal maturity. The commonest site of fracture is distal radius with a relative frequency of 23.3% including physeal injuries.

Ref:
Wilkins KE, Aroojis AJ. Incidence of fracture in children. In Rockwood & Wilkins. *Fracture in Children.* 6th ed. (2006) Philadelphia. Lippincott Williams & Wilkins.

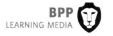

33.  **E**
With a physeal injury, the treatment considerations undertaken to avoid the risk of iatrogenic growth disturbance of the physis are:

- Avoidance of repeated manipulation attempts as this may increase the incidence of growth disturbance
- Physeal fractures do not generally require anatomical reduction unless intra-articular which should be treated with internal fixation.
- Internal fixation when required should not cross the physis when possible. In events requiring crossing of the physis, a smallest feasible pin should be used.
- For intra-articular fracture, the congruity should be maintained by use of a compression screw inserted parallel to the physis.

Ref:

Rathjen KE, Birch JG. Physeal Injury and growth disturbance. In Rockwood & Wilkins. *Fracture in Children.* 6th ed. (2006) Philadelphia. Lippincott Williams & Wilkins.

34.  **C**
Partial arrest of the Physis occurs in 3 patterns: peripheral bars (commonest), central bar and linear bar. The hallmark radiographic sign of partial arrest is blurring and narrowing of the Physis or an area of sclerosis resulting from bone condensation seen typically 3–6 months following Physeal injury. Arrest affecting more than 20 percent of the Physis has a poor prognosis, but post traumatic arrest and arrest following Blount's disease has good prognosis compared to other causes of partial arrest. Treatment options include – conversion to complete arrest and this procedure prevents further angulation but causes leg length discrepancy. Bar resection procedures have shown good results when performed for bars involving less than 20% of Physis with at least 2 years of potential remaining Physeal growth is present.

Ref:

Broughton NS, Dickens CR, Cole WG, *et al.* Epiphysiolysis for partial growth plate arrest: results after four years or at maturity. *JBJS Br.* 1989; 71: 13–16
Rathjen KE, Birch JG. Physeal injury and growth disturbance. In Rockwood & Wilkins. *Fracture in Children.* 6th ed. (2006) Philadelphia. Lippincott Williams & Wilkins.

35.  **B**
The distal femoral Physis is the largest and the fastest growing Physis. Injury to the distal femoral Physis is rare and results from sports or motor vehicle accidents. The most common complication following a distal femoral Physeal injury is leg length discrepancy. Other complications include – angular deformity, Physeal bar formation, neurovascular injuries and extensive knee contractures.

Ref:

Beaty JH, Kumar A. Fractures about the knee in children. *JBJS Am* 1994; 76: 1870–1880.

36.  **D**
Menisci are completely vascularised at birth. With maturation, the vascular supply to the inner 2/3rd diminishes. Meniscal injuries generally affect the adolescent group, its rare in prepubescent children. Indications for non-operative management include tears 10mm or

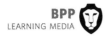

less in the outer 30% of the meniscus, radial tears less than 3 mm and stable partial tears. Tears requiring surgical treatment are managed with partial meniscectomy or repair.

Ref:

Greis PE, Holstrum LC, Bardana DD, *et al.* Meniscal Injury II. Management. *J Am Acad Orthop Surg.* 2002; 10: 177–187.

37.  **D**

Compartment syndrome is a grave complication commonly seen following open or closed tibial fractures. Clinical presentation involves poorly controlled pain as the earliest sign, increased discomfort on passive stretch of the involved muscles. Treatment includes splitting of the cast and padding; this may reduce the pressure by 50%. Four-compartment fasciotomy using two-incision technique is the treatment of choice. Partial fibular resection can decompress all the four compartments; however this is contraindicated in children due to the complication of valgus deformity following the resection.

Ref:

Heinrich SD, Mooney JF. Fractures of the shaft of the tibia & fibula. In Rockwood & Wilkins. *Fracture in Children.* 6th ed. (2006) Philadelphia. Lippincott Williams & Wilkins.

38.  **D**

In children, closed tibial diaphyseal fractures can be successfully managed conservatively with a long leg cast. An acceptable alignment of the fracture in the cast includes: at least 50% apposition of the fragments, up to 10 degrees of anterior angulation and up to 5 degrees of posterior angulation (recurvatum). Up to 5–10 degrees of varus or valgus deformity and up to 1cm of shortening. The fractures that fail to satisfy these criteria or fail conservative management on weekly review should be stabilised operatively or re-manipulated.

Ref:

Heinrich SD, Mooney JF. Fractures of the shaft of the tibia & fibula. In Rockwood & Wilkins. *Fracture in Children.* 6th ed. (2006). Philadelphia. Lippincott Williams & Wilkins.

39.  **C**

A bucket handle fracture, or metaphyseal avulsion fracture of the tibia is pathognomic of child abuse. The injury is sustained by sudden twisting of the limb. A mild variant of bucket handle fracture is called 'corner' fracture. This commonly occurs at the junction of metaphysis and physis.

Bicycle spokes injury is a soft tissue injury to the foot following entrapment in the spokes of the bicycle wheel. The patient should be monitored for compartment syndrome of the foot; surgical debridement should be undertaken as guided by the wound.

Ref:

Green NE, Swiontkowski MF. *Skeletal trauma in children.* 2nd ed. 1998. Philadelphia. WB Saunders.

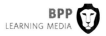

**40.    C**

The distal tibial physis begins to close at 12–13 years. The physeal closure occurs at the central portion earliest followed by medial portion and finally lateral portion. Injury sustained during this time of closure results in tillaux and triplanar fractures. An external rotation force, leading to a lateral physeal and an epiphyseal injury is described as a tillaux fracture. Triplanar fracture has a multiplanar pattern. Both fractures require operative intervention with open or closed reduction. CT scan helps to assess the configuration of the fracture.

Ref:

Cummings JR. Distal tibial and fibular fractures. In Rockwood & Wilkins. *Fracture in Children.* 6th ed. (2006) Philadelphia. Lippincott Williams & Wilkins.

**41.    B**

A tillaux fracture is described as an equivalent to a Salter-Harris Type III injury, as it involves the lateral tibial epiphysis. A triplanar fracture is multiplanar and involves the epiphyses and the metaphysis along with the physis. This is described as equivalent to a Salter-Harris Type IV injury.

Ref:

Dias L, Giegerich C. Fractures of the distal tibial epiphysis in adolescence. *JBJS Am* 1983; 65: 438–444.

**42.    C**

Talar fracture results from a forced dorsiflexion of the foot in either inversion or eversion. The blood supply to the talus is precarious and hence these fractures run a high incidence of avascular necrosis. A Talar fracture commonly involves the talar neck and is rarely seen in children. Closed reduction and conservative treatment with a non weight-bearing cast for 6 weeks is accepted with up to 5mm of fracture displacement. All talus fractures should be monitored with periodic radiographic assessments for evidence of avascular necrosis. AVN is the most common complication and usually is seen during the first 6 months following injury. A 'Hawkins sign', subchondral lucency seen on plain radiographs signifies intact blood supply and not AVN of the talus. However, in children the absence of Hawkins sign does not indicate AVN. MRI is the investigation of choice for AVN of the talus.

Ref:
1.    Hawkins LG. Fractures of the neck of talus. *JBJS Am* 1970; 52: 991–995.
2.    Jarvis JG, Moroz PJ. Fractures and dislocation of Foot. In Rockwood & Wilkins. *Fracture in Children.* 6th ed. (2006) Philadelphia. Lippincott Williams & Wilkins.

**43.    E**

Puncture wounds of the foot are commonly seen in children. A general presentation is one with a nail on the wooden plank injuring the sole of the feet through the sneaker. The concern following these types of injuries to the sole of the foot is cellulitis, osteomyelitis or septic arthritis. The commonest organism following such injury is Pseudomonas aeruginosa; however this generally does not cause superficial infection. Cellulitis around the puncture site is caused by Staphylococcus aureus. Osteochondritis is caused by Pseudomonas and treatment is debridement with use of intravenous anti-pseudomonal antibiotics for 6–12 weeks. Piperacillin is an anti-pseudomonal antibiotic.

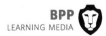

Ref:
1.    Verdile VP, Freed H, Gerard J. Puncture wounds to the foot. *J Emerg Med* 1989; 7: 193–199.
2.    Jarvis JG, Skipper J. Pseudomonas osteochondritis complicating puncture wound in children. *J Pediatr Orthop* 1994; 14: 755–759.

**44.    A**

In a normal elbow the long axis of the radius extends to the centre of the capitellum. This can be appreciated radiologically and this is described as the radiocapitellar relation. This relation remains intact with a supracondylar fracture, as the fracture is above the condyles. In a transphyseal humeral fracture, there is entire distal humeral epiphyseal separation, the ossification centre of the capitellum migrates and is posteromedial to the humeral metaphysis, and the radiocapitellar relationship is intact. The radiocapitellar relation is lost with lateral condylar fracture, where the capitellum lies laterally to the long axis of radius or dislocation of the elbow.

Ref:
Delee JC, Wilkins KE, Rogers LF, *et al.* Fracture separation of distal humeral epiphysis. *JBJS Am* 1980; 62: 46–51.

**45.    D**

Supracondylar fractures are commonly associated with injury to the median and radial nerve as the commonest pattern is a posteromedial or posterolateral displacement in an extension type fracture. Incidence of ulnar nerve injury is been reported more frequently with the use of medial pins to stabilise the fracture. A flexion angulation displacement of the supracondylar fracture is associated with incidence of ulnar nerve injury.

Ref:
Royle SG, Burke D. Ulna neuropathy after elbow injury in children. *J Pediatr Orthop* 1990; 10(4): 495–496.

**46.    C**

The most stable construct with percutaneous pinning of supracondylar fracture is achieved by using a medial and lateral pin. The pins need to be bicortical and extending through the corresponding columns. A mini-open approach is used for the medial pin to avoid injury to the ulnar nerve. Cadaveric study determines this to be the most stable construct to tensional force. The use of two lateral pins required significantly less torque to produce 10 degrees of rotation (37% less for parallel pins and 80% less for lateral pins crossing near the fracture as compared to medial and lateral pins). The lateral pins used in divergence are more stable than the lateral pins inserted in parallel.

Ref:
1.    Zionts LE, Mckellop HA, Hathway R. Torsional strength of pin configuration used to fix supracondylar fractures of the humerus in children. *JBJS Am* 1994; 76(2): 253–256.
2.    Lee SS, Mahar AT, Miesen D, *et al.* Displaced pediatric supracondylar fracture: biomechanical analysis of percutaneous pinning techniques. *J Pediatr Orthop* 2002; 22(4): 440–443.

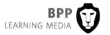

47.   C
Medial epicondylar fracture occurs between the ages of 9 and 14 years. Approximately 50% are associated with elbow dislocation. The mechanism of injury is valgus stress to the elbow, direct blow to the elbow or a flexion-pronation muscle contraction leading to avulsion. This is an apophyseal fracture and not epiphyseal and hence no growth disorders are seen. Open reduction internal fixation is required if the displacement is > 5mm and rotation of 90 degrees, incarceration of fracture fragment in the joint, elbow instability and ulnar nerve injury. These fractures are extra-articular and hence are not associated with haemarthrosis. Presence of a haemarthrosis indicates towards an associated radial neck, olecranon or coronoid process fracture.

Ref:
Wilson NIL, Ingran R, Rymaszewski L, *et al.* Treatment of fracture of the medial epicondyle of the humerus. *Injury* 1988; 19: 342–344.


48.   C
The fracture of the lateral condyle of the elbow is classified into two types by Milch classification based on the position of the fracture line. A Milch Type I fracture is described when the fracture line is lateral to the trochlear (through the capitulotrochlear groove). This is a Salter-Harris Type IV fracture and the elbow joint remains stable. Type I fractures can be safely treated non operatively. The fracture is commonly associated with nonunion; however, a cubitus varus deformity commonly results following malunion.

Ref:
Herring JA. Lateral Condylar fracture of the elbow. *J Pediatr Orthop* 1986; 6: 724–727.

Milch H. Fractures and fracture dislocation of humeral condyles. *J Trauma* 1964; 4: 592–607.


49.   B
The lateral condyle is largely intra-articular. A small portion of the lateral condyle at its posterior aspect is extra-articular. The extraosseous blood supply of the lateral condyle is from the nutrient vessel entering the lateral condyle from this posterior extra articular region. Therefore a posterolateral approach runs the risk of damage to this nutrient vessel leading to avascular necrosis of the lateral condyle.

Ref:
Haraldsson S. On osteochondrosis deformans juvenilis capituli humeri including investigation of intra-osseous vasculature in distal humerus. *Acta Orthop Scand* 1959; 38 (suppl).


50.   C
Olecranon fracture in children is classified according to Wilkins classification into four types. This is based on the mechanism of injury.

1.   Type A – flexion injury
2.   Type B – extension injury. This is divided into the varus and valgus type. The valgus type pattern is associated with a radial neck fracture and avulsion of medial epicondyle. The varus pattern is associated with dislocation of the radial head and posterior interosseous nerve injury.
3.   Type C – shear injury

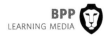

Ref:
Eilert RE, Erickson MA. Fractures of the proximal radius and ulna. In Rockwood & Wilkins. *Fracture in Children.* 6th ed. (2006) Philadelphia. Lippincott Williams & Wilkins.

**51.** **C**

Monteggia fracture-dislocation is a fracture of the ulna with dislocation of the radiocapitellar joint. The Monteggia fracture dislocation has been classified by Bado into four types.

a. Type I – fracture of ulna, anterior dislocation of the radial head (commonest)
b. Type II – fracture of the ulna with apex posterior, posterior dislocation of the radial head
c. Type III – fracture of the ulna, with lateral dislocation of the radial head
d. Type IV – fracture of the ulna, radial shaft fracture and anterior dislocation of radial head

Ref:
Bado JL. The Monteggia lesion. *Clin Orthop* 1967; 50: 71–86.

**52.** **A**

Avulsion fractures are common in children. These occur around the secondary ossification centre because of the elasticity present in the pediatric pelvis and the powerful contraction of the attached muscles. The most commonest avulsion fractures occurs at ischium (38%), anterior superior iliac spine (32%), anterior inferior iliac spine (18%), iliac crest and lesser trochanter.

Ref:
Fernbach SK, Wilkinson RH. Avulsion injuries of the pelvis and proximal femur. *Am J Roentgenol* 1981; 137(3): 581–584.

**53.** **B**

Fractures of the pelvis in children are divided into avulsion fractures, fracture of the pubis or ischium, iliac wing fracture (Duverney fracture), sacral fractures, single ring fractures and double ring fractures.

Fractures of the pubis and ischium are stable fractures due to intact pelvic ring. They result from high-energy trauma and are associated with multiple life threatening injuries like head injury and long bone fractures.

Iliac wing fracture is common with 15% of pediatric pelvic fractures. They are commonly associated with motor vehicle accidents.

Sacral fractures and coccygeal fractures may be associated with pelvic ring break. When combined with anterior pelvic ring break are classified as double ring fractures.

Single breaks of pelvic rings include – ipsilateral pubic rami fractures, pubic symphysis fractures and sacro-iliac joint fractures.

The most dangerous fractures are the double break ring fractures. These include: straddle fracture or double vertical pubic rami fractures. They are associated with bladder or urethral disruption.

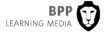

Malgaigne fracture – posterior arch fracture with ipsilateral or contralateral anterior arch fracture.

Multiple pelvic crushing injuries – massive hemorrhage is common, survival is rare.

Ref:
Rieger H, Brug E. Fractures of the pelvis in children. *Clin Orthop* 1997; 336: 226–239.

**54.  C**

Patients admitted following a fall, complaining of hip pain commonly reveal an occult femoral neck fracture. The physical examination only reveals pain with no deformity. The radiographs of the hip are generally normal with no evidence of fracture. MR scan of the hip is the most sensitive investigation to reveal occult fracture within the first day following an injury to the hip. Bone scan is sensitive at 72 hours.

Ref:
Rizzo PF, Gould ES, Lyden JP, *et al.* Diagnosis of occult fracture about the hip: magnetic resonance imaging compared with bone scanning. *JBJS Am* 1993; 75: 395–401.

**55.  C**

The mechanism of internal fixation with cannulated screws for femoral neck fractures has been described by many, but the preferred method is the use of a triangle or an inverted triangle. The configuration of the screw should be achieved with the first screw running along the calcar inferiorly preventing inferior displacement of the head by having the shaft of the screw resting on the calcar. The second screw should be placed posteriorly in the neck close to the posterior cortex preventing posterior displacement of the head. The third screw can be positioned anywhere in the neck for further support.

Ref:
Leighton RK. Fractures of the neck of femur. In Rockwood & Wilkins. *Fracture in Adults*, Vol 2. 6th ed. (2006) Philadelphia. Lippincott Williams & Wilkins.

**56.  C**

Patients with chronic renal failure have poor bone quality and are not suitable for internal fixation. Even in the case of an undisplaced fractures, these patients should undergo femoral head replacement. Patients with Paget's disease are prone to femoral deformity and bleeding, both complicate femoral head replacement and these patients should be considered for total hip replacement. Severe dementia, parkinsonism are not a contraindication for the use of internal fixation. Femoral head replacement in these patients should be performed using antero-lateral approach to prevent dislocation and wound contamination.

Ref:
Leighton RK. Fractures of the neck of femur. In Rockwood & Wilkins. *Fracture in Adults*, Vol 2. 6th ed. (2006) Philadelphia. Lippincott Williams & Wilkins.

**57.  D**

A prospective randomised controlled study performed on patients with femoral fractures with multiple injuries showed best treatment was early stabilisation. The results compared

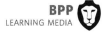

early stabilisation within 24 hours to late stabilisation after 48 hours. They showed a lower incidence of ARDS, fat embolism and pulmonary dysfunction in patients with Injury Severity Score of >18. Length of intensive care stay and overall health care cost were also reduced in early treatment in patients with ISS >18.

In groups with an ISS <18, only the hospital cost and length of stay were lower following early stabilisation. No difference was seen in complications related to ARDS, fat embolism and pulmonary dysfunction or duration of intensive stay.

Ref:
Bone LB, Johnson KD, Weigelt J, Scheinberg R. Early versus delayed stabilisation of femoral fractures. A prospective randomised study. *JBJS Am* 1989; 71(3): 336–340.

**58.  C**

Femoral nails are at a risk of breakage when used for stabilisation of fractures within 5cm from the most proximal distal locking screw. The peak stress on the nail exceeds the nail fatigue endurance limits in these circumstances.

The risk of breakage is reduced by using larger diameter nail and by limiting weight bearing until 50% femoral stiffness is regained. Use of steel instead of titanium increases stiffness of the nail. Use of interlocking nails increases the bending stiffness of the nail and should be preferred.

Ref:
Bucholz RW, Rose SE, Lawrence KL. Fatigue fracture of the interlocking nail in the treatment of fractures of the distal part of the femoral shaft. *JBJS Am* 1987; 69(9): 1391–1399.

**59.  A**

Piriform fossa is the ideal entry point for IM nail as it coincides with the neutral axis of the femoral canal. However > 6mm displacement anterior from this point of entry causes high hoop stress which result in bursting of the proximal femur, femoral neck or peri-trochanteric fractures. Lateral and medial displacement of the starting point does not increase the hoop stress.

Ref:
Johnson KD, Tencer AF, Shearman MC. Biomechanical factors affecting fracture stability and femoral bursting in closed intramedullary nailing of femoral shaft fractures, with illustrative case presentation, *J Orthop Trauma* 1987; 1(1): 1–11.

**60.  B**

Angular femoral malunion is commonly associated with closed treatment of femoral fractures. Intramedullary nailing of the femoral fractures is associated with rotational deformity and shortening resulting in leg length discrepancy. Correction of this deformity is considered if > 15 degrees of rotation or >2cm of shortening is present.

Ref:
Nork SE. Fractures of the shaft of femur. In Rockwood & Wilkins. *Fracture in Adults*, Vol 2. 6th ed. (2006) Philadelphia. Lippincott Williams & Wilkins.

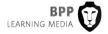

**61.** **C**

Knee dislocations can be placed into five types based on the joint position following dislocation. This can be anterior, posterior, medial, lateral and rotatory.

Rotatory dislocations are further divided into anteromedial, anterolateral, posteromedial and posterolateral dislocation. Posterolateral dislocation is the least common and the most described form. The hallmark of this dislocation is its irreducibility by closed methods. The medial femoral condyle button holes through the medial capsule and the medial collateral ligament invaginates into the knee joint preventing reduction.

Ref:
1.  Kennedy J. Complete dislocation of the knee joint. *JBJS Am* 1963; 45: 889–904
2.  Hill JA, Rana NA. Complications of poster lateral dislocation of the knee: case report and review of literature. *Clin Orthop* 1981; 154: 212–215.

**62.** **D**

The popliteal artery is rigidly fixed at the adductor hiatus and the soleus arch. Knee dislocation leads to traction or direct tearing of the artery. Limb loss is imminent if the re-vascularisation is not performed within 6–8 hours from the time of the popliteal injury. The overall incidence of arterial injury occurs in a third of the patients with knee dislocation.

Ref:
1.  Schenck RC Jr, Stannard JP, Wascher DC. Dislocations and fracture-dislocations of the knee. In Rockwood & Wilkins. *Fracture in Adults*, Vol 2. 6th ed. (2006) Philadelphia. Lippincott Williams & Wilkins.
2.  Green Ne, Allen BL. Vascular injuries associated with dislocation of the knee. *JBJS Am* 1977; 59: 236–239.

**63.** **B**

The anatomic classification of the knee dislocation (KD), classifies dislocations based on the ligamentous injuries around the knee joint. A KD-IIIM is a dislocation associated with rupture of ACL, PCL and medial collateral ligament or medial corner. The treatment includes a medial approach to the joint with stabilisation of PCL and MCL followed by late reconstruction of ACL. Alternatively, after an initial period of ROM exercises, both the ACL and PCL can be considered for reconstruction simultaneously, However PCL should be tensioned first as tensioning of ACL first results in a posterior tibio-femoral subluxation.

Ref:
Schenck RC Jr, Stannard JP, Wascher DC. Dislocations and fracture-dislocations of the knee. In Rockwood & Wilkins. *Fracture in Adults*, Vol 2. 6th ed. (2006) Philadelphia. Lippincott Williams & Wilkins.

**64.** **D**

Proximal tibio-fibular dislocation principally occurs with knee injury in flexion. Flexion results in the relaxation of the fibular collateral ligament, which is the most important constraint for the tibio-fibular joint. The dislocation of the joint is classified into four types, however the most common type being the anterolateral dislocation. Reduction is performed

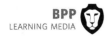

with the knee in flexion and application direct pressure. Chronic tibio-fibular dislocation is associated with peroneal nerve irritation and treatment is fibular head resection.

Ref:
Ogden JA. Dislocation of proximal fibula. *Radiology* 1972; 105: 547–549.


**65. C**

A fracture dislocation of the knee is associated with ligamentous injury along with a fracture of either the tibial side or the femoral side. Repair of both the fracture and the ligament is necessary for appropriate surgical management of this condition. Moore detailed the classification of the tibial side of the fractures into five types:

Type 1 – coronal split of the medial condyle

Type 2 – complete condylar fracture (medial or lateral)

Type 3 – enlarged lateral joint rim fracture, either avulsion of Gerdy's tubercle or enlarged Segond's fracture (lateral capsular sign). This injury are also called 'rim avulsion' fracture

Type 4 – compression of the lateral tibial plateau edge and tearing of MCL. Also called 'rim compression' injuries.

Type 5 – four-part fracture involving both tibial plateau, tibial eminence and tibial shaft.

Knee instability is seen in 60% of type 1 and 2 fractures, and 90% of type 3–5 fractures.

Ref:
Moore TM. Fracture dislocation of the knee. *Clin Orthop* 1981; 156:128–140.


**66. D**

Patellar dislocation is more common in females. The mechanism of injury is valgus load applied to a flexed, weight bearing and externally rotated knee. Anatomical and radiological findings that may predispose a knee to patellar dislocation include:

1. Q angle > 20 degrees
2. Genu valgus
3. A shallow patellofemoral sulcus, patellofemoral sulcus angle of >144 degrees
4. Lateralisation of tibial tubercle > 9mm
5. Merchant's congruence angle of + 16
6. Generalised hyperlaxity syndromes
7. Patella alta

Ref:
Maenppa H, Lehto MUK. Patellar dislocation. *Am J Sports Med* 1997; 25(2): 213–217.


**67. B**

The medial patellofemoral ligament (MPFL) spans from the medial epicondyle to medial patella. This is a distinct structure and is located in the second layer of the medial aspect of

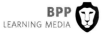

the knee. This has additional attachments to VMO and adductor tubercle and forms a major medial patella constraint. Rupture of MPFL is associated with patellar dislocation.

The knee has three layers of both medial and lateral structure. The layer 1 contains sartorius and fascia medially, illiotibial tract, biceps and fascia laterally. The layer 2 contains superficial MCL, semimembranosus, posterior oblique ligament and patellofemoral ligament medially, patellar retinaculum laterally. The third layer contains deep MCL and capsule medially, LCL, arcuate ligament, capsule and fabellofibular ligament laterally.

Ref:
Warren LF, Marshal JL. The supporting structures and the layers on the medial side of the knee. *JBJS Am* 1979; 61: 56–62.

68. **C**
Tibial plateau fracture is based on the position of the leg in relation to the direction of the force. Young patients have strong bones and hence present with split fractures associated with ligamentous injuries, older patients have poor quality bones and are associated with depression or depression-split type fracture with no ligamentous injuries. Association of ligamentous injuries with tibial plateau fracture is around 30%. The association of meniscal injury following a tibial plateau fracture is up to 50%, as the mechanism of injury is an axial compressive force.

Ref:
Egol KA, Koval KJ. Fractures of the proximal tibia. In Rockwood & Wilkins. *Fracture in Adults*, Vol 2. 6ᵗʰ ed. (2006) Philadelphia. Lippincott Williams & Wilkins.

69. **A**
The Schatzker classification of the tibial plateau fracture is most widely accepted and used. This classification divides the tibial shaft fracture in six types. The type I is a split wedge fracture of the lateral plateau without joint depression. These are commonly seen in young patients with good bone quality and are associated with lateral meniscal tear or incarceration of the lateral meniscus. Hence arthroscopy may be required to exclude this when undertaking percutaneous screw fixation.

Ref:
Schatzker J, Mcbroom R, Bruce D. The tibial plateau fracture: the Toronto experience 1968–1975. *Clin Orthop* 1979; 138: 94–104.

70. **D**
The technique for Schatzker Type VI fractures is reduction of metaphyseal component followed by reduction and stabilisation of the metaphyseal fragment to the diaphysis. This achieved by the use of double plates inserted with minimum dissection, single plates for transverse fractures, single plate with contralateral external fixator or hybrid fixators.

The complications of the treatment include infection, peroneal neuropathy, skin slough, malunion and nonunion. Malunion and nonunion are rarely seen but has been seen in Schatzker Type VI fractures treated by hybrid external fixator.

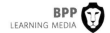

Ref:
Young MJ, Barrack RL. Complications of internal fixation of tibial plateau fractures. *Orthop Rev* 1994; 23: 149–154.

71.    **C**
Soft tissue injury associated with closed fractures has been classified based on its severity by Tscherne. The grading for soft tissue injury includes:

Grade 0 – negligible soft tissue injury

Grade 1 – closed fracture with superficial abrasion or contusion of the overlying soft tissue

Grade 2 – closed fracture with significant contusion to the muscle and/or deep contaminated skin abrasion

Grade 3 – closed fracture, severe soft tissue injury with degloving, crushing, compartment syndrome or vascular injury

Soft tissue injury influences the overall treatment of the fracture with consideration appropriate stabilisation technique and need for flap coverage and decompression of compartment syndrome.

Ref:
Tscherne H, Gotzens L. *Fractures with soft tissue injuries.* 1984. Springer-Verlag, Berlin.

72.    **D**
Closed reduction and stabilisation in a long leg cast of tibial shaft fractures is associated with good results provided length, alignment and rotational stability is maintained. Closed reduction and immobilisation of the tibial shaft fractures should be reviewed with weekly radiographs for 3–4 weeks and loss of alignment, length and rotation should warrant a re-manipulation.

The parameters warranting a re-manipulation include: > 10 degress in sagittal plane and >5 degrees in coronal plane. Wedging of the plaster cast should be undertaken to correct higher angulations than more than 10 degrees in sagittal plane and more than 5 degress in coronal plane.

Ref:
Littenberg B, Weinstein LP, McCarren M, *et al.* Closed fractures of the tibial shaft: A meta-analysis of three methods of treatment. *JBJS Am*; 80: 174–183.

73.    **B**
The indication for operative treatment of the tibial shaft fracture can be divided into absolute and relative indications

The absolute indication requiring operative fixation of the tibial shaft fracture includes open fractures, fractures with vascular injury, compartment syndrome and patients with multiple injuries.

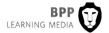

The relative indication for operative stabilisation includes significant shortening, significant comminution, same level fracture of the tibia and fibula and tibial fracture with intact fibula. These fractures run a high risk of malunion or nonunion and hence usually warrant operative stabilisation.

Ref:
Court-Brown CM. Fractures of the tibia and fibula. In Rockwood & Wilkins. *Fracture in Adults*, Vol 2. 6th ed. (2006) Philadelphia. Lippincott Williams & Wilkins.

74. **C**

The stability of an external fixator to the tibia can be increased by placement of the half pins perpendicular to the anteromedial tibial surface with bicortical purchase of the pins. The most important factor in increasing the stability is by allowing contact of the fracture ends. The stiffness is directly proportional to the fourth power of the radius of the pins and hence increasing the diameter of the half pins, increases stiffness of the construct. The stiffness is inversely proportional to the third power of the distance between the bar and the bone, hence decreasing the distance between the bar and the bone increases stiffness. Increasing the number of half pins can also increase the stiffness of the external fixator. Use of lag screw to supplement the external fixation increases the risk of nonunion and re-fractures as a result of devitalisation of the bone during reduction and fixation.

Ref:
Tencer AF, Biomechanics of fixation and fracture. In Rockwood and Green's. *Fracture in Adults*. 6th ed. (2006) Philadelphia. Lippincott Wilkins & Saunders

75. **C**

The most important complication of tibial shaft fracture is compartment syndrome. Diagnosis of compartment syndrome warrants an urgent four-compartment fasciotomy for decompression. These four compartments include the superficial and deep posterior, the anterior and the lateral compartment. A two-incision fasciotomy uses a medial longitudinal incision 1.5 cm posterior to the posterior crest of the tibia. This incision decompresses the superficial and the deep posterior compartment. The lateral longitudinal incision is undertaken 1.5 cm anterior to the fibula. This incision decompresses the lateral and the anterior compartment.

Ref:
McQueen MM. Acute compartment syndrome. In Rockwood & Wilkins. *Fracture in Adults*, Vol 1. 6th ed. (2006) Philadelphia. Lippincott Williams & Wilkins.

76. **B**

The direction of the force applied to the distal tibia and the position of the foot and ankle at the time of injury determines the injury pattern. Extensive posterior comminution of the tibial plafond occurs on axial loading with ankle in plantar flexion. while extensive anterior comminution occurs on axial loading with ankle in dorsiflexion, rotation force or shear force causes large articular tibial plafond fragment with no cortical comminution.

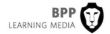

Ref:
Marsh JL, Saltzman CL. Ankle Fracture. In Rockwood & Wilkins. *Fracture in Adults*, Vol 2. 6<sup>th</sup> ed. (2006) Philadelphia. Lippincott Williams & Wilkins.

**77.    E**
Displaced tibial plafond fracture requires surgical reconstruction. Low energy injuries lead to a small number of large articular fragments and can be treated by open reduction internal fixation. High energy injury leads to a large number of small articular fragments and are best treated with the use of external fixator. Use of interfragmentary screws for the diaphyseal fragments is associated with high risk of re-fracture.

Ref:
Marsh JL, Saltzman CL. Ankle Fracture. In Rockwood & Wilkins. *Fracture in Adults*, Vol 2. 6<sup>th</sup> ed. (2006) Philadelphia. Lippincott Williams & Wilkins.

**78.    B**
Weber classified ankle fractures according to the level of the fibular fracture. Weber classification divides fibulae fractures in three groups labelled A, B and C. A classification of ankle fracture based on the mechanism of the injury was described by Lauge-Hansen. As Weber's classification is widely used for description of the ankle fracture, its corresponding Lauge-Hansen classifications are described as follows:

1.    Weber A = Lauge Hansen – supination – adduction injury
2.    Weber B = Lauge Hansen – supination – external rotation injury
3.    Weber C = Lauge Hansen – pronation – external rotation injury

Ref:
Lauge-Hansen N. Fractures of the ankle. Combined experimental-surgical and experimental roentgenological investigation. *Arch Surg*. 1950; 60: 957–985.

**79.    C**
The NASCIS III study concluded the following:

1.    No difference in the neurological recovery was seen in the patients treated with bolus dose of methyl prednisolone within three hours of injury in all the three groups.
2.    Significant statistical improvement in the neurological recovery of the patients treated within 3–8 hours with a bolus dose Methyl prednisolone followed by a 48 hour infusion of methyl prednisolone was seen compared with the group treated with 24 hour infusion and 6 hourly tirilazad mesylate infusion for 48 hours.
The study stressed on the importance of initiating a bolus dose of 30mg/kg of methyl prednisolone within 3–8 hours following the spinal cord injury followed by a 48 hour infusion of methyl prednisolone at the rate of 5.4mg/kg/hr.

Ref:
Bracken MB, Shepard MJ, Holford TR *et al.* Administration of methylprednisolone for 24 or 48 hours or tirilazad mesylate for 48 hours in the treatment of acute spinal cord injury: Results of the Third National Acute Spinal Cord Injury Randomised Controlled Trial, National Acute Spinal Cord Injury Study. *JAMA* 1997; 277: 1597–1604.

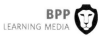

80.   **D**
      Bending load causes the fracture to start at the tensile cortex with a crack. As the bone weakens the compression cortex begins to fail. Compression force drives together the ends of the failing bone causing development of a third fragment (butterfly fragment).

      Ref:
      Tencer AF, Biomechanics of fixation and fracture. In Rockwood & Wilkins. *Fracture in Adults*, Vol 1. 6th ed. (2006) Philadelphia. Lippincott Williams & Wilkins.

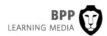

BPP
LEARNING MEDIA

# Hands and Upper Limb

## Question Bank

Fahad G Attar & Talal Ibrahim

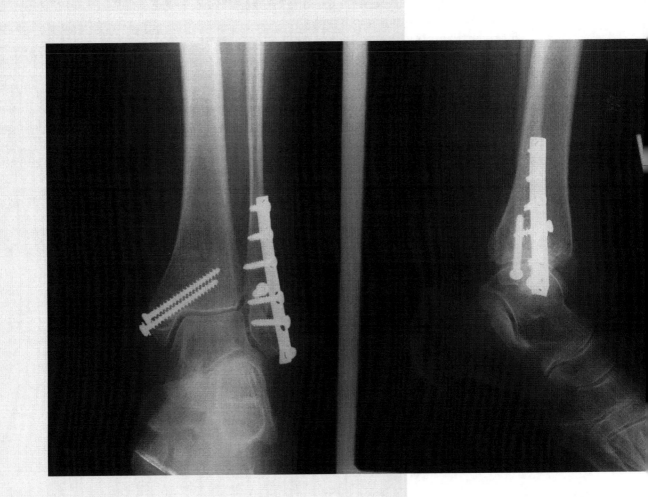

1. The IFSSSH classification system of congenital hand and upper limb anomalies has all the following categories except:
   A. Failure of differentiation
   B. Duplication
   C. Defect malformation
   D. Undergrowth (hyperplasia)
   E. Congenital constriction band syndrome

2. The three most common defects seen in amniotic constriction band is:
   A. Digit amputations, constriction rings and acrosyndactyly
   B. Cleft lip, cleft palate and hemangiomas
   C. Scoliosis, short umbilical cord and constriction rings
   D. Gastroschisis, cleft lip and digit amputations
   E. Complete absence of upper limb, hemangiomas and cranial defects

3. Trigger finger is associated with all of the following except:
   A. Hyperthyroidism
   B. De Quervain's disease
   C. Rheumatoid arthritis
   D. Amyloidosis
   E. Carpal tunnel syndrome

4. All of the following statements regarding trigger finger are **true** except:
   A. Females more commonly affected
   B. Fibrocartilaginous metaplasia of retinacular sheath
   C. Poor diabetic control increases the risk
   D. Lifetime risk is 2–3%
   E. No evidence to suggest that repeated finger movements and local trauma are risk factors

5. In a patient with symptoms of trigger finger in a single digit, of less than 6 months duration, the best first line of management would be:
   A. Night splinting with MCP at 15 degrees of flexion and DIP and PIP joints free
   B. Splinting with activity modification
   C. Corticosteroid injection
   D. Percutaneous A1 pulley release
   E. Open A1 pulley release

6. With regards to complex regional pain syndrome type 1, all the following statements apply except:
   A. Twice as common in women than men
   B. Men and women are equally affected
   C. Known to occur more commonly in the elderly
   D. No specific measures are known to prevent CRPS after trauma or surgery
   E. No relationship with cigarette smoking has been shown

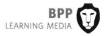

7.    In Kienbock's disease, which of the following treatment options is not recommended for individuals who do heavy manual work?
      A.    Ulna lengthening procedures
      B.    Radial shortening procedures
      C.    Lunate revascularisation procedures
      D.    Radial closing wedge osteotomy
      E.    Simple excision of lunate

8.    All the following are implicated as common causes in the pathophysiology of 'snapping scapula syndrome' except:
      A.    Lushka's tubercle
      B.    Absence of spine of scapula
      C.    Osteochondroma
      D.    Cosmetic breast procedures
      E.    Scapular muscle overuse

9.    With regards to shoulder resurfacing all these statements are **true** except:
      A.    Contraindicated in cuff tear arthropathy
      B.    Indications include rheumatoid arthritis
      C.    Use is precluded in patients with a Hill Sachs lesion
      D.    More than 60% bone stock should be present pre-operatively for a successful outcome
      E.    Partial resurfacing can be used for lesions affecting < 20% of the humeral head

10.   Which of the following do not contribute to the rocking-horse mechanism of glenoid component loosening?
      A.    Inferior placement of glenoid component
      B.    Superior placement of humeral component
      C.    Massive cuff tear
      D.    Separation of polyethylene from metal back of prosthesis
      E.    Eccentric loading of glenoid component

11.   With regards to acromio-plasty which statement is **false**?
      A.    If pain relief is used as an outcome measures, open acriomio-plasty has similar results as arthroscopic acromio-plasty
      B.    If range of motion is used as an outcome measures, open acriomio-plasty has similar results as arthroscopic acromio-plasty
      C.    If strength is used as an outcome measure, open acromio-plasty has similar results as arthroscopic acromio-plasty
      D.    Acromio-plasty does not significantly influence outcomes in cuff repair (DASH, Constant scores)
      E.    Acromio-plasty significantly influences outcomes in cuff repair (DASH, Constant scores)

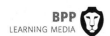

12. In the clinical tests used to assess impingement and rotator cuff pathology, which statement is **not true**:
    A. Neer and Hawkins test are more sensitive than specific for subacromial bursitis
    B. Jobe's and the empty can test for supraspinatous tears are less specific than sensitive
    C. Gerber's lift off test for subscapularis pathology is highly specific, but with lower sensitivity
    D. Neer test has high sensitivity and specificity
    E. For long head of biceps tendon pathology, no test has high sensitivity or specificity


13. In an elderly low demand patient who has cuff tear arthropathy, with an intact deltoid but incompetent coraco-acromial arch, the best line of treatment would be:
    A. Reverse total shoulder arthroplasty
    B. Hemiarthroplasty
    C. Arthroscopic debridement
    D. Deltoid incorporation exercise
    E. Arthrodesis


14. The following are all radiographic signs suggestive of cuff tear arthropathy except:
    A. Osteopenia of the acromion and humerus
    B. Sourcil sign – sclerosis of the superior aspect of the humerus
    C. An acromion to humeral head space of less than 7 mm
    D. Acetabulisation of the acromion
    E. Stress fractures of the acromion.


15. A more specific test for antero-superior cuff tears would be:
    A. Belly press test
    B. Lift off test
    C. Horn blowers test
    D. External rotation lag test
    E. None of the above


16. For a young patient with an irreparable antero-superior rotator cuff tear whose main complaint is weakness, the most appropriate treatment method could be:
    A. Physiotherapy and re-education of muscle recruitment
    B. Arthroscopic debridement of torn edges of rotator cuff and bursectomy
    C. Partial repair of rotator cuff
    D. Pectoralis major tendon transfer
    E. Complete repair with tendon substitutes (allograft)


17. All the following are branches of the medial cord except:
    A. Medial pectoral nerve
    B. Medial cutaneous nerve of arm
    C. Medial cutaneous nerve of forearm
    D. Ulna nerve
    E. Musculocutaneous nerve

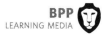

18. All the following are branches of the lateral cord except:
    A. Lateral pectoral nerve
    B. Musculocutaneous nerve
    C. Lateral root of median nerve
    D. Lower subscapular nerve
    E. Lateral cutaneous nerve of forearm

19. In pathology of the sternoclavicular joint, SAPHO is an unusual condition associated with all these except:
    A. Pustulosis
    B. Hyperostosis
    C. Synovitis
    D. Friedrich's disease
    E. Acne

20. A middle aged woman with bilateral sternoclavicular swelling and pain, associated with pustular or psoriatic lesions is most likely suffering from:
    A. Friedrich's disease
    B. SAPHO
    C. Condensing osteitis
    D. Inflammatory arthritis
    E. Psoriatic arthritis

21. In relation to the development of neuralgic amyotrophy, the following are all implicated except:
    A. Post surgical
    B. Infections
    C. Pregnancy
    D. Hereditary
    E. Drugs

22. Dupuytren's disease is associated with all the conditions listed below except:
    A. Alcoholism
    B. HIV
    C. Smoking
    D. Hypercholesterolemia
    E. Hyperthyroidism

23. Which of the following is **false** regarding the central aponeurosis in Dupuytren's disease?
    A. Its longitudinal fibres form 'pre-tendinous bands'
    B. The transverse ligament is distal and parallel to the natatory ligament
    C. The transverse ligament is deep to the pre-tendinous bands
    D. The transverse fibres form the natatory ligament
    E. The middle layer of the bifurcated pre-tendinous bands forms the spiral band

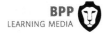

24. The neurovascular bundle in the digit is surrounded by all the following fascial structures except:
   A. The Grayson ligament
   B. The Cleland ligament
   C. The Gosset lateral digital sheet
   D. The Thomine retro vascular fascia
   E. The natatory ligament

25. In the pathophysiology of Dupuytren's disease tissue, which of the following statements is **true**?
   A. The spiral cord is most frequently seen in Dupuytren's disease
   B. The Grayson's ligament does not contribute to the formation of the spiral cord
   C. Spiral cord is most commonly encountered in the little finger
   D. The spiral cord causes flexion contracture at the metacarpophalangeal joint
   E. The lateral cord does not contribute to flexion contracture of the proximal interphalangeal joints

26. Non Dupuytren's disease is characterised by:
   A. Preponderance in African races
   B. Bilateral involvement
   C. Involvement of lower limbs
   D. Exclusively associated with trauma
   E. Spontaneously improves

27. Which of the following is **not true** regarding the clinical manifestations of Dupuytren's disease?
   A. Vertical bands are the first structures to be affected
   B. Skin pitting isn't a reliable early sign
   C. Nodules are fixed both to skin and deep fascia
   D. Knuckle pads most commonly affect the index finger
   E. Nodules regress spontaneously

28. Weakness of flexion at the thumb interphalangeal joint and distal interphalangeal joints of the index finger are most commonly associated with:
   A. Parsonage-Turner syndrome
   B. Pronator syndrome
   C. Anterior interosseous syndrome
   D. Carpal tunnel syndrome
   E. Cubital tunnel syndrome

29. According to the Millender and Nalebuff staging of Boutonniere deformity in rheumatoid arthritis, what stage does a patient fit into with a 30 degree extensor lag in the PIP joint, passively correctable:
   A. Stage I
   B. Stage II
   C. Stage III
   D. Stage IV
   E. Stage V

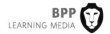

30. According to the Millender and Nalebuff staging of swan-neck deformities in rheumatoid arthritis, what stage does a patient fit into with a limited flexibility of the PIP joint in all positions of the MCP joint (articular/para-articular problems):
    A. Stage I
    B. Stage II
    C. Stage III
    D. Stage IV
    E. None of the above

31. According to the Millender classification of rheumatoid thumb deformities, a patient with a MCP joint in fixed flexion (with joint destruction), IP joint in hyperextension and passively correctable, but no CMC joint involvement belongs to:
    A. Stage I
    B. Stage II
    C. Stage III
    D. Stage IV
    E. Stage V

32. The inheritance pattern in Dupuytren's disease is believed to be:
    A. Autosomal recessive
    B. Autosomal dominant
    C. Sex linked
    D. Familial
    E. As a result of acquired gene mutation

33. A lesion in the proximal metaphysis of the proximal phalanx of the hand which is expansile and eccentric is most likely to be:
    A. Giant cell tumour
    B. Osteoid osteoma
    C. Enchondroma
    D. Giant cell tumour
    E. Anuerysmal bone cyst

34. In radial tunnel syndrome which statement is most appropriate?
    A. Middle finger extension test is usually positive in radial tunnel syndrome and tennis elbow
    B. 5% of patients with tennis elbow have radial tunnel syndrome
    C. 50% of patients with radial tunnel syndrome may have concomitant tennis elbow
    D. All of the above
    E. None of the above

35. A firm swelling on the palmar aspect of the proximal phalanx of the thumb of the dominant hand which is mobile transversely but not longitudinally is a:
    A. Bowlers thumb
    B. Ganglion
    C. Osteoid osteoma
    D. Lipoma
    E. Giant cell tumour

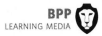

36.  Which is the commonest primary malignant bone tumour which occurs in the hand?
     A.  Osteosarcoma
     B.  Chondrosarcoma
     C.  Chondroblastoma
     D.  Enchondroma
     E.  Giant cell tumour


37.  The second most common swelling encountered in the hand following a ganglion is:
     A.  Lipoma
     B.  Enchondroma
     C.  Pigmented villonodular synovitis
     D.  Pyogenic granuloma
     E.  Carpometacarpal boss


38.  A patient in the fourth decade presents with intermittent pain and local swelling in the metacarpal bone of the hand. X-rays show an eccentric, bony lesion with central lucency, fine trabeculation, expasile, no marginal sclerosis. The likely lesion is;
     A.  Enchondroma
     B.  Anuerysmal bone cyst
     C.  Intraosseous bone cyst
     D.  Giant cell tumour
     E.  Eosinophillic granuloma


39.  A simple ganglion in the hand is most commonly seen in all these sites except:
     A.  Distal phalanx overlying the nail bed
     B.  Proximal digital crease of the middle finger
     C.  Anterior aspect of the wrist just lateral to the flexor carpi radialis
     D.  Dorsal aspect of the wrist from the scapho-lunate ligament
     E.  Dorsal aspect of the wrist over the ulna styloid


40.  According to the classification adopted by the International Federation of Hand Societies for congenital hand abnormalities, all these are failure of differentiation of parts except:
     A.  Clasped thumb
     B.  Phocomelia
     C.  Syndactyly
     D.  Radio-ulnar synostosis
     E.  Arthrogryphosis


41.  Kanaverel's four classic signs for tendon sheath infections include all the following except:
     A.  Tenderness over the involved tendon sheath
     B.  Pain on passive extension
     C.  Parasthesia in the affected finger
     D.  Fusiform swelling of the digit
     E.  Flexed attitude of the finger

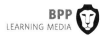

42. A dumbbell or 'collar-button-shaped' abscess is characteristic of
    A. Tendon sheath infection
    B. Felon
    C. Web space infection
    D. Radial bursal infection
    E. None of the above


43. A common organism which grows in culture, specific to human hand bites is:
    A. Streptococcus pyogenes
    B. Staphylococcus aureus
    C. Pasteurella multicoda
    D. Eikenella corrodens
    E. Pseudomonas aeroginousa


44. With regards to carpal instability, all the statements below are **true** except:
    A. Lunotriquetral instability is the commonest form volar intercalated segment instability
    B. Scapholunate instability is the commonest form of dorsal intercalated segment instability
    C. Terry Thomas sign is suggestive of volar intercalated segment instability
    D. For a SLAC wrist a salvage procedure is indicated
    E. Dorsal intercalated segment instability is the commonest form of carpal instability


45. With regards to the triangular fibrocartilage complex (TFCC) which statement is **not true**?
    A. Ulnar collateral ligament is part of TFCC
    B. Incorporates the extensor carpi ulnaris sheath
    C. Volar radioulnar ligament is part of TFCC
    D. Arises from ulna aspect of lunate fossa of radius
    E. Inserts into triquetrum, hamate and pisiform


46. In radial nerve palsy which of the following is tendon transfers is indicated:
    A. Extensor carpi ulnaris to abductor pollicis longus
    B. Pronator teres to extensor carpi radialis brevis
    C. Pronator teres to extensor carpi ulnaris
    D. Extensor carpi ulnaris to flexor carpi ulnaris
    E. Flexor digitorum profundus to extensor digitorum superficialis


47. Which of the following can be used as donor tendons in tendon transfer for a median nerve palsy for improving thumb apposition?
    A. Flexor digitorum superficialis of the ring finger
    B. Extensor indices proprius
    C. Extensor digitorum quinti proprius
    D. All the above
    E. None of the above

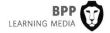

48. Which of the following is **false** regarding the extensor compartments at the wrist?
    A. The 2$^{nd}$ compartment is composed of extensor carpi radialis longus and brevis
    B. The 1$^{st}$ compartment is abductor pollicis longus and extensor pollicis brevis
    C. The 5$^{th}$ compartment is extensor digiti minimi
    D. The 3$^{rd}$ compartment is extensor pollicis longus
    E. The 4$^{th}$ compartment is extensor digitorum communis

49. With regards to Triangular fibrocartilage complex (TFCC) of the wrist, which statement is **false**?
    A. Palmer classification TFCC Class 1 is traumatic
    B. Palmer classification TFCC Class 2 is degenerative
    C. Essex Lopresti lesion may be an acquired cause of ulnar impaction syndrome
    D. Infiltration of local anaesthetic may help localise pain source
    E. Arthrographic findings of TFCC perforation correlate well with clinical findings

50. For Ulna impaction syndrome all the following are recognised surgical treatments except:
    A. Ulnar shortening osteotomy
    B. Combined radio-ulna joint shortening osteotomy
    C. Darrachs procedure
    D. Hemiresection interposition arthroplasty
    E. Wafer resection

51. With regards wrist fusion, choose the **false** statement:
    A. Indications include Volkmann ischaemic contracture, spastic cerebral palsy, and tuberculosis
    B. Wrist is fused in 10 to 20 degrees of flexion
    C. Fusion is done with long axis of third metacarpal aligned with long axis of radial shaft
    D. In children operation is usually postponed until 12 years of age
    E. Addition of AO type plate and screw systems yields fusion rates of close to 100%

52. In carpal instability, which statement is **not true**?
    A. Radiographic intercarpal relationships is important to assess static from dynamic instability
    B. Dissociative carpal instability occurs when extrinsic radiocarpal ligaments are disrupted
    C. The scapholunate angle on a lateral radiograph is increased in DISI
    D. The normal scapholunate angle is between 30–80 degrees
    E. The normal capitolunate angle is less than 20 degrees

53. With regards to the vascularity of the hand which of the following is **true**:
    A. The radial artery forms the superficial palmar arch
    B. The ulnar artery forms the deep palmar arch
    C. The deep arch is incomplete in 25% of individuals
    D. Aneurysms are usually due to trauma
    E. Allen's test is not a reliable clinical test

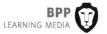

54. In frostbite injuries to the hand, treatment protocol includes all of the following except:
    A. Blisters should not be aspirated to prevent secondary infection
    B. Aloe vera topically
    C. Triple phase bone scan at 48 hours for deep frostbites
    D. Penicillin
    E. Daily hydrotherapy and hand therapy

55. In proximal row carpectomy:
    A. Indicated in patients with low demands who would like to preserve some wrist motion
    B. Excision of the lunate, triquetrum and entire scaphoid is recommended
    C. Distal pole of scaphoid can be left behind
    D. Radial styloidectomy is not a part of this procedure
    E. Arthrosis of the capitolunate joint is an absolute contraindication to the procedure

56. In intrinsic claw hand:
    A. Intrinsic metacarpophalangeal joint flexors are paralysed
    B. Intrinsic interphalangeal joint extensors are paralysed
    C. The long extensor of the thumb is unopposed causing abduction
    D. Thumb interphalangeal joint is flexed
    E. Abductor pollicis brevis is a thumb intrinsic which is paralysed

57. In planning tendon transfers in the hand:
    A. Pronator teres could be made available for thumb abduction
    B. Palmaris longus could be made available for thumb extension
    C. Flexor carpi ulnaris could be made available for finger extension
    D. All of the above
    E. None of the above

58. In tendon transfers for restoration of pinch, all of the following are **true** except:
    A. The abductor pollicis brevis is single most important muscle contributing to pinch
    B. The long thumb extensor aids thumb adduction as a substitute to opposition
    C. Arthrodesis of the metacarpophalangeal joint of the thumb may be necessary, if available muscle power is inadequate
    D. A pulley is never usually required during tendon transfer
    E. The flexor digitorum sublimis of the ring finger is the harvested tendon of choice

59. Opposition of the thumb during pinch grip is a combination of all these movements except:
    A. Pronation of thumb
    B. Adduction of thumb from palmar surface of index finger
    C. Flexion of the metacarpophalangeal joint of the thumb
    D. Radial deviation of the proximal phalanx of the thumb on the metacarpal
    E. Movement of thumb towards the fingers

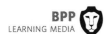

60. In cerebral palsy of the hand which of the following statements is **not true** regarding treatment:
    A. Night splinting at an early age is routinely used and is very effective
    B. Hand therapy helps in control of exaggerated reflexes
    C. Under correction rather than overcorrection is always preferred
    D. Myotomy, tenotomy, tenodesis and excisional arthroplasty are all recognised forms of surgical treatment
    E. Tendon lengthening does not require strict post operative compliance

61. With regards the arthritic hand:
    A. Bouchards nodes affect the distal interphalangeal joints in OA
    B. Almost 95% of patients with psoriatic arthritis have asymmetrical peripheral joint involvement.
    C. The metacarpophalangeal and proximal interphalangeal joints are usually spared in SLE
    D. Tapering of the phalanges and metacarpals is seen radiographically in SLE
    E. Heberdens nodes affect the proximal interphalangeal joints in OA

62. Which of the following statements is **false** regarding arthritis in the hand?
    A. Aspiration of a joint in gout show positively birefringent crystals
    B. Nail pitting is seen in 15% of patients with psoriatic arthritis
    C. Erosion of terminal phalangeal tufts is a radiographic finding in psoriatic arthritis
    D. Reiters syndrome is a triad of conjunctivitis, urethritis and synovitis
    E. Only 5–10% of patients suffering from psoriatic arthropathy have distal interphalangeal joint involvement.

63. Which of the statements is **not true** regarding carpal tunnel syndrome?
    A. Commonly occurs in 30–60 years of age
    B. Female: Male ratio is 3:1
    C. Obesity is not a risk factor
    D. Smoking is a risk factor
    E. Elevation of carpal tunnel pressure over 30 mm of mercury predisposes to nerve impairment

64. Which of the following are not factors involved in pathogenesis of carpal tunnel syndrome:
    A. Diabetes mellitus
    B. Eclampsia
    C. Scleroderma
    D. Osteoporosis
    E. Raynauds phenomena

65. In clinical testing for carpal tunnel syndrome:
    A. Phalen's test has high specificity
    B. Tinel's test has high sensitivity
    C. Tourniquet test is extremely sensitive but not specific
    D. Durkan's test is more sensitive and specific than Phalen's and Tinel's
    E. Tinel's test is more sensitive than Durkan's

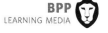

66. Nerve conduction studies for carpal tunnel syndrome, which of the statements is **not true**:
    A. A distal motor latency of more than 4.5ms is abnormal
    B. A distal sensory latency of more than 3.5ms is abnormal
    C. Nerve conduction studies are 90% specific for diagnosis of carpal tunnel syndrome
    D. Positive sharp waves are a sign of nerve damage
    E. Fibrillation at rest is a sign of nerve damage

67. In carpal tunnel syndrome decompression surgery:
    A. If palmar sensory branch of median nerve is cut, it should be sectioned at its origin
    B. Superficial palmar arch is not at risk
    C. Palmar sensory branch lies medial to palmaris longus tendon
    D. The recurrent branch of median nerve is predominantly subligamentous
    E. The recurrent branch of median nerve is predominantly transligamentous

68. In de Quervains disease all of the following are **true** except:
    A. Typically a disease of overuse
    B. Typical age group is 30–50 years old
    C. Women are typically affected up to 10 times more frequently than men
    D. Affects the first dorsal compartment tendons abductor pollicis brevis and extensor pollicis longus
    E. Steroid injection into tendon sheath is most successful within 6 weeks of onset of symptoms

69. In tendon repairs:
    A. Vicryl is routinely used because of high resistance to disrupting forces
    B. Braided polyester sutures are routinely used
    C. Smooth juncture of tendon ends does not influence for tendon repair
    D. Interrupted suture technique is found to have similar results as continuous four strand repairs
    E. Minimal gapping at repair site does not influence healing

70. In flexor tendon repairs choose the **false** statement:
    A. Zone I injury involves repair of FDP only
    B. Zone II injuries have a risk of adhesions and scarring
    C. Zone V repairs usually do not need wound extension
    D. Zone III repairs lumbrical bellies are not usually repaired
    E. A Z plasty of the flexor retinaculum may be needed in Zone IV repairs

71. In the treatment of medial epicondylitis of the elbow (Golfers elbow), choose the **false** statement:
    A. Surgery is indicated in only 10% of patients due to success of conservative treatment.
    B. In Type IA, only epicondylar debridement is an established form of treatment
    C. In Type IB, epicondylar debridement along with cubital tunnel decompression is an established form of treatment
    D. Percutaneous medial epicondylar release is an established form of treatment
    E. The focus of pathology musculotendinous rather than osseous

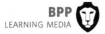

72. In the principles of Continuous passive movement (CPM) following elbow surgery, choose the **false** statement:
    A. CPM causes a sinusoidal oscillation in intra-articular pressure
    B. Prior to starting CPM all circumferential dressings should be removed
    C. It is necessary that full range of motion be utilised
    D. CPM requires close supervision by someone skilled with its use
    E. CPM should never be used continuously in the immediate post operative period

73. In elbow arthroscopy:
    A. Patient position is either prone, lateral or supine
    B. Proximal anteromedial portal poses risks to ulnar nerve, medial antebrachial cutaneous nerve, median nerve and brachial artery
    C. Distal anteromedial portal poses risks to medial antebrachial nerve, median nerve and brachial artery
    D. Proximal postero-lateral portal has highest risk of damage to neurovascular structures
    E. Portals should be created with a fully distended joint following injection

74. The ideal candidate for interpositional arthroplasty of the elbow joint is:
    A. Incapacitating pain in a 27-year-old non manual worker with rheumatoid arthritis
    B. A 35-year-old heavy manual labourer with post traumatic arthritis, currently employed
    C. A wheelchair bound patient with rheumatoid arthritis
    D. A patient with a grossly unstable elbow from rheumatoid arthritis
    E. A 65-year-old patient with osteoarthritis with loss of flexion motor power at the elbow

75. Substance(s) used in interpositional arthroplasty of the elbow:
    A. Fascia lata
    B. Autogenous skin
    C. Achilles tendon
    D. All the above
    E. None of the above

76. With regards elbow joint stability and the medial collateral ligament, which of the following statements is **false**:
    A. The anterior oblique portion of the medial collateral ligament is stronger than the posterior oblique portion
    B. The posterior oblique portion of the medial collateral ligament is taut only in fixed flexion
    C. The anterior oblique fibres of the medial collateral are taught in the entire flexion arc
    D. The posterior oblique fibres are the primary stabiliser of the elbow in valgus stress
    E. Absence of radial head does not affect valgus stability in the presence of the medial collateral ligament.

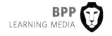

77.  Which of the following statements is **not true** with regards to heterotrophic ossification around the elbow joint?
     A.   May completely surround the ulnar nerve
     B.   May produce radial ulnar synostosis
     C.   May occur in 90% of cases of combined head and elbow trauma
     D.   Excision is not recommended until most motor neurologic recovery has occurred
     E.   Persistent spasticity following head injury is not associated with recurrence

78.  A 16-year-old boy complains of some pain in his shoulder following a fall. The X-ray shows a lytic lesion in the proximal humerus with cortical thinning. Histology reveals giant cells, inflammatory cells and haemosiderin deposits. The likely diagnosis is:
     A.   Eosinophillic granuloma
     B.   Ewing's sarcoma
     C.   Unicameral bone cyst
     D.   Chondroblastoma
     E.   Osteosarcoma

79.  A 12-year-old presents with local tenderness in the shoulder region. X-rays reveal a lucent lesion in the epiphyseal region sharply delimited from surrounding bone by a thin margin of increased bony density. Histology reveals giant cells, polygonal cells with a grooved nucleus, mitotic figures and little stroma. The most likely diagnosis is:
     A.   Aneurysmal bone cyst
     B.   Giant cell tumour
     C.   Osteoblastoma
     D.   Chondroblastoma
     E.   Clear cell chondrosarcoma

80.  With regards to tumours of the proximal humerus, which statement is **false**?
     A.   It is the most frequent site for unicameral bone cysts
     B.   Pathological fracture is rare except for unicameral bone cysts
     C.   Chondroblastomas rarely occur at this site
     D.   Delto-pectoral interval should always be avoided for biopsy
     E.   Bony metastases are common in the adult

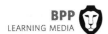

BPP
LEARNING MEDIA

# Hands and Upper Limb

## Answers

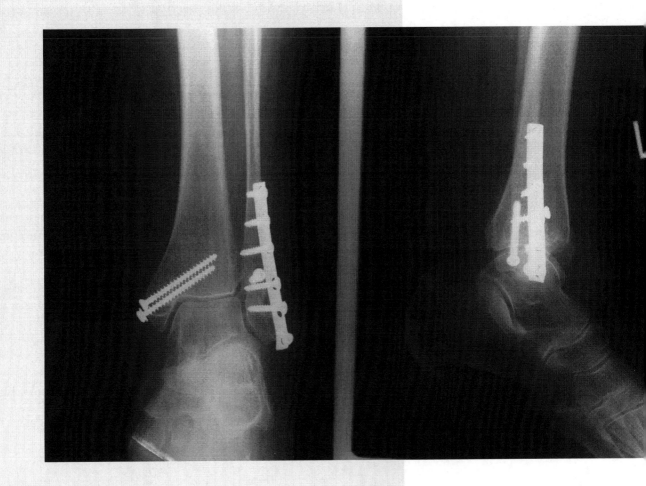

1.  **C**

    The IFSSH (International Federation and Society for Surgery of the Hand) classification is the most widely used. It is as follows :

    I.   Failure of formation
    II.  Failure of differentiation
    III. Duplication
    IV.  Overgrowth (gigantism)
    V.   Undergrowth (hypoplasia)
    VI.  Congenital constriction band syndrome
    VII. Generalised skeletal abnormalities

    Defect malformation is not part of the classification.

    Ref:

    Manske PR. (2009) Classification and developmental biology of congenital anomalies of the hand and upper extremity. *Journal of Bone and Joint Surgery*. Vol 91–3.

2.  **A**

    Amniotic bands are associated with three types of anomalies – disruptions, deformations and malformations. Cleft lip, anal atresia and ventricular septal defects are also found to be associated with this condition in 5–15% of cases in a study.

    Ref:

    Goldfarb CA. (2009) Amniotic constriction band: A multidisciplinary assessment of aetiology and clinical presentation. *Journal of Bone and Joint Surgery*, Vol 91-A. Supplement 4.

3.  **A**

    Also found to be associated with renal disease. Hypothyroidism, (not hyperthyroidism) is associated with it.

    Ref:

    Makkouk AH. (2008) Trigger finger: aetiology, evaluation and treatment. *Curr Rev Musculoskel Med* 1: 92–96.

4.  **C**

    Incidence of trigger finger is related to duration of disease and not actual glycaemic control in diabetics. Lifetime risk of developing it increases up to 10% in diabetics.

    Ref:

    Makkouk AH. (2008) Trigger finger: aetiology, evaluation and treatment. *Curr Rev Musculoskel Med* 1: 92–96.

5.  **C**

    In a study, splints of the MCP joint at 15 degrees of flexion (leaving the PIP and DIP joints free) were shown to provide resolution of symptoms in 65% of patients at 1-year follow-up. Splinting yields lower success rates in patients with severe triggering or longstanding duration of symptoms.

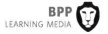

Ref:

Makkouk AH. (2008) Trigger finger: aetiology, evaluation and treatment. *Curr Rev Musculoskel Med* 1: 92–96.

6. **B**

Complex regional pain syndrome type 1 (CRPS, formerly reflex sympathetic dystrophy) is a descriptive term for a complex of symptoms and signs, including pain, swelling and regional vasomotor instability (changes in colour, temperature and sweating) which are accompanied by significant functional impairment of the hand or whole extremity. It is usually caused by trauma or surgery. The hypotheses that CRPS is related to hormonal changes in the postmenopausal period remains unproven. The effects of generalised diseases such as hyperlipidaemia, hypercholesterolaemia, diabetes, gout and excessive alcohol intake on the development of CRPS have been evaluated, but no associations have been proven.

Ref:

Zyluk A. (2004) Complex regional pain syndrome type 1. Risk factors, prevention and risk of recurrence, *Journal of Hand Surgery (British and European Volume)* 29B: 4: 334–337.

7. **E**

Keinbock's disease is osteonecrosis of the lunate. Classification is by the Lichtman staging. Simple excision of the lunate is controversial but has been shown to produce satisfactory results in studies. However it is not recommended for heavy manual workers. Radial shortening osteotomies are preferred over ulna lengthening to reduce the risk of ulna non union, need for bone graft and removal of metalwork.

Lichtman's Classification of Kienbock's disease: Stage 1: normal except for the possibility of either a linear or a compression fracture; Stage 2: definite density changes apparent in the lunate; Stage 3a: collapse of entire lunate without fixed scaphoid rotation; Stage 3b: collapse of entire lunate with fixed scaphoid rotation; Stage 4: stage 3 with generalised degenerative changes in the carpus.

Ref:

Canale, S Terry ed. *Campbell's Operative Orthopaedics* (2008); 11<sup>th</sup> ed. p. 4040.

8. **B**

Also known as scapulothoracic bursitis may occur following a single traumatic insult or as a result of a series of repetitive motions of the scapulothoracic joint. In most cases, the bursitis is believed to be caused by abnormal motion between the anterior surface of the scapula and the thoracic cage. Symptoms include activity related pain and crepitus. Majority of patients can be managed successfully by non operative means. Mainstay of treatment includes improving muscle strength and balance, addressing postural conditions (such as excessive thoracic kyphosis), and core strengthening.

Ref:

Lazar MA. (2009) Snapping scapula syndrome. *Journal of Bone and Joint Surgery* 91: 2251–2262.

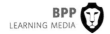

9.   **A**

Resurfacing can be used in patients with cuff tear arthropathy, OA, osteonecrosis. It is contraindicated in 4 part fractures of the humerus. Its main advantages include resurfacing arthroplasty, the humeral neck and >50% of the humeral head are retained, which is beneficial with regard to restoration of the biomechanics of the shoulder, easier operation compared to total arthroplasty and success rates comparable to total shoulder arthroplasty in mid and long term studies.

Ref:
Burgess DL. (2009) Shoulder resurfacing. *Journal of Bone and Joint Surgery* 91: 1228–1238.

10.   **D**

Component mal-position can give rise to the rocking-horse loosening mechanism, in which loading of one edge of the glenoid component causes the opposite edge to lift off of the glenoid bone.

Ref:
Matsen FA. (2008) Glenoid component failure in total shoulder arthroplasty. *Journal of Bone and Joint Surgery* 90: 885–896.

11.   **E**

A systematic review of one Level II and four Level I randomised controlled prospective studies have confirmed the first three statements. A randomised prospective study has confirmed the fourth statement.

Ref:
Ramsey ML. (2008) What's new in shoulder and elbow surgery. *Journal of Bone and Joint Surgery* 90: 677–687.

12.   **D**

Cuff tear arthropathy is the end stage of the disease continuum, which is caused by a tear of the supraspinatus or rotator cuff. It is characterised by proximalisation of the humerus and acetabulisation of the acromion.

Ref:
Feeley BT. (2009) Cuff tear arthropathy: current trends in diagnosis and surgical management. *J Shoulder Elbow Surg* 18: 484–494.

13.   **A**

Cuff tear arthropathy is the end stage of the disease continuum, which is caused by a tear of the supraspinatus or rotator cuff. It is characterised by proximalisation of the humerus and acetabulisation of the acromion. Reverse total shoulder arthroplasty is based on the principle of elongating the deltoid lever arm, which aids in ease of shoulder abduction. Hence an intact deltoid is essential. Arthroscopic debridement is used in low demand elderly patients, with multiple co-morbidities in whom a major procedure may not be tolerated.

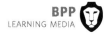

Ref:
Feeley BT (2009) Cuff tear arthropathy: current trends in diagnosis and surgical management. *J Shoulder Elbow Surg* 18: 484–494.

14. **B**

Sourcil sign is sclerosis of the inferior border of the acromion and not humerus. It is highly suggestive of cuff tear arthropathy. All the other mentioned are also signs of this condition.

Ref:
Feeley BT (2009) Cuff tear arthropathy: current trends in diagnosis and surgical management *J Shoulder Elbow Surg* 18: 484–494.

15. **A**

Belly press test assesses the upper portion of the subscapularis while the lift off test assesses the lower portion of this muscle. Hence belly press test is more likely to be abnormal in an antero-superior cuff tear. Horn blower's sign assesses the teres minor muscle.

Ref:
Neri BR (2009) Management of massive and irreparable rotator cuff tears. Review article. *J of Shoulder Elbow Surg* 18: 808–818.

16. **D**

Conservative means are used for elderly patients in whom pain is not a major symptom. Debridement and bursectomy is useful in patients with pain as a major symptom, particularly in the elderly. Complete repair with substitutes has not been validated by clinical trials.

Ref:
Neri BR (2009) Management of massive and irreparable rotator cuff tears. Review article. *J of Shoulder Elbow Surg* 1, 808–818.

17. **E**
Ref:
Snell RS. (2003) *Clinical Anatomy*. Lippincott Williams, Philadelphia, p. 481.

18. **D**
Ref:
Snell RS. (2003) *Clinical Anatomy*. Lippincott Williams, Philadelphia, p. 481.

19. **B**

SAPHO is characterised by synovitis, acne, pustulosis, hyperostosis and osteitis.

Ref:
Robinson CM. (2008) Disorders of the sternoclavicular joint c. *JBJS Br*; 90-B: 685–96.

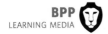

20. **B**

Friedrich's disease is osteonecrosis of the medial head of the clavicle. SAPHO syndrome is a site specific condition usually affecting middle aged adults with a slight female preponderance. It is characterised by synovitis, acne, pustulosis, hyperostosis and osteitis.

Ref:
Robinson CM. et al. (2008) Disorders of the sternoclavicular joint. *JBJS Br*; 90-B: 685–96.

21. **E**

Aetiology is unknown, but it is thought to that various antecedent factors may trigger an immune mediated response which can predispose to it.

Ref:
Sathasivam S. (2008) Neuralgic amyotrophy. Aspects of current management. *JBJS Br*; 90-B: 550–3.

22. **E**

Dupuytren's is also associated with diabetes. It also has a strong association with genetic disposition. There is controversy regarding its association with seizures. Rheumatoid arthritis is the only condition with which there is a reduced incidence.

Ref:
Rayan MG. (2007) Dupuytren's disease: anatomy, pathology, presentation and treatment. *Journal of Bone and Joint Surgery* 89: 189–198.

23. **B**

The central aponeurosis is the core of Dupuytrens disease activity. Its fibres are oriented longitudinally, transversely, and vertically. The longitudinal fibres fan out as pre-tendinous bands. The transverse fibres make up the natatory ligament located in the distal part of the palm and the transverse ligament of the palmar aponeurosis. The transverse ligament of the palmar aponeurosis is proximal and parallel to the natatory ligament and deep to the pre-tendinous bands.

Ref:
Rayan MG. (2007) Dupuytren's disease: anatomy, pathology, presentation and treatment, *Journal of Bone and Joint Surgery* 89: 189–198.

24. **E**

The transverse fibres of the central aponeurosis make up the natatory ligament located in the distal part of the palm. The distal fibres of the natatory ligament contribute to the formation of the lateral digital sheet.

Ref:
Rayan MG. (2007) Dupuytren's disease: anatomy, pathology, presentation and treatment. *Journal of Bone and Joint Surgery* 89: 189–198.

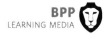

25. **C**

The spiral cord is most commonly seen in the little finger followed by the ring finger. It has four origins: the pre-tendinous band, the spiral band, the lateral digital sheet, and the Grayson ligament. It causes contractures at the proximal interphalangeal joint.

Ref:
Rayan MG. (2007) Dupuytren's disease: anatomy, pathology, presentation and treatment. *Journal of Bone and Joint Surgery* 89: 189–198.

26. **E**

Non-Dupuytren's disease occurs mostly in a diverse ethnic group. It is unilateral, usually involving a single digit, and it is frequently associated with trauma, including surgery. Patients with this disease rarely need surgical treatment.

Ref:
Rayan MG. (2007) Dupuytren's disease: anatomy, pathology, presentation and treatment. *Journal of Bone and Joint Surgery* 89: 189–198.

27. **B**

Skin pitting is a reliable early sign. Nodules are often painless but may enlarge and cause pain particularly if they are associated with stenosing tenosynovitis as a result of direct pressure on flexor tendons and the A1 pulley. Palmar nodules are usually adjacent to the distal palmar crease, often in line with the ring and little fingers. Knuckle pads commonly affect the proximal interphalangeal joints.

Ref:
Rayan MG. (2007) Dupuytren's disease: anatomy, pathology, presentation and treatment. *Journal of Bone and Joint Surgery* 89: 189–198.

28. **C**

Anterior interosseous syndrome is commonly associated with motor symptoms, while pronator syndrome causes mainly pain and parasthesia which may be confused with carpal tunnel syndrome. Parsonage-Turner syndrome is brachial neuritis, characterised by transient shoulder pain followed by weakness or parasthesia in the upper limb usually after a viral illness or immunisation.

Ref:
Tsai P. (2008) Median and radial nerve compression about the elbow. *Journal of Bone and Joint Surgery* 90: 420–428.

29. **B**

The staging system is I,II,III. Stage I (mild) is the earliest stage and is the result of PIP joint synovitis with mild extensor lag that still can be corrected passively. The metacarpophalangeal (MP) joint usually is normal, and the DIP may or may not be hyper extended. Stage II (moderate) is characterised by 30–40 degrees of flexion contracture at the PIP joint and hyperextension of the MP joint as a compensatory mechanism. The finger has increased functional loss. Early passive extension still is possible. With time, soft-tissue contractures develop, and passive extension becomes restricted. Stage III (severe) begins when the PIP

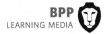

joint can no longer be extended passively. Radiographs demonstrate destruction of the joint surfaces.

Ref:
Nalebuff EA. (1975) Surgical treatment of the boutonniere deformity in rheumatoid arthritis. *Orthop Clin North Am* 6(3): 753–63.

30. **C**
Stages are of IV types, based on the flexibility of the PIP joint, the amount of intrinsic tightness and radiographic changes. Stage I is PIP joint being flexible in all positions. Stage II is limited PIP joint flexibility with MCP joint extension (intrinsic tightness). Stage III is limited PIP joint flexibility in all positions of the MCP joint and Stage IV is a stiff PIP joint with advanced radiographic changes.

Ref:
Dee R, Hurst LC. (1997) *Principles of orthopaedic practise*. McGraw Hill, International edition. 1135–1137.

31. **A**
Stage I has no CMC joint involvement. Stage III is a swan neck deformity. Stage IV is a gamekeeper's deformity.

Ref:
Dee R, Hurst LC. (1997) *Principles of orthopaedic practise*. McGraw Hill, International edition. 1135–1137.

32. **B**
Ref:
Shaw RB. (2007) Dupuytren's disease: History, diagnosis and treatment. *Plastic and Reconstructive Surgery* 120(3).

33. **C**
Enchondromas commonly occur in this location. They are the most common destructive primary bone tumours of the hand. Pathological fracture is a common complication and fractures are allowed to heal prior to tumour excision to reduce the risk of complications.

Ref:
Canale, S Terry ed. *Campbell's Operative Orthopaedics* (2008); 11th ed. p. 4320.

34. **D**
Radial tunnel syndrome is characterised by pain over dorsal proximal aspect of the forearm. Motor symptoms are usually minimal. It occurs due to compression of posterior interosseous nerve in proximal part of forearm and differential diagnosis is lateral epicondylitis and compression neuropathy of the lateral antebrachial cutaneous nerve. Mainstay of treatment is non-operative initially in the form of elbow splints, avoidance of provocative activities and NSAIDs. If there is no improvement after 3 months, surgical decompression can be considered.

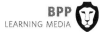

Ref:
Tsai P. (2008) Median and Radian nerve compression about the elbow. *Journal of Bone and Joint Surgery* 90: 420–428.

35.   **A**

A bowler's thumb is a neuroma of the digital nerve with the above description.

Ref:
Lister G. (1993) *The Hand diagnosis and indications.* Churchill Livingstone, Singapore. p. 406.

36.   **B**

One quarter of chondrosarcomas arise secondary to multiple enchondroma. Peak incidence in the hand is in the seventh decade.

Ref:
Lister G. (1993) *The Hand diagnosis and indications.* Churchill Livingstone, Singapore. p. 414.

37.   **C**

PVNS also called giant cell tumour is a swelling of unknown aetiology. But it is always found in the presence of synovial tissue, commonly arising from the flexor tendon sheath or interphalangeal joints.

Ref:
Lister G. (1993) *The Hand diagnosis and indications.* Churchill Livingstone, Singapore. p. 438.

38.   **D**

Enchondromas are central lesions, while GCT is classically eccentric. Intraosseous bone cysts are mainly seen in the carpal bones. Aneurysmal bone cyst is typically seen in the second decade, metaphyseal and with a characteristic soap bubble experience.

Ref:
Lister G. (1993) *The Hand diagnosis and indications.* Churchill Livingstone, Singapore. pp. 412–423.

39.   **E**

The first four are the most common sites for the location of ganglionic cysts.

Ref:
Lister G. (1993) *The Hand diagnosis and indications.* Churchill Livingstone, Singapore. pp. 435–436.

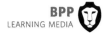

**40.    B**

Phocomelia is an intercalary deficiency (failure of formation of a part). It is either complete, where hand attaches to the trunk, proximal where forearm attaches to trunk or distal where the hand attaches to the humerus.

Ref:
Lister G. (1993) *The Hand diagnosis and indications*. Churchill Livingstone, Singapore. p. 459.

**41.    C**

Tendon sheath infections are usually due to Coagulase positive Staph. Aureus. Antibiotic therapy alone may be curative if instituted early, but incision and drainage should be done if there is no improvement within 24 hours.

Ref:
Dee R, Hurst L. (1997) *Principles of orthopaedic practice*. McGraw Hill. p. 1194.

**42.    C**

The boundary of the web space is defined dorsally by the webbed skin, volarly by the transverse palmar fascia, radially and ulnarly by the vertical septae. A sagittal section through the web space shows a collection dorsally and volarly with a communicating channel like a collar button.

Ref:
Dee R, Hurst L. (1997) *Principles of orthopaedic practice*. McGraw Hill. p. 1194.

**43.    D**

This is the commonest bacteria which is found in human hand bites. Pseudomonas is found in abscesses in IVDU patients.

Ref:
Lister G. (1993) *The Hand diagnosis and indications*. Churchill Livingstone, Singapore. p. 459.

**44.    C**

The Terry Thomas sign is suggestive of a DISI. An AP X-ray shows a scapholunate gap of more than 3mm. it is named after the British actor who had a large space between his front two teeth.

Ref:
Dee R, Hurst L. (1997) *Principles of orthopaedic practise*. McGraw Hill. p. 1194.

**45.    E**

The TFCC also incorporates the dorsal radioulnar ligament, the meniscus homologue, anatomically definable disk and inserts distally into triquetrum, hamate and base of 5th metacarpal.

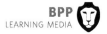

Ref:
Dee R, Hurst L. (1997) *Principles of orthopaedic practise*. McGraw Hill. p. 1203.

46.   **B**
In EPL deficit – brachioradialis, FCR split tendon transfer and palmaris longus can be considered. In wrist extension deficit – pronator teres transfer to ECRB is commonly used.

Ref:
Dee R, Hurst L. (1997) *Principles of orthopaedic practise*. McGraw Hill. pp. 1154–1155.

47.   **D**
FDS of ring finger is most commonly used.

Ref:
Dee R, Hurst L. (1997) *Principles of orthopaedic practise*. McGraw Hill. pp. 1154–1155.

48.   **C**
Ref:
Dee R, Hurst L. (1997) *Principles of orthopaedic practise*. McGraw Hill. p. 11.

49.   **E**
Arthrography does not correlate to clinical findings in TFCC tears. Initial management is splintage and analgesia. If symptoms persist surgical repair should be considered.

Ref:
Canale, S Terry ed. *Campbell's Operative Orthopaedics*, (2008); 11th ed., p. 4043.

50.   **B**
Hemiresection interposition arthroplasty is indicated for un-reconstructable fractures of ulnar head, rheumatoid arthritis of DRUJ and chronic painful tear of TFCC besides ulna impaction syndrome.

Ref:
Canale, S Terry ed. *Campbell's Operative Orthopaedics*, (2008); 11th ed., p. 4059.

51.   **B**
Wrist fusion is normally done in 10–20 degrees of extension. This is the functional position. Fusion of the wrist is difficult to achieve in children because of the amount of cartilage in the wrist joint, and if possible should be delayed until 12 years.

Ref:
Canale, S Terry ed. *Campbell's Operative Orthopaedics*, (2008); 11th ed., p. 4070.

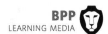

**52.**  **B**

Carpal instability is considered as static if there is no change in intercarpal relationships and dynamic if there is change in intercarpal relationships on radiographs with manipulation and motion. Dissociative carpal instability occurs when intrinsic carpal ligaments of the proximal row are disrupted. When the extrinsic ligaments are disrupted it is called non dissociative instability.

Ref:
Canale, S Terry ed. *Campbell's Operative Orthopaedics*, (2008); 11<sup>th</sup> ed., p. 4074.

**53.**  **D**

The radial artery forms the deep palmar arch, which is complete in 98% of individuals. The ulnar artery forms the superficial palmar arch which is complete in 80% of individuals. Although anerurysms are due to atherosclerosis, mycotic, metabolic and congenital causes, trauma is usually the implicating factor in hands and wrist.

Ref:
Canale, S Terry ed. *Campbell's Operative Orthopaedics*, (2008); 11<sup>th</sup> ed., p. 4103.

**54.**  **A**

Frostbite injury treatment protocol of McCauley is widely accepted. In resuscitation and re-warming – blisters are aspirated, topical aloe vera 6 hourly, extremity elevation and splinting tetanus prophylaxis is indicated.

Ref:
Canale, S Terry ed. *Campbell's Operative Orthopaedics*, (2008); 11<sup>th</sup> ed., p. 4114.

**55.**  **E**

Although excision of the lunate, triquetrum and entire scaphoid is recommended, the distal pole of the scaphoid can be left to provide a stable base to the thumb. If this is done, then a radial styloidectomy is done to prevent impingement of the distal pole of scaphoid on the radius. The pisiform is not usually excised as it is a sesamoid bone.

Ref:
Canale, S Terry ed. *Campbell's Operative Orthopaedics*, (2008); 11<sup>th</sup> ed., p. 4026

**56.**  **C**

The intrinsic minus or claw hand occurs because the lumbricals and interrosei which are the intrinsic are paralysed. The usual action of these muscles is flexion of the MCP joints and extension at the interphalangeal joints. This action is lost causing MCP joint hyperextension and flexion of the interphalangeal joints. The long finger extensors are not able to extend the interphalangeal joints because the stabilisation effect afforded by the MCP joints in neutral or slight flexed position is lost.

Ref:
Canale, S Terry ed. *Campbell's Operative Orthopaedics*, (2008); 11<sup>th</sup> ed., p. 4126.

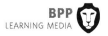

**57.** **D**

The most important points while considering a muscle transfer is its expendibility and strength. Restoring a major function should not be at the cost of sacrificing another.

Ref:

Canale, S Terry ed. *Campbell's Operative Orthopaedics*, (2008); 11<sup>th</sup> ed., p. 4127.

**58.** **D**

A pulley is a usually needed for this procedure. The basic principle is that a healthy extrinsic, expendable muscle tendon unit is required. Usually the flexor digitorum sublimis of the ring finger is the first choice and in its absence, the sublimis tendon of the middle finger is used. If fusion of the MCP joint is needed it is done in 15 degrees of flexion and slight internal rotation.

Ref:

Canale, S Terry ed. *Campbell's Operative Orthopaedics*, (2008); 11<sup>th</sup> ed., p. 4129.

**59.** **B**

Opposition of the thumb is a complex movement involving the long and short muscles of the thumb. But the abductor pollicis brevis is the single most important muscle involved in this movement. It rotates internally and *abducts* the thumb away from the 2<sup>nd</sup> metacarpal, internally rotates and abducts the proximal phalanx of the thumb on its metacarpal.

Ref:

Canale, S Terry ed. *Campbell's Operative Orthopaedics*, (2008); 11<sup>th</sup> ed., p. 4129.

**60.** **A**

Although night splinting was routinely used, it is not very effective. This is because fixed contractures rarely occur at an early age. Also during sleep, the hand is relaxed and supple which precludes the need for night splinting.

Ref:

Canale, S Terry ed. *Campbell's Operative Orthopaedics*, (2008); 11<sup>th</sup> ed., p. 4175.

**61.** **B**

Bouchard's nodes affect PIP joints and Heberden's nodes affect the DIP joints in OA. The MCP and PIP joints are commonly involved in SLE and hand manifestations may be the first sign of the disease. Tapering of the phalanges and metacarpals with cupping of the proximal ends of these bones (pencil-in-cup deformity) is radiographic finding in psoriatic arthritis.

Ref:

Canale, S Terry ed. *Campbell's Operative Orthopaedics*, (2008); 11<sup>th</sup> ed., p. 4198.

**62.** **A**

On polarised microscopy, negatively birefringent crystals are normally seen in gout.

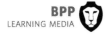

Ref:
Canale, S Terry ed. *Campbell's Operative Orthopaedics*, (2008); 11<sup>th</sup> ed., p. 4199.

**63.** **C**

Female gender, age, obesity and use of vibratory tools are all some of the risk factors implicated in this condition.

Ref:
Canale, S Terry ed. *Campbell's Operative Orthopaedics*, (2008); 11<sup>th</sup> ed., p. 4285.

**64.** **D**

Osteoarthritis, menopause, amyloidosis, rheumatoid arthritis, gout, thyroid disorders and long term haemodialysis are some of the others.

Ref:
Canale, S Terry ed. *Campbell's Operative Orthopaedics*, (2008); 11<sup>th</sup> ed., p. 4286.

**65.** **D**

Phalens test has high sensitivity compared to specificity. Tinels has high specificity compared to sensitivity, Durkan's compression test was found to have high sensitivity and specificity compared to Phalen's and Tinel's.

Ref:
Canale, S Terry ed. *Campbell's Operative Orthopaedics*, (2008); 11<sup>th</sup> ed., p. 4286.

**66.** **C**

Nerve conduction tests are 90% sensitive and 60% specific for diagnosis of carpal tunnel syndrome. These studies are occasionally normal when clinical signs of carpal tunnel are present and abnormal in asymptomatic patients.

Ref:
Canale, S Terry ed. *Campbell's Operative Orthopaedics*, (2008); 11<sup>th</sup> ed., p. 4286.

**67.** **A**

Palmar sensory branch of median nerve is at risk at the proximal extent of the incision. It lies between tendons of Palmaris longus and flexor carpi radialis. When cut, it can cause a painful neuroma and repair should not be attempted. The recurrent branch of median nerve is predominantly extra-ligamentous (46%).

Ref:
Canale, S Terry ed. *Campbell's Operative Orthopaedics*, (2008); 11<sup>th</sup> ed., p. 4290.

**68.** **D**

De Quervain's tenovaginitis is inflammation, thickening and fibrosis of the synovium sheath of the first extensor compartment and not the tendons themselves. Commonly seen in women between third and fifth decade. Differential diagnosis includes arthritis of first CMC and Wartenburg syndrome (neuritis of superficial radial nerve).

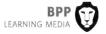

Ref:

Canale, S Terry ed. *Campbell's Operative Orthopaedics*, (2008); 11th ed., p. 4290.

69.  **B**

Vicryl becomes weak too early after surgery to be effective. Braided polyester is routinely used due to sufficient resistance to disrupting forces and gap formation, handle easily and satisfactory knot characteristics.

Ref:

Canale, S Terry ed. *Campbell's Operative Orthopaedics*, (2008); 11th ed., p. 3854.

70.  **C**

Zone V repairs frequently need proximal wound extension to search for the retracted tendons. Lumbrical bellies are not repaired in Zone III to prevent the 'lumbrical plus' finger – paradoxical proximal interphalangeal extension on attempted finger flexion.

Ref:

Canale, S Terry ed. *Campbell's Operative Orthopaedics*, (2008); 11th ed., p. 3870.

71.  **D**

Percutaneous medial epicondylar release is contraindicated due to risk to medial antebrachial cutaneous nerve and ulnar nerve. The origin of the pronator teres from the medial conjoint tendon is the focus of pathology. It is only 15–20% as common as lateral epicondylitis.

Ref:

Morrey BF. (2000) *The elbow and its disorders*. Saunders, Philadelphia. pp. 537–41.

72.  **E**

CPM works on the principle of preventing collection of blood and fluid in the joint and surrounding tissues immediately post-op, by ensuring continuous motion of the joint through its full range of motion. In the immediate post operative period, its continuous use is advocated with only bathroom privileges being allowed. Its use is contraindicated in an unstable elbow or an inadequate fracture fixation.

Ref:

Morrey BF. (2000) *The elbow and its disorders*. Saunders, Philadelphia. pp. 147–48.

73.  **D**

The postero-lateral portal has the largest area of anatomical safety. It is made 3cm proximal to the olecranon and lateral to the triceps tendon.

Ref:

Morrey BF. (2000) *The elbow and its disorders*. Saunders, Philadelphia. p. 505.

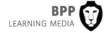

74. **A**

The ideal candidate for interpositional arthroplasty of the elbow is an individual less than 30 years of age with rheumatoid arthritis, and less than 60 years of age with osteoarthritis or traumatic arthritis with low levels of manual activity. A heavy manual labourer may not have as satisfactory an outcome as with a painless arthrodesis in a functional position. A patient who uses his upper limbs for transfer and ambulation is a relative contraindication, as excessive loading will destabilise the joint. Loss of motor flexion power is an absolute contraindication.

Ref:
Morrey BF. (2000) *The elbow and its disorders.* Saunders, Philadelphia. p. 505.

75. **D**

Fascia lata is the preferred choice but the others have also been used.

Ref:
Morrey BF. (2000) *The elbow and its disorders.* Saunders, Philadelphia. p. 718.

76. **D**

The MCL consists of anterior oblique, posterior oblique and transverse fibres. It is the primary stabiliser of the elbow for range of movement between 20–120 degrees. Humeral origin of MCL lies behind the axis of elbow flexion, due to this anterior fibres are taught in extension and posterior fibres are taught in flexion.

Ref:
Dee R, Hurst L. (1997), *Principles of orthopaedic practice.* McGraw Hill. p. 1108.

77. **E**

Poor neurologic recovery and persistent spasticity is associated with recurrence. Excision should be delayed until motor neurologic recovery has taken place and further delayed if there is ongoing improvement in neurologic status.

Ref:
Dee R, Hurst L. (1997) *Principles of orthopaedic practice*, McGraw Hill, p. 1112.

78. **C**

Proximal humerus is the commonest site for unicameral bone cysts. Lesions are asymptomatic until a pathological fracture occur. Histology reveals giant cells haemosiderin deposits and inflammatory cells. Surgery is not indicated in the initial management of this condition.

Ref:
Dee R, Hurst L. (1997) *Principles of orthopaedic practice.* McGraw Hill. p. 278.

79. **D**

Chondroblastoma occurs in the immature skeleton in the epiphysis. Proximal humerus is one of the commonest sites for this tumour. It is a locally aggressive benign tumour. Chondroid matrix is also seen along with multinucleated giant cells on microscopy.

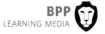

Clear cell chondrosarcoma is the rarest form of chondrosarcoma and is slow growing. It is frequently confused with chondroblastoma. Histologically consist of sheets of vague lobules composed of round clear cells.

Ref:
Dee R, Hurst L. (1997) *Principles of orthopaedic practice*. McGraw Hill. p. 263.

**80.  C**
Chondroblastoma and unicameral bone cysts most commonly occur at the proximal humerus. The delto-pectoral interval should always be avoided for biopsy, as this approach guarantees contamination of subscapularis and pectorals, which in turn could involve the entire brachial plexus region.

Ref:
Dee R, Hurst L. (1997) *Principles of orthopaedic practice*. McGraw Hill. p. 277.

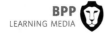

BPP
LEARNING MEDIA

# Paediatrics

## Question Bank

Ibrar Majid, Assad A Qureshi,
Haroon A Mann & Talal
Ibrahim

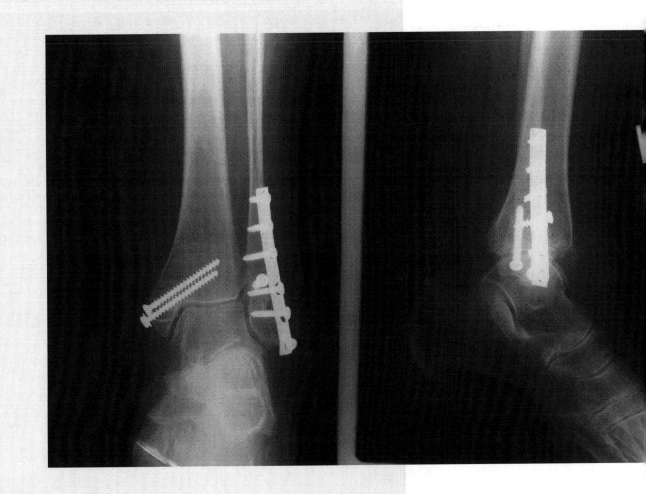

1. A young boy with Down syndrome requires cervical spine clearance before undertaking sporting activity. Flexion-extension lateral radiographs of the cervical spine show an atlantodens interval of 7mm. Neurological examination is unremarkable. What is the next most appropriate step in management?
   A. MRI scan of cervical spine
   B. Posterior spinal fusion
   C. No further action required
   D. Annual radiographs and neurological examination and no contact sports
   E. Traction and bracing

2. An autosomal recessive inheritance pattern according to Sillence classification is seen in osteogenesis imperfecta type:
   A. IVB
   B. III
   C. IA
   D. IVA
   E. IB

3. A 14-year-old girl presents with a 3-month history of bilateral knee pain, stiffness and swelling, and eye pain. Blood investigations reveal the presence of anti-nuclear antibodies (ANA). Rheumatoid factor is negative. Appropriate first line management would be
   A. Splinting
   B. Non-steroidal anti-inflammatory drugs (NSAIDs)
   C. Methotrexate
   D. Physical therapy
   E. Arthroscopy and synovectomy

4. Hip subluxation secondary to cerebral palsy in the presence of a normal acetabulum is best treated by:
   A. Pelvic osteotomy
   B. Soft tissue release
   C. Femoral and acetabular osteotomy
   D. Femoral osteotomy
   E. Soft tissue release and femoral osteotomy

5. Hip dislocation secondary to spina bifida is most common with a defect at
   A. L3/4
   B. L2/3
   C. L1/2
   D. L4/5
   E. L5/S1

BPP
LEARNING MEDIA

6. The following organism as a cause of septic arthritis is seen almost only in the neonate
   A. S. aureus
   B. E. coli
   C. N. gonorrhoeae
   D. Salmonella
   E. Group A Streptococcus

7. An 8-year-old boy presents to the Emergency Department with a 2-day history of gradual onset painful left hip, following a sore throat a few days previously. There is no history of trauma. On examination he is pyrexial and unable to weight bear on that side. What is the next most appropriate step in management?
   A. Blood cultures
   B. Radiographs of the pelvis
   C. Serum C-reactive protein (CRP)
   D. Ultrasound scan of the hip
   E. Hip aspiration

8. A deficiency in vitamin C leads to abnormal bone formation most markedly in the:
   A. Metaphysis
   B. Epiphysis
   C. Diaphysis
   D. Physis
   E. Articular surface

9. The following are risk factors for developmental dysplasia of the hip, except:
   A. Polyhydramnios
   B. Family history
   C. Breech delivery
   D. Female
   E. Oligohydramnios

10. The Herring classification of Perthes' disease is based on involvement of the lateral pillar of the capital femoral epiphysis in which stage of the disease?
    A. Osteonecrosis
    B. Reossification
    C. Final healing
    D. Fragmentation
    E. Segmental

11. The most common musculoskeletal sequlae associated with achondroplasia is:
    A. Lumbar spinal stenosis
    B. Trident hand
    C. Radial head subluxation
    D. Champagne glass pelvis
    E. Genu valgus

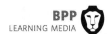

12. In hereditary multiple exostosis, the following are all indications for excision of an exostosis, except:
    A. Significant pain
    B. Limb length discrepancy
    C. False aneurysm
    D. Rapid increase in size
    E. Significant valgus deformity

13. A ten-year-old boy falls off a swing and lands on his elbow. He complains of pain and has a tender and swollen elbow. Radiographs taken would most likely show ossification of all the following ossification centres, except:
    A. Radial head
    B. Lateral epicondyle
    C. Trochlea
    D. Capitellum
    E. Olecranon

14. In the normally developing child, the tibiofemoral angle is neutral at a mean age of:
    A. 6 months
    B. 12 months
    C. 24 months
    D. 36 months
    E. 72 months

15. The most abundant collagen in the physeal growth plate is type:
    A. II
    B. XI
    C. VII
    D. IX
    E. X

16. In the Salter-Harris classification of physeal fractures, presence of the Thurston Holland fragment is seen in which type of injury?
    A. I
    B. II
    C. III
    D. IV
    E. V

17. A 9-month-old boy presents to the Emergency Department with a painful left arm. Radiographs reveal a fracture of the scapula. You note he has bruising around the buttock and arm. What is the most appropriate next step in management?
    A. CT head
    B. Bone scan
    C. Skeletal survey
    D. Repeat radiograph in two weeks
    E. CT shoulder

BPP
LEARNING MEDIA

18. In the paediatric forearm, in one year, remodeling can correct angulation deformity up to:
    A. 5 degrees
    B. 7 degrees
    C. 10 degrees
    D. 12 degrees
    E. 15 degrees

19. The following statements regarding Galeazzi fractures in children are all **true**, except:
    A. Involves a distal radius fracture and a distal ulnar physeal injury
    B. Is less common than a Monteggia fracture
    C. Can be successfully treated by closed reduction in a long arm cast
    D. Rarely require intramedullary fixation
    E. When treated in cast the forearm should be cast in slight supination

20. The most common nerve palsy associated with the Monteggia fracture type involves the:
    A. Anterior interosseous nerve
    B. Posterior interosseous nerve
    C. Median nerve
    D. Ulnar nerve
    E. Superficial radial nerve

21. A posterior fat pad sign on plain radiographs, in the absence of any other radiological findings, is predictive of an occult fracture in what percentage of cases following trauma to the elbow in children?
    A. 10%
    B. 25%
    C. 50%
    D. 75%
    E. 90%

22. A five-year-old girl has fallen off a climbing frame and presents with a painful elbow. Examination reveals a closed injury, and a good radial pulse. The child is unable to flex the thumb interphalangeal joint (IPJ) when asked to do so. This is most likely to represent an injury to the:
    A. Radial nerve
    B. Anterior interosseous nerve
    C. Ulnar nerve
    D. Posterior interosseous nerve
    E. Median nerve

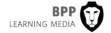

23.    Initial treatment of a closed supracondylar fracture of the humerus with no neurovascular deficit, and in which radiographs show the capitellum to be behind the anterior humeral line with no associated medial collapse, would involve:
    A.    Splinting in a plaster cast for a total of three weeks
    B.    Manipulation under anaesthesia
    C.    Closed reduction and K-wire fixation
    D.    Open reduction and K-wire fixation
    E.    Collar and cuff sling for a total of three weeks

24.    The following is an important and well recognised complication of lateral condyle fractures of the humerus:
    A.    Avascular necrosis of the capitellum
    B.    Volkmann's ischaemia
    C.    Ulnar nerve plasy
    D.    Cubitus varus
    E.    Loss of terminal elbow extension

25.    A 13-year-old boy sustains an isolated closed fracture of the femur following a road traffic accident (RTA). Radiographs show a simple spiral fracture, with an open distal femoral growth plate. The most appropriate management would be:
    A.    Retrograde intramedullary nailing
    B.    Intramedullary elastic nailing
    C.    Spica cast
    D.    Piriform fossa antegrade intramedullary nailing
    E.    Trochanteric antegrade intramedullary nailing

26.    A young child presents in agony with a painful knee following trauma. Radiographs reveal a displaced Salter-Harris type II injury of the proximal tibia. What is the most appropriate next step in management?
    A.    MRI of the knee
    B.    Application of an above knee cast
    C.    Doppler studies
    D.    Immediate fasciotomies
    E.    Reduction under anaesthesia and immobilisation

27.    In fractures of the tibial and fibular shafts, all of the following deformities do not remodel well, except:
    A.    Valgus angulation
    B.    Varus angulation
    C.    Recurvatum
    D.    Internal rotation
    E.    Shortening

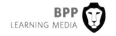

28    Spinal cord injury without radiographic abnormality (SCIWORA):
      A.   Often occurs after low energy trauma
      B.   Commonly occurs at the cervicothoracic junction
      C.   Is a compression injury of the immature spinal column
      D.   Is always a complete spinal cord injury
      E.   Is more common in children over the age of ten

29.   Osteochondritis dissecans most commonly affects the:
      A.   Elbow
      B.   Ankle
      C.   Hip
      D.   Shoulder
      E.   Knee

30.   In the treatment of osteochondritis dissecans, stage IV disease with mechanical symptoms
      due to a large fragment is best treated with:
      A.   Adjusting activity levels
      B.   Immobilisation with cast bracing
      C.   Removal of loose body and microfracture
      D.   Removal of loose body, and bone and cartilage grafting
      E.   Bone grafting

31.   Stress fractures of the proximal tibia are best diagnosed by:
      A.   Clinical examination
      B.   Plain radiography
      C.   Single photon emission CT
      D.   MRI
      E.   Bone scan

32.   Regarding triplane fractures of the ankle:
      A.   They occur in children at all ages
      B.   The injury propagates through the medial distal tibial physis
      C.   Plain AP radiographs of the ankle joint show an appearance similar to the tillaux type
           fracture
      D.   Plain lateral radiographs of the distal tibia have the appearance of a Salter-Harris type
           III injury
      E.   CT scan is not useful in managing such injuries

33.   Radial deficiency is associated with the all of following, except:
      A.   Septal cardiac defects
      B.   Thromobocytopaenia
      C.   Chest wall deformity
      D.   Trachoesophageal fistula
      E.   Aplastic anaemia

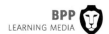

34. In the Ponseti method of treatment of clubfoot:
    A. Manipulations and castings occur every three months
    B. Rotation of the foot is controlled by a below knee cast
    C. Percutaneous tenotomy is required in 10% of cases
    D. Night time splintage is rarely required after initial treatment
    E. Lateral transfer of the tibialis anterior tendon is required to balance the foot in refractory cases

35. The 'C' sign on weight bearing plain lateral radiographs of the ankle is associated with:
    A. Talocalcaneal coalition
    B. Congenital vertical talus
    C. Freiberg's disease
    D. Calcaneonavicular coalition
    E. Tarsonavicular coalition

36. A four-year-old girl presents to the paediatric outpatients with parents reporting a long history of a limp and toe walking, with no preceding trauma. Examination reveals a positive Trendelenburg sign and a positive Galeazzi test. All blood investigations are within normal parameters. Plain AP radiographs of the pelvis show a broken Shenton's line. What is the most appropriate next step in management?
    A. Ultrasound of the hip
    B. MRI of the hip
    C. Open reduction plus femoral shortening
    D. Traction followed by closed reduction
    E. Application of a Pavlik harness

37. The most important prognostic factor for Perthes' disease is:
    A. Extent of involvement of capital femoral epiphysis
    B. Age of onset
    C. Duration of disease
    D. Herring classification
    E. Presence of the Gage sign

38. Regarding the Loder classification of slipped upper femoral epiphysis:
    A. A child with an unstable slip is unable to weight bear pain free
    B. It is not useful for predicting prognosis
    C. In the stable slip children can only weight bear, pain free, with crutches
    D. There is no difference in the prevalence of AVN between unstable and stable slips
    E. Patients with stable slips present with sudden onset, severe, fracture like pain

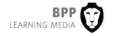

39. An obese 12-year-old girl presents to the Emergency Department (ED) with a sudden onset severe pain in both hips. There is no history of trauma. On examination she is apyrexial, unable to weight bear pain free on either side and has global reduction in movement around both hip joints. Plain AP radiographs reveal no abnormalities. Blood investigations are all within normal parameters. The next most appropriate line of investigation would be:
   A. Frog leg lateral radiographs
   B. Ultrasound scan of the hips
   C. Bone scan
   D. CT of the pelvis
   E. MRI of the pelvis

40. Scheuermann's kyphosis:
   A. Is an increased thoracic kyphosis characterised by vertebral wedging of 5 degrees or more at three adjacent levels
   B. Demonstrates radiographic changes early in childhood, before age five years
   C. Has a female predominance
   D. Has no place for bracing in treating structural deformity
   E. Has surgery as its mainstay of treatment

41. The following are all **true** in relation to torticollis, except:
   A. Head tilt occurs towards the affected side, and rotatory deviation is away from the affected side
   B. A palpable mass may be felt in the sternocleidomastoid muscle
   C. Stretching is successful in a minority of cases
   D. Refractory cases can be treated with surgical release of the sternocleidomastoid muscle
   E. The most common form presents in the first few months of life

42. The best modality for investigating possible osteomyelitis in the paediatric pelvis is:
   A. Plain radiographs
   B. Ultrasound
   C. CT
   D. MRI
   E. Isotope bone scan

43. In paediatric musculoskeletal infection:
   A. Septic arthritis is less common than osteomyelitis
   B. Osteomyelitis more commonly occurs in the first five years of life
   C. Streptococcus pyogenes is the most common causative organism
   D. Simultaneous bone and adjacent joint infection has been reported in up to 30% of cases
   E. Dual involvement of both bone and joint is most common around the hip

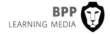

44. Short limb dwarfism with disproportionate involvement of the arms and thigh is known as:
    A. Microcormia
    B. Micromelia
    C. Rhizomelia
    D. Mesomelia
    E. Acromelia

45. Osteogenesis imperfecta is associated with a defect in which type of collagen?
    A. I
    B. II
    C. V
    D. VII
    E. X

46. An undisplaced fracture of the proximal humerus through a unicameral bone cyst is best treated, in the first instance with:
    A. Collar and cuff
    B. Injection of bone marrow
    C. Injection of bone graft substitutes
    D. Elastic intramedullary nailing
    E. Curettage and bone grafting

47. Aneurysmal bone cysts occur most commonly in the;
    A. Humerus
    B. Spine
    C. Pelvis
    D. Femur
    E. Tibia

48. With regards to lower limb length inequality in a child:
    A. Tibial corticotomies heal faster than femoral
    B. Patients younger than 14 years require significantly longer time for bone healing
    C. Patients less than 14 years old have fewer complications
    D. The use of circular frames compared with a unilateral external fixator is associated with more complications in lengthening greater than 20% of the original bone
    E. Femoral lengthening is associated with more complications than tibial

49. The following are all inherited in an autosomal dominant pattern, except:
    A. Osteogenesis imperfecta
    B. Hurler's syndrome
    C. Achondroplasia
    D. Multiple epiphyseal dysplasia
    E. Cleidocranial dysplasia

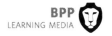

50. The Erb Duchenne palsy occurs as a result of damage to nerve roots:
    A. C5–T1
    B. C8–T1
    C. C5–C8
    D. C5–C7
    E. C5–C6

51. At what point in development does the femoral ossific nucleus normally appear?
    A. Third trimester
    B. Within the first 2 months
    C. 2–8 months
    D. 6–9 months
    E. 9–12 months

52. The normal range for the centre edge angle of Wiberg on a radiograph of the paediatric hip is:
    A. Less than 15 degrees
    B. 10–20 degrees
    C. 25–45 degrees
    D. 10–60 degrees
    E. > 60 degrees

53. Which of the following is not a packaging disorder?
    A. Torticollis
    B. Metatarsus varus
    C. Calcaneovalgus
    D. Knee dislocation
    E. Lateral tibial torsion

54. What is the incidence of clubfoot?
    A. 1 in 100
    B. 1 in 1000
    C. 1 in 5000
    D. 1 in 10,000
    E. 1 in 20,000

55. Varus angulation in infants usually resolves:
    A. Within the first 6 months
    B. Within the first year
    C. Between 12–18 months
    D. Between 18–24 months
    E. Between 2–3 years

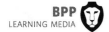

56. Which investigations are mandatory in the investigation of pes cavus?
    A. Serum CK and LDH
    B. Weightbearing AP and lateral views of both feet
    C. Sural nerve biopsy
    D. Genetic testing
    E. MRI, electromyography and nerve conduction studies

57. Which of the following statements is **false** regarding infantile tibia vara?
    A. The condition is more common in obese toddlers
    B. Standard plain radiographs of proximal tibia demonstrate a sharp varus angulation in the metaphysis
    C. Rarely presents before 18 months
    D. Corrective osteotomy should not be performed before 8 years
    E. The Langenskiold classification describes 6 progressive stages

58. Which of the following is **not** a cause for paediatric genu valgum?
    A. Proximal tibial fracture
    B. Renal osteodystrophy
    C. Idiopathic
    D. Spondyloepiphyseal dysplasia
    E. Infantile rickets

59. Tibial torsion is defined as:
    A. Abnormal tibial rotation within 1 standard deviation of the mean value for the age group of the affected child
    B. Abnormal tibial rotation greater than 1 standard deviation from the mean value for the age group of the affected child
    C. Abnormal tibial rotation greater than 2 standard deviations from the mean value for the age group of the affected child
    D. Abnormal tibial rotation greater than 3 standard deviations from the mean value for the age group of the affected child
    E. Abnormal tibial rotation greater than 5 standard deviations from the mean value for the age group of the affected child

60. Which of the following statements regarding tibial torsion is incorrect
    A. Tibial torsion is the most common cause of intoeing or out-toeing gait up to the age of 4 years
    B. Medial tibial torsion is usually not evident until the age of 12 months
    C. Bracing is ineffective in improving alignment
    D. If surgery is indicated, the preferred site of a rotational osteotomy is in the proximal tibia
    E. Surgery is only indicated if there is significant cosmetic or functional impairment persisting after the age of 8 years

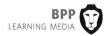

61.  Which of the following statements regarding anterolateral tibia bowing is **false**?
     A.  Anterolateral bowing carries a worse prognosis than posteromedial bowing
     B.  The condition is associated with neurofibromatosis.
     C.  The condition is associated with fibrous dsyplasia of the tibia
     D.  Most cases have only unilateral involvement
     E.  Fractures occurring before walking age are likely to heal without intervention

62.  Which of the following statements regarding posteromedial bowing of the tibia is **true**?
     A.  The condition is associated with pes cavus
     B.  Parents should be advised that the deformity will take at least 5 years to correct
     C.  The main concern is residual limb length disparity
     D.  There is no role for splinting
     E.  Angulation of the deformity rarely exceeds 20 degrees

63.  At what point in development does the navicular commonly ossify?
     A.  30<sup>th</sup> week in utero
     B.  Within the first 6 months of life
     C.  Between 6 months and 2 years
     D.  Between 2–5 years
     E.  Between 6–7 years

64.  Which of the following statements regarding Kohler's disease is **false**?
     A.  Characteristic radiographic findings include sclerosis, flattening and irregularity of the navicular
     B.  The condition is more common in girls and usually presents between 2–7 years
     C.  The condition may be an incidental radiographic finding in an asymptomatic child.
     D.  The condition has a good prognosis with spontaneous resolution during childhood
     E.  A walking cast is indicated in symptomatic patients

65.  Which of the following statements regarding Freiberg's disease is **true**?
     A.  The condition only ever affects the second metatarsal
     B.  The disorder commonly presents at 10–13 years
     C.  The frequency is higher in boys
     D.  A bone scan may reveal increased uptake in the metatarsal head
     E.  The mainstay of treatment is excision of the affected metatarsal head

66.  Which of the following is not a characteristic feature of metatarsus adductus?
     A.  Associated with torticollis and developmental hip dysplasia
     B.  The sole has a characteristic bean shape
     C.  There is increased space between the first and second toes
     D.  The medial border of the foot is concave with a high arch
     E.  The hindfoot may be in valgus or varus

67.  Which of the following statements regarding talipes calcaneovalgus is **false**?
     A.  The condition is associated with developmental hip dysplasia
     B.  The forefoot is dorsiflexed and the heel is in equinus
     C.  The condition usually improves within 3–6 months
     D.  The condition is associated with metatarsus adductus
     E.  The condition is more common in girls and firstborn children

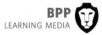

68.  Which of the following best describes the deformity in skewfoot?
     A.  Forefoot varus, midfoot abduction and hindfoot valgus
     B.  Forefoot valgus, midfoot abduction and hindfoot valgus
     C.  Forefoot valgus, midfoot abduction and hindfoot varus
     D.  Forefoot valgus, midfoot abduction and hindfoot valgus
     E.  Forefoot varus, midfoot aligned and hindfoot valgus


69.  Which of the following statements regarding clubfoot is **false**?
     A.  The deformity is associated with arthrogryposis
     B.  Treatment is highly effective with minimal risk of recurrence
     C.  Milder forms of the condition may relate to inutero positioning
     D.  The condition is associated with Down syndrome
     E.  Tarsal dysplasia is most marked in the talus


70.  Which of the following is not a category of deformity in the Pirani classification of talipes equinovarus?
     A.  Midfoot medial crease
     B.  Medial rotation of calcaneopedal 'block'
     C.  Talar head coverage
     D.  Posterior crease
     E.  Equinus rigidity


71.  Which of the following statements regarding Ponseti treatment of clubfeet is **false**?
     A.  The results are better if the condition is treated earlier
     B.  The order of deformity correction is: adductus, cavus, varus, equinus
     C.  Serial casts are applied which extend above the knee and are changed every 5–7 days
     D.  Percutaneous heel tenotomy may need to be performed to correct the equinus deformity
     E.  After removal of the last cast, the parents are advised that Denis Browne boots and bar need to be worn for at least 23 hours a day for the first 3–4 months then at nap and nighttimes for 2–4 years.


72.  A child with bilateral clubfeet is commenced on the Ponseti regime shortly after birth and full correction is achieved. The child is followed up at 6 months and the deformity has recurred. The next appropriate step in management is:
     A.  Abduction foot orthosis prescribed 23 hours a day for the next 3 months
     B.  Repeat serial manipulation and casting
     C.  Posteromedial release
     D.  Posteromedial-lateral release
     E.  Talectomy

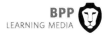

73. Which of the following is not associated with developmental dysplasia of the hip (DDH)?
    A. Breech delivery
    B. Family history of affected relatives with DDH
    C. Female sex
    D. Metatarsus adductus
    E. Coxa vara

74. Which of the following structures is least likely to become interposed in a dysplastic dislocated hip and lead to difficulties in attempts at closed reduction?
    A. Iliopsoas
    B. Adductor longus
    C. Gluteus medius
    D. Inverted limbus
    E. Ligamentum teres

75. A normal α angle in the Graf grading of developmental dysplasia is considered to be:
    A. < 10 degrees
    B. 10–20 degrees
    C. 20–30 degrees
    D. 30–50 degrees
    E. > 60 degrees

76. A 2-month-old child is diagnosed with developmental dysplasia of the hip on ultrasound. Treatment with a Pavlik harness is commenced and repeat ultrasound demonstrates reduction in the abducted position in the harness. The patient is followed up at 4 weeks and the hip is found to be dislocated. The next most appropriate step in management is:
    A. Further trial with Pavlik harness for 4 weeks
    B. CT scan to delineate position of head relative to acetabulum
    C. Proceed to open reduction and spica cast
    D. Arthrogram, attempted closed reduction and spica cast
    E. Open reduction and pelvic osteotomy

77. Which of the following is not a recognised complication of treatment in a Pavlik harness?
    A. Brachial plexopathy
    B. Femoral nerve palsy
    C. Avascular necrosis of femoral head
    D. Skin rashes
    E. Knee dislocation

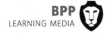

78. In the Kalanchi-MacEwen classification of avascular necrosis of the femoral head, which type is characterised by the presence of a lateral physeal bridge causing tethering of growth?
    A. Type I
    B. Type II
    C. Type III
    D. Type IV
    E. Type V

79. Which of the following pelvic osteotomies produces a fibrocartilage surface for weightbearing articulation with the femoral head?
    A. Chiari
    B. Pemberton
    C. Dega
    D. Salter
    E. Ganz

80. Which of the following is not a recognised cause of femoral head avascular necrosis in the paediatric population?
    A. Gaucher's disease
    B. Von Willebrand's disease
    C. Sickle cell anaemia
    D. Mucopolysaccharidoses
    E. Hypothyroidism

BPP
LEARNING MEDIA

# Paediatrics

## Answers

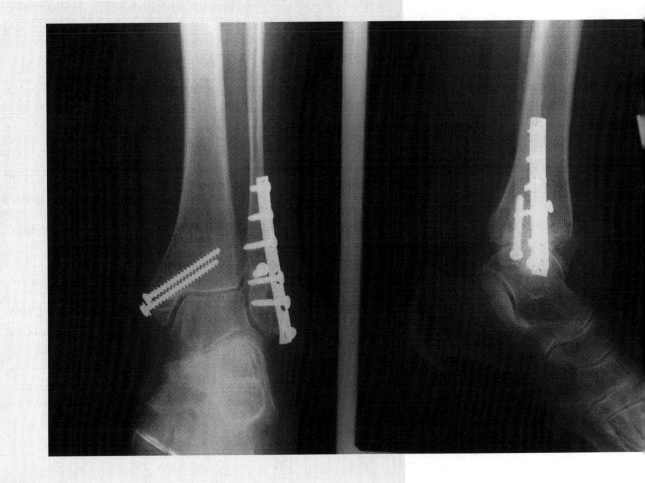

1.  **D**

    Atlantoaxial instability is a potentially fatal sequlae of Down syndrome. The atlantodens interval (ADI) is measured on flexion-extension lateral radiographs of the cervical spine, and an ADI between 5 and 10mm with no neurologic symptoms can be observed with annual radiographic and neurologic examinations. Surgical stabilisation is indicated in asymptomatic ADI of more than 10mm or symptomatic ADI between 5mm and 10mm. Traction and bracing can be used for rotatory atlantoaxial instability, but is not a recognised treatment for anterior-posterior instability.

    Ref:
    Chin, K. and Mehta, S. (ed.) (2007) *Orthopaedic Key Review Concepts*, Lippincott Williams & Wilkins, Philadelphia.

2.  **B**

    Osteogenesis Imperfecta is inherited in an autosomal dominant fashion in types IA, IB, IVA and IVB and an in an autosomal recessive fashion in types II and III.

    Ref:
    Chin, K. and Mehta, S. (ed.) (2007) *Orthopaedic Key Review Concepts*, Lippincott Williams & Wilkins, Philadelphia.

3.  **B**

    Nonsteroidal anti-inflammatory agents such as aspirin are the mainstay of therapy in juvenile rheumatoid arthritis, and methotrexate is used as a second-line drug. Physical therapy, splinting, and occasionally synovectomy, are all helpful in selected cases. Progressive inflammation with joint destruction may require arthrodesis or joint arthroplasty.

    Ref:
    Chin, K. and Mehta, S. (ed.) (2007) *Orthopaedic Key Review Concepts*, Lippincott Williams & Wilkins, Philadelphia.

4.  **E**

    The most common procedure in a subluxed hip in cerebral palsy with a normal acetabulum is a soft tissue release followed by a varus derotational proximal femoral osteotomy. In the presence of coexisting acetabular dysplasia (Acetabular Index [AI] > 25 to 27 degrees), a volume reducing pelvic osteotomy may also be required. Solitary soft tissue procedures are only indicated for the 'at risk' hip. Acetabular osteotomy is indicated for reconstruction of the dislocated hip.

    Ref:
    Chin, K. and Mehta, S. (ed.) (2007) *Orthopaedic Key Review Concepts*, Lippincott Williams & Wilkins, Philadelphia.

5.  **A**

    In spina bifida, hip dislocation is most common at the L3/4 level. A functional level above L4 allows independent quadriceps function, and its presence is an indication for treatment.

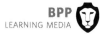

Ref:

Chin, K. and Mehta, S. (ed.) (2007) *Orthopaedic Key Review Concepts*, Lippincott Williams & Wilkins, Philadelphia.

6.     **B**

Acute bacterial septic arthritis due to *S. aureus* is seen in all age groups from neonate to adolescent. *Salmonella* species and *N. gonorrhoeae* are mostly seen in the neonate and children over 4 years old. *Group A Streptococcus* seems to be more common in the infant and young child.

Ref:

Chin, K. and Mehta, S. (ed.) (2007) *Orthopaedic Key Review Concepts*, Lippincott Williams & Wilkins, Philadelphia.

7.     **C**

Serum CRP begins to rise within 6 hours of infection and increases several hundredfold, reaching a peak within 36–50 hours of onset. Blood cultures yield positive results in only 30%–50% of cases. Bony changes on plain radiographs may take up to 14 days to become apparent from the onset of infection.

Ref:

Chin, K. and Mehta, S. (ed.) (2007) *Orthopaedic Key Review Concepts*, Lippincott Williams & Wilkins, Philadelphia.

8.     **A**

Scurvy is caused by a nutritional deficiency of vitamin C which is necessary for the hydroxylation of lysine and proline. The deficiency results in primitive collagen formation, and bone that forms is lacking in tensile strength and is defective in structural arrangement. The greatest effect on bone formation is observed in the metaphysis. The deficiency in the metaphysis is most probably related to the large amount of Type I collagen normally found in this region.

Ref:

Chin, K. and Mehta, S. (ed.) (2007) *Orthopaedic Key Review Concepts*, Lippincott Williams & Wilkins, Philadelphia.

9.     **D**

Female gender, family history, breech presentation and oligohydramnios are all risk factors for DDH.

Ref:

Chin, K. and Mehta, S. (ed.) (2007) *Orthopaedic Key Review Concepts*, Lippincott Williams & Wilkins, Philadelphia.

10.    **D**

The Herring classification, a radiological classification, is based on involvement of the lateral pillar of the capital femoral epiphysis in the fragmentation stage.

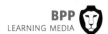

Ref:

Chin, K. and Mehta, S. (ed.) (2007) *Orthopaedic Key Review Concepts*, Lippincott Williams & Wilkins, Philadelphia.

**11.    A**

Achondroplasia is the most frequent short-limb dwarfism and is transmitted as an autosomal dominant trait. Features include limitation of elbow extension, trident hand, radial head subluxation, kyphosis at the thoracolumbar junction and a champagne glass pelvis. Knees are most commonly in varus alignment, but can sometimes be in excessive valgus. Lumbar spinal stenosis is the most common and disabling problem, and spinal decompression may be indicated in these circumstances.

Ref:

Chin, K. and Mehta, S. (ed.) (2007) *Orthopaedic Key Review Concepts*, Lippincott Williams & Wilkins, Philadelphia.

**12.    E**

In hereditary multiple exostosis, reasonable indications for excision of exostosis include pain, growth disturbance leading to limb-length discrepancy, **false** aneurysm produced by an osteochondroma, and a rapid increase in the size of a lesion. Significant valgus deformities of the knee and ankle are treated by osteotomy or hemiepiphyseodesis in young patients or corrective varus osteotomy in older patients.

Ref:

Chin, K.and Mehta, S. (ed.) (2007) *Orthopaedic Key Review Concepts*, Lippincott Williams & Wilkins, Philadelphia.

**13.    B**

The ossification centres around the elbow ossify according to the acronym CRITOL, starting in the first year of life and after two successive years for each subsequent ossification centre.

C – Capitellum (year 1)
R – Radial head (year 3)
I – Internal (medial) epicondyle (year 5)
T – Trochlea (year 7)
O – Olecranon (year 9)
L – Lateral epicondyle (year 11)

Ref:

Dormans, J. (ed.) (2005) *Pediatric Orthopaedics: Core Knowledge in Orthopaedics*, Elsevier Mosby, Philadelphia.

**14.    C**

At birth the tibiofemoral angle is in marked varus. Between 18–24 months the knee straightens to neutral tibiofemoral alignment. Refer to Salenius curve for physiological tibiofemoral alignment with age.

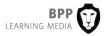

Ref:
Dormans, J. (ed.) (2005) *Pediatric Orthopaedics: Core Knowledge in Orthopaedics*, Elsevier Mosby, Philadelphia.

15. **A**

The growth plate contains primarily Type II collagen.

Ref:
Dormans, J. (ed.) (2005) *Pediatric Orthopaedics: Core Knowledge in Orthopaedics*, Elsevier Mosby, Philadelphia.

16. **B**

The Thurston Holland fragment is the eponymous name of the metaphyseal triangle fragment seen in Salter-Harris Type II physeal plate injuries.

Ref:
Dormans, J. (ed.) (2005) *Pediatric Orthopaedics: Core Knowledge in Orthopaedics*, Elsevier Mosby, Philadelphia.

17. **C**

Non-accidental injury (NAI) most commonly occurs in children under one year of age. Orthopaedic injuries are seen in 30–50% of cases, and include bucket handle fractures, scapular fractures, posterior rib fractures, multiple fractures of different ages and spinous process fractures. Suspicion of NAI should prompt the performing of a skeletal survey, which includes the following radiographs: AP or lateral skull; lateral cervical, thoracic and lumbar spine, AP pelvis and extremities, and AP chest. A CT scan of the head should be reserved for those cases where fractures of the skull or neurological abnormalities are equivocal. Bone scan is an option to determine subtle fractures.

Ref:
Dormans, J. (ed.) (2005) *Pediatric Orthopaedics: Core Knowledge in Orthopaedics*, Elsevier Mosby, Philadelphia.

18. **C**

Typically, in the forearm of a child, remodeling can correct angulation of about 10 degrees per year.

Ref:
Dormans, J. (ed.) (2005) *Pediatric Orthopaedics: Core Knowledge in Orthopaedics*, Elsevier Mosby, Philadelphia.

19. **E**

Galeazzi fractures in the child are a relatively rare injury and are a less common than the Monteggia type injury. They involve a distal radius fracture with a distal ulnar physeal injury, and most can be treated in a long arm cast for six weeks. If casted, the forearm should be splinted in slight pronation. They rarely require intramedullary fixation.

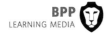

Ref:
Dormans, J. (ed.) (2005) *Pediatric Orthopaedics: Core Knowledge in Orthopaedics*, Elsevier Mosby, Philadelphia.

**20.** **B**

Nerve injuries occur in up to 11% of Monteggia lesions in childhood. The most common are those involving the posterior interosseous nerve and are associated with a Bado III lesion. Most resolve without operative intervention.

Ref:
Olney, BW. Menelaus, MB. (1989) Monteggia and equivalent lesions in childhood, *J Pediatr Orthop*, 9(2): 219–223.

**21.** **D**

In the presence of normal AP, lateral and oblique radiographs of the elbow, following trauma, the posterior fat pad sign is predictive of a non displaced fracture in 76% of children.

Ref:
Skaggs, DL. Mirzayan, R. (1999) The posterior fat pad sign in association with occult fracture of the elbow in children, *J Bone Joint Surg (Am)*, 81(10): 1429–1433.

**22.** **B**

Supracondylar fractures of the humerus occur most frequently in children younger than 8 years old. The most common nerve injury is to the anterior interosseous nerve, and this is evaluated by checking flexion of the thumb and index finger distal phalanges.

Ref:
Dormans, J. (ed.) (2005) *Pediatric Orthopaedics: Core Knowledge in Orthopaedics*, Elsevier Mosby, Philadelphia.

**23.** **C**

Supracondylar fractures in which the anterior humeral line intersects the capitellum, and in which there is no collapse of the medial column can be treated in plaster cast immobilisation. All other fractures should be treated with closed reduction and K-wire fixation.

Ref:
Dormans, J. (ed.) (2005) *Pediatric Orthopaedics: Core Knowledge in Orthopaedics*, Elsevier Mosby, Philadelphia.

**24.** **C**

Lateral condyle fractures of the humerus can proceed to non union, and this is thought to be due to the tenuous blood supply of the largely cartilaginous fracture fragment. This may lead to a cubitus valgus deformity and an associated tardy ulnar nerve plasy may develop. Loss of terminal elbow extension is a common complication following fractures to the medial epicondyle.

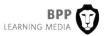

Ref:

Dormans, J. (ed.) (2005) *Pediatric Orthopaedics: Core Knowledge in Orthopaedics*, Elsevier Mosby, Philadelphia.

**25. E**

In children older than 11 years, femoral fractures treated with trochanteric antegrade intramedullary nailing allow for earlier weigh bearing and return to function. Trochanteric nails are favoured over piriformis fossa entry nails to minimise the risk of AVN. There is no place for the use of hip spica or elastic nails in this age group. Retrograde intramedullary nailing should only be used in the presence of a closed distal femoral growth plate.

Ref:

Dormans, J. (ed.) (2005) *Pediatric Orthopaedics: Core Knowledge in Orthopaedics*, Elsevier Mosby, Philadelphia.

**26. C**

Proximal tibial physeal fractures are the paediatric equivalent of a traumatic knee dislocation. The most important aspect of this injury is to recognise the presence of an associated vascular injury to the popliteal artery, and this may require the use of doppler studies or an arteriogram. In the absence of vascular injury non displaced fractures can be treated in an above knee cast. MRI is usually not indicated. Displaced fractures will require closed reduction and immobilisation.

Ref:

Green. NE. Swiontkowski, MF. (ed.) (1998) *Skeletal Trauma in Children*, Saunders, Philadelphia.

**27. B**

Deformities of the tibial shaft that do not remodel well include valgus angulation, recurvatum, and all rotations. Shortening can be compensated for by growth acceleration.

Ref:

Shannak, AO. (1988) Tibial fractures in children: Follow up study. *J Pediatr Orthop*, 8(3): 306–310.

**28. B**

SCIWORA is a traumatic high energy distraction injury to the relatively immature spinal column of the younger child, normally less than eight years old. It occurs in the absence of any abnormality on radiographs and CT, and can be either a complete or an incomplete lesion, most commonly occurring at the cervicothoracic junction.

Ref:

Pang, D. and Wilberger, JE. (1982) Spinal cord injury without radiographic abnormalities in children. *J Neurosurg*, 57: 114–129.

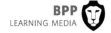

**29.  E**

OCD most commonly affects the knee joint. The elbow, ankle, shoulder, wrist, hand and hip are less commonly affected.

Ref:

Dormans, J. (ed.) (2005) *Pediatric Orthopaedics: Core Knowledge in Orthopaedics*, Elsevier Mosby, Philadelphia.

**30.  D**

Stage IV OCD involves the presence of a displaced loose body. If associated with mechanical symptoms, large lesion fragmentations should be removed and consideration be given to bone and cartilage grafting.

Ref:

Ganley, TJ. Pill, SG. Flynn, JM. Gregg, JR. (2003) Treatment of massive osteochondritis dissecans lesions of the capitellum: Arthroscopic assisted debridement and bone grafting for large full-thickness defects. *Arthroscopy*, 19(2): 222–225.

**31.  E**

Diagnosis of extremity stress fractures are best diagnosed by bone scan. Radiographs may be helpful in some cases, demonstrating a radiolucent line suggestive of a stress fracture. CT scan is most precise when evaluating the spine.

Ref:

Dormans, J. (ed.) (2005) *Pediatric Orthopaedics: Core Knowledge in Orthopaedics*, Elsevier Mosby, Philadelphia.

**32.  C**

Triplane fractures of the ankle are seen in children with partially closed growth plates. In such individuals the lateral distal tibial physis fuses after the medial, and it is this part which is then vulnerable to injury. On AP radiographs the appearance is of a Salter-Harris Type III injury, similar to that seen in a Tillaux fracture. Lateral radiographs show a Salter-Harris Type II injury with involvement of the posterior distal metaphysis. CT scan is a valuable tool in evaluating articular incongruity and planning for surgery.

Ref:

Dormans, J. (ed.) (2005) *Pediatric Orthopaedics: Core Knowledge in Orthopaedics*, Elsevier Mosby, Philadelphia.

**33.  C**

Radial deficiency is associated with Holt Oram syndrome (commonly manifesting as cardiac septal defects), thrombocytopenia-absent-radius syndrome (TAR) syndrome, VACTERL syndrome (which includes tracheoesophageal fistula), and Fanconi anaemia (aplastic anaemia). Chest wall deformities are common in Poland's syndrome which is associated with atypical cleft hand.

Ref:

Dormans, J. (ed.) (2005) *Pediatric Orthopaedics: Core Knowledge in Orthopaedics*, Elsevier Mosby, Philadelphia.

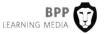

**34.   E**

The Ponseti method for the treatment of clubfoot is a programme of four to six weekly manipulations and castings, supplemented by night time bracing for up to five years. Rotation is controlled by the use of a long leg cast with the knee flexed at 90 degrees. Percutaneous tenotomy is required in 90% of cases. Lateral transfer of the tibialis anterior tendon is required to balance the foot in up to one third of cases.

Ref:

Ponseti IV. (1996) *Congenital Clubfoot: Fundamentals of Treatment*, Oxford University Press, Oxford.

**35.   A**

Talocalcaneal coalition is evident by the presence of the 'C' sign on weight bearing plain lateral radiographs of the ankle, and is due to an area of increased sclerosis at the obliterated joint space. The 'C' sign associated with Freiberg's Disease is due to subchondral bone collapse at the metatarsal head.

Ref:

Lateur, LM. Van Hoe, LR. Van Ghillewe, KV. Gryspeerdt, SS. Baert, AL. (1994) Subtalar coalition: Diagnosis with the C sign on lateral radiographs of the ankle. *Radiology*, 193. 3, 847–851.

**36.   C**

Dislocation of the hip secondary to developmental dysplasia in children older than three years usually requires open reduction. Femoral shortening is an essential component of managing such cases, and is associated with a lower rate of proximal femoral growth disturbances. Ultrasound and MRI scanning are of limited use in such instances. The use of the Pavlik harness is limited to those children less than six months old. Traction followed by closed reduction is indicated in children between the ages of six and 24 months.

Ref:

Herring, JA. (2002) *Tachdjian's Pediatric Orthopaedics*, WB Saunders, Philadelphia.

**37.   B**

Age of onset, deformity and congruity at maturity are the main prognostic factors for Perthes' disease. Children developing symptoms before five years of age tend to recover without residual problems, while those over nine usually have a poor prognosis. Other factors associated with poor prognosis include the extent of the capital femoral epiphysis involvement, the duration of the disease process and those in Herring group C. The Gage sign is a radiolucency in the lateral epiphysis and metaphysis, and is a radiographic 'at risk' sign identified by Catterall. It is present when the changes are reversible with treatment.

Ref:

1.   Thompson, GH. Price, CT. Roy, D. Meehan, PL. Richards BS. (2002) Legg-Calve-Perthes' disease. *Instr Course Lect*, 51: 367–384.
2.   Catterall, A. (1971) The natural history of Perthes' disease. *J Bone Joint Surgery (Br)* 53(1): 37–53.

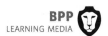

**38.** **A**

The Loder classification for slipped upper femoral epiphysis separates patients based on their ability to weight bear pain free, with or without the aid of crutches. In stable slips the child presents with intermittent pain in the groin or thigh and is able to fully weight bear pain free with or without crutches. In the unstable slip, presentation is usually with the sudden onset of a severe, fracture like, pain and weight bearing is painful irrespective of the use of crutches. The prevalence of AVN is up to 50% in unstable slips and close to 0% in stable slips.

Ref:

Loder, RT. Richards, BS. Shapiro, PS. Reznick, LR. Aronson, DD. (1993) Acute slipped capital femoral epiphysis: The importance of physeal stability. *J Bone Joint Surgery (Am)* 75(8): 1134–1140.

**39.** **E**

Slipped upper femoral epiphysis is often diagnosed with the use of plain radiography only. In the presence of an unstable slip, frog legs lateral views should be avoided because of the risk of increasing physeal displacement. If plain radiographs appear normal, MRI would be the modality of choice to confirm a slip, exposing the child to less radiation than CT.

Ref:

Dormans, J. (ed.) (2005) *Pediatric Orthopaedics: Core Knowledge in Orthopaedics*, Elsevier Mosby, Philadelphia.

**40.** **A**

Scheuermann's kyphosis is characterised by increased kyphosis in adolescence, with vertebral wedging of 5 degrees or more at three adjacent levels, and occurs more commonly in males. Radiographic changes are not seen before ten years of age. Treatment is based on the degree of deformity, and include bracing and casting. Surgery is reserved for cases in which curves progress beyond 70 degrees despite bracing.

Ref:

Sorensen, KH. (1964) *Scheuermann's Juvenile Kyphosis: Clinical Appearances, Radiography, Aetiology, and Prognosis*, Munksgaard, Copenhagen.

**41.** **C**

Torticollis is clinically identified by head tilt towards and rotatory deviation away from the affected sternocleidomastoid muscle. Congenital muscular torticollis is the most common aetiology and present in the first few months of life, sometimes with a palpable mass in the muscle body. Radiographs of the cervical spine are useful to rule out congenital cervical anomalies. Stretching is the mainstay of treatment and is successful in 90% of cases. Recalcitrant cases may be treated with surgical release of either one or both (proximal and distal) attachments of the sternocleidomastoid muscle

Ref:

Dormans, J. (ed.) (2005) *Pediatric Orthopaedics: Core Knowledge in Orthopaedics*, Elsevier Mosby, Philadelphia.

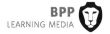

**42.    D**

MRI has been shown to be highly sensitive (97%) and specific (92%) in evaluating musculoskeletal infection. In particular, it is useful in identifying infection in the spine, pelvis and foot. Isotope bone scans are useful when infection has not been localised, but do have a high rate of false positives (32%) and false negatives (30%) and can be difficult to interpret around the spine and pelvis. Ultrasound is most useful in evaluating septic arthritis of the hip, in the presence of excess fluid in the joint.

Ref:

Kothari, NA. Pelchovitz, DJ. Meyer, JS. (2001) Imaging of musculoskeletal infections. *Radiol Clin North Am*, 39(4): 653–671.

**43.    D**

Septic arthritis in the child is twice as common as osteomyelitis, and occurs at an earlier age (during the first five years). Staphylococcus aureus is the most commonly isolated organism in all age categories. Simultaneous bone and adjacent joint involvement is reported in up to 30% of cases, and is most common around the knee joint (in 31% of cases).

Ref:

Perlman, MH. Patzakis, MJ. Kumar, PJ. Holtom, P. (2000) The incidence of joint involvement with adjacent osteomyelitis in pediatric patients. *J Pediatr Orthop*, 20: 40–43.

**44.    C**

Microcormia refers to short trunk dysplasias where there is disproportionate involvement of the trunk relative to the limbs. Micromelia refers to short limb dysplasias where the extremities are disproportionately short compared with the trunk, and this can be divided into the segments of the limb which are most affected: rhizomelia (proximal limb segments); mesomelia (middle limb segments); acromelia (distal limb segments)

Ref:

Dormans, J. (ed.) (2005) *Pediatric Orthopaedics: Core Knowledge in Orthopaedics*, Elsevier Mosby, Philadelphia.

**45.    A**

Osteogenesis Imperfecta is associated with a defect in type I collagen formation

Ref:

Herring, JA. (2002) *Tachdjian's Pediatric Orthopaedics*, WB Saunders, Philadelphia.

**46.    A**

Most fractures of the proximal humerus associated with unicameral bone cysts can be treated conservatively in the first instance. After fracture healing, injection of bone marrow and bone graft substitutes can be considered for extensive or active lesions. Elastic intramedullary nailing is indicated in fractures of the femur, where there is higher risk of subsequent complication. There is no place for open curettage with bone grafting.

Ref:

Dutoit, M. (2007) Unicameral and aneurysmal bone cysts. *Eur Instr Course Lect*, 8: 49–55.

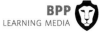

47. **D**

Aneurysmal bone cysts occur most commonly in the femur, then the tibia, spine and pelvis

Ref:

De Dios, Am. Bond, JR. Shives, TC. McLeod RA. Krishan Unni, K. (1992) Aneurysmal bone cyst: a clinicopathologic study of 238 cases. *Cancer*, 69: 2921–31.

48. **C**

In the treatment of lower limb length inequality in children, femoral lengthening is associated with fewer complications than tibial, and femoral corticotomies also heal faster than tibial. Children less than 14 years of age heal much quicker and with fewer complications. Unilateral external fixators cause more complications than circular devices when lengthening is more than 20% of the original bone length.

Ref:

Ippolito, E. Mancini, F. Savarese, E. (2007) Management of limb length inequality. *Eur Instr Course Lect*, 8: 63–83.

49. **B**

Almost all major forms of dwarfism are inherited in an autosomal dominant pattern. Osteogenesis imperfecta types IA, IB, IVA and IVB are all inherited in an autosomal dominant fashion. Hurler's syndrome is a mucopolysaccharidosis which follows an autosomal recessive inheritance.

Ref:

Miller, MD. (ed.) (2008) *Review of Orthopaedics*, Saunders Elsevier, Philadelphia.

50. **E**

The classic Erb's palsy affects nerve roots C5–6 and presents with absence of shoulder abduction and external rotation, elbow flexion and forearm supination. This is the mildest clinical group of brachial plexus palsies, with spontaneous recovery occurring in up to 90% of cases

Ref:

Miller, MD. (ed.) (2008) *Review of Orthopaedics*, Saunders Elsevier, Philadelphia.

51. **C**

The femoral head usually ossifies between the 2$^{nd}$ to 8$^{th}$ months of life. Ossification of all three pelvic bones, femoral shaft and distal epiphysis occurs before birth. Therefore, radiographic evaluation of the hip is usually not undertaken in the first three months of life with ultrasound being the preferred imaging modality.

Ref:

Staheli LT (4$^{th}$ ed.) (2007). *Fundamentals of Pediatric Orthopaedics*, Lippincott Williams & Wilkins, Philadelphia.

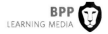

52.    **C**
The optimum age for plain radiographs as a screening tool in the evaluation of the paediatric hip is the second to third month of life when the femoral head first starts to ossify. A single antero-posterior radiograph is usually adequate. There are several important relationships and angles to be mindful of when scrutinising these images:

- Hilgrenreiner's line is a line drawn through both tri-radiate cartilages.
- Perkins line is a vertical line perpendicular to Hilgrenreiner's line which intersects the lateral border of the acetabulum.
- After construction of these two lines and divisions into quadrants, the medial beak of the femoral metaphysis should lie within the infero-medial quadrant if the joint is reduced
- The acetabular index is the inclination of a line drawn from the tri-radiate cartilage to the supero-lateral edge of the acetabulum with respect to Hilgrenreiner's line. Less than 30 degrees can be considered as normal, 30–40 degrees suspicious of acetabular dysplasia and greater than 40 degrees abnormal although development of the angle with time is equally clinically relevant.
- The centre edge angle of Wiberg is the angle between a vertical line through the centre of the head and perpendicular to Hilgrenreiner's line and a line from the centre of the head to the supero-lateral margin of the acetabulum. It is a measure of acetabular dysplasia and the acceptable range for this angle is 25–45 degrees but it increases as the joint ossifies.

Ref:
Staheli LT (4th ed.) (2007). *Fundamentals of Pediatric Orthopaedics*, Lippincott Williams & Wilkins, Philadelphia.


53.    **E**
Medial tibial torsion may be due to in utero malpositioning. However, lateral tibial torsion has not been shown to be related to in utero position.

Ref:
Staheli LT (4th ed.) (2007). *Fundamentals of Pediatric Orthopaedics*, Lippincott Williams & Wilkins, Philadelphia.


54.    **B**
Clubfoot is the most common congenital orthopaedic condition requiring treatment. The incidence is around 1 to 2 in 1000 live births.

Ref:
Herring JA (4th Ed) (2008). *Tachdjian's Pediatric Orthopaedics*, Saunders, Philadelphia.

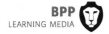

**55.** **D**

Development of the tibio-femoral angle with growth has been extensively documented by several investigators (Heath and Staheli, Salenius). Normal children typically display maximal varus at 6 to 12 months of age and neutral alignment by 18–24 months. Maximum valgus angle is usually achieved around the age of 4 years thereafter a gradual decrease in the angle to adult alignment occurs up to the age of 11 years. Generally varus alignment persisting after the age of 2 years is regarded as abnormal and merits further investigation although some children may be slightly late in the transition from varus to valgus alignment.

Ref:

Heath CH, Staheli LT. Normal limits of knee angle in white children-genu varum and genu valgum. *Journal of Pediatric Orthopaedics* 1993; 13: 259.

**56.** **E**

Bilateral pes cavus deformity may occur within the spectrum of normality. However, it is essential to exclude neuromuscular disorders which give rise to this deformity as it may be the first presentation of serious disease or may be associated with a genetically transmissible condition. The important causes can be grouped according to the site of pathology:

- Neuromuscular disorders
  - Muscular dystrophy
  - Charcot Marie Tooth disease
  - Friedriech's ataxia
  - Roussy-Levy syndrome
- Central nervous system disorders
  - Cerebral palsy
  - Poliomyelitis
- Spinal pathology
  - Spinal dysraphism
  - Diastematomyelia
  - Spina bifida
  - Myelomeningocele
  - Syringomyelia
  - Spinal cord tumour
- Muscle pathology
  - Crush injury
  - Burns
  - Compartment syndrome

Thus, it is essential to exclude the serious causes which may have an occult presentation such as spinal pathology or a neuromuscular condition. This is best done by undertaking magnetic resonance imaging of the spine as well as nerve conduction studies and electromyography. Genetic studies may be indicated if the results of the above investigations suggest a transmissible cause such as hereditary sensorimotor neuropathy although these are not indicated as a primary investigation.

Ref:

Staheli LT (4th ed.) (2007). *Fundamentals of Pediatric Orthopaedics*, Lippincott Williams & Wilkins, Philadelphia.

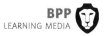

57. **D**

Infantile tibia vara is commonly referred to as Blount's disease (Blount, 1937); although in fact the condition was described much earlier by Erlacher in 1922. The condition is generally regarded as a developmental rather than congenital disorder as the characteristic radiographic features have not been observed for children younger than 17 months of age. Thus is can be very difficult to differentiate from physiologic bowing and the importance of follow up in this regard cannot be understated. The patients are frequently above the 95th centile for body weight suggesting that the growth disturbance may relate to compressive forces. Radiographs are essential to establishing the diagnosis. However, normal radiographs do not exclude the condition. The characteristic radiographic changes are:

- Sharp varus angulation of the metaphysic
- Medial physis widened and irregular
- Medially sloped epiphysis with irregular calcification
- Medial metaphysis beaking

Many different geometric measurements from radiographs have been used to grade and predict progression of the disease process. These include the metaphyseal-diaphyseal angle (Levine and Drennan) and the epiphyseal-metaphyseal angle. However, such measurements have been shown to be influenced by limb rotation on X-ray limiting their potential usefulness.

Langenskiold (1952) classified the radiographic changes seen in infantile tibia vara into six progressive stages with prognostic implications. Although its application for descriptive purposes allows comparison between different cases, subsequent studies have shown that recurrence can occur despite treatment in the early stages and that certain demographic groups, in particular non- Caucasian groups, can manifest more progressive disease with poorer outcomes, than that predicted by this classification. Earlier treatment has a better prognosis. Surgical treatment should ideally be undertaken before 4 years of age and should involve overcorrection of the mechanical axis to valgus alignment with lateral translation of the distal osteotomy fragment.

Ref:
Herring JA (4th ed.) (2008). *Tachdjian's Pediatric Orthopaedics*, Saunders, Philadelphia.

58. **E**

Valgus alignment is common between the ages of 2 to 8 years with the peak occurring between 2 to 4 years. After the age of 8, there is very little change in alignment. Idiopathic genu valgum is thought to exist at the extreme of the spectrum of normality and may give rise to knee problems, awkward gait and difficulty in running. Corrective surgery is usually undertaken after the age of 8 and is achieved through hemi-epiphyseodesis procedures which may be temporary (using staples) or permanent. Other causes of genu valgum include:

- Post-traumatic – post proximal tibial fracture
- Renal osteodystrophy – renal failure through acquired causes frequently leads to metabolic bone disease during the years of valgus alignment. This is in contrast to infantile rickets where the metabolic bone effects take place during the period when physiologic varus exists.
- Spondyloepiphyseal dysplasia/metaphyseal dysplasia

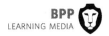

- Multiple hereditary exostoses
- Fibrous dysplasia

Ref:
Herring JA (4<sup>th</sup> ed.) (2008). *Tachdjian's Pediatric Orthopaedics*, Saunders, Philadelphia.

**59.  C**

Version describes a normal variation in limb rotation which is defined as within 2 standard deviations of the mean rotation in that particular age group. Torsion describes a deformity and is classed as abnormal limb rotation greater than 2 standard deviations from the mean rotation in the age group of the child. With respect to the tibia, outward or lateral rotation occurs with development. In utero, the medial malleolus lies posterior to the lateral malleolus. The malleoli are almost level in the coronal plane at birth and by the time walking age is reached the medial malleolus is in front of the lateral.

Ref:
Staheli LT (4<sup>th</sup> ed.) (2007). *Fundamentals of Pediatric Orthopaedics*, Lippincott Williams & Wilkins, Philadelphia.

**60.  D**

Tibial torsion is the most common lower limb rotational abnormality producing an intoeing or out-toeing gait up to the age of 3–4 years. After this age, the rotational profile of the femur assumes dominance in determining gait. A torsion profile should include examination of the hips, femora, tibia and feet.

Most newborns demonstrate out-toeing due to lateral hip contracture which resolves during early infancy. Medial tibial torsion is therefore not usually evident until about 1 year of age when the infant first starts to walk. Parents may assume the affected side is the normal one and the foot that demonstrates out-toeing is the abnormal side.

As the tibia develop, they rotate laterally and most cases of medial tibial torsion resolve without treatment. Bracing has been shown to be ineffective and possibly harmful to the maturing lower limb joints. Surgery is only indicated if there is a significant cosmetic defect or problems relating to function such as fatigue due to muscles acting through abnormal lever arms. Such cases of persistent deformity causing symptoms are quite rare. As the condition demonstrates progressive improvement with time, surgery is never considered before the age of 8 years.

Rotational tibial osteotomies are best performed in the supramalleolar region as proximal tibial osteotomies carry risks of iatrogenic common peroneal nerve injury, compartment syndrome and possible deleterious effects on the proximal tibial growth plate.

Ref:
Herring JA (4<sup>th</sup> ed.) (2008). *Tachdjian's Pediatric Orthopaedics*, Saunders, Philadelphia.

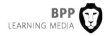

**61.   E**

Anterolateral tibia bowing is usually associated with formation of a pseudoarthrosis and has a more unfavourable natural history in comparison to posteromedial bowing. The condition is associated with both neurofibromatosis, fibrous dysplasia and more rarely, amniotic band syndrome. The diagnosis is usually made at birth with an anterolateral prominence of the tibia which in the vast majority of cases is unilateral. A pseudoarthrosis may also be evident at this time due to abnormal motion at the site of deformity. Once a fracture has occurred, the likelihood of spontaneous healing is low especially if the fracture occurs before walking age. Many surgical treatments have been advocated to correct the deformity and fuse the pseudoarthrosis site with varying success. These include resection of the pseudoarthrosis and intramedullary fixation, vascularised fibula grafting and distraction osteogenesis with a circular frame.

Ref:
Herring JA (4th ed.) (2008). *Tachdjian's Pediatric Orthopaedics*, Saunders, Philadelphia.

**62.   C**

Posteromedial bowing, unlike anterolateral bowing, follows quite a benign course with spontaneous resolution over time. The appearance at birth may be quite dramatic with up to 60 degrees of angulation but the deformity usually resolves within 2 years. The condition is not associated with dysplasia or deformity elsewhere and is highly likely to be due to a packaging disorder. Treatment is usually directed at stretching the deformity and in more severe cases; serial casting and splintage may be employed. Rarely, corrective osteotomy has to be undertaken for severe deformities persisting after growth has begun to tail off around 3–4 years of age. The main concern is an eventual limb length disparity which is usually managed by contralateral epiphysiodesis.

Ref:
Herring JA (4th ed.) (2008). *Tachdjian's Pediatric Orthopaedics*, Saunders, Philadelphia.

**63.   D**

The talus, calcaneus, cuboid, metatarsals and phalanges are all ossified at birth. The lateral cuneiform usually ossifies between 4 and 20 months, the intermediate cuneiform at 3 years and the medial cuneiform around 2 years. The navicular is usually the last to ossify somewhere between 2–5 years.

Ref:
Herring JA (4th ed.) (2008). *Tachdjian's Pediatric Orthopaedics*, Saunders, Philadelphia.

**64.   B**

Kohler's disease, described in 1908, is a benign osteochondritis of the navicular. The precise aetiology is not understood but may relate to avascular necrosis due to mechanical compression in a tarsal bone made vulnerable by its late ossification compared to its neighbours. The disorder is usually more common in boys than girls and it is theorised that this is due to the later ossification of the tarsal navicular in boys. Symptoms usually include pain in the midfoot and a painful gait although some studies have shown up to a fifth of cases to be asymptomatic. The condition usually spontaneously resolves and treatment is directed at symptomatic relief and walking casts have been shown to be beneficial in this regard.

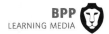

Ref:
Herring JA (4<sup>th</sup> ed.) (2008). *Tachdjian's Pediatric Orthopaedics*, Saunders, Philadelphia.

**65.   D**

Freiberg's infarction is most common in the head of the second metatarsal although other metatarsals may be involved. The condition is more common in girls and usually presents after 13 years of age. Conventional radiographs are usually all that is required to establish the diagnosis with characteristic findings of lucency and collapse. Bone sans also reveal increased uptake at the involved site. All cases should initially be managed conservatively with a walking cast or a shoe with a metatarsal bar. Surgery is usually reserved for refractory cases as the resection of the head or shortening of the affected metatarsal may leave residual symptoms.

Ref:
Herring JA (4<sup>th</sup> ed.) (2008). *Tachdjian's Pediatric Orthopaedics*, Saunders, Philadelphia.

**66.   E**

The terms metatarsus adductus and metatarsus varus are frequently used interchangeably although some describe a distinction with adductus describing a flexible deformity whereas the varus condition has a rigid deformity. Kite described 6 characteristic features:

- Spontaneous active medial deviation of the foot by the child.
- High arch
- Concave medial border of the foot
- Separation of the first and second toes
- Fixed adductus of the forefoot when the hind foot is in neutral
- Bean shaped sole of the foot.

The hind foot is always in valgus and dorsiflexes easily. The condition is thought to be a packaging disorder due to in utero malposition. Most mild deformities correct spontaneously although serial casting may be used if the deformity is not passively correctible. Surgery is indicated in refractory cases and usually takes the form of soft tissue releases with osteotomies advocated for children older than 3 years.

Ref:
Herring JA (4<sup>th</sup> ed.) (2008). *Tachdjian's Pediatric Orthopaedics*, Saunders, Philadelphia.

**67.   D**

Talipes calcaneovalgus is a packaging disorder and examination of these patients should include the hip to rule out dysplasia especially if a contralateral metatarsus adductus is present. The condition is differentiated from the more pathologic vertical talus by the heel being in valgus rather than equinus as both conditions involve dorsiflexion of the forefoot. Spontaneous resolution is the norm with serial casting reserved for severe cases.

Ref:
Herring JA (4<sup>th</sup> ed.) (2008). *Tachdjian's Pediatric Orthopaedics*, Saunders, Philadelphia.

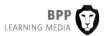

68.  **A**

Skewfoot or serpentine deformity resembles metatarsus adductus in that there is forefoot varus. However, the equinus element tends to be more rigid and there is associated lateral subluxation of the navicular on the talus producing the characteristic 'S' shaped deformity. The condition cannot be discretely categorised as there are elements of both flatfoot and metatarsus adductus present to a varying degree. Indeed, skewfoot can be considered within the spectrum of these conditions depending on the prevailing deformity. Treatment frequently consists of stretching and serial casting to convert the deformity into flatfoot. However, more rigid deformities may require surgical intervention.

Ref:

Herring JA (4th ed.) (2008). *Tachdjian's Pediatric Orthopaedics*, Saunders, Philadelphia.

69.  **B**

Talipes equinovarus occurs in conjunction with several neuromuscular diseases and syndromes such as arthrogryposis, Freeman-Sheldon syndrome, Mobius syndrome and Down syndrome. The condition is known to be present in utero very early on during development and is thus not a **true** packaging disorder. However, a mild postural variant which is easily correctible may be as a result of in utero positioning. Unlike DDH the condition is very prone to recurrence despite seeming resolution with early satisfactory treatment. Successful treatment does not produce a foot identical to the unaffected side with the affected foot usually shorter with some residual deformity although the functional results are usually excellent.

Imaging studies have shown varying amounts of dysplasia of the tarsal bones. The talus usually has a short, medially and plantarward directed neck with the navicular and cuboid displaced medially at their mid foot articulations. This produces the characteristic mid foot abduction. The talus and calcaneum are parallel in all three planes due to plantar and medial rotation of the calcaneum producing hind foot varus. The metatarsals like the navicular are also deviated medially and plantarward producing a cavus deformity. Finally triceps shortening and posterior capsule contracture produce ankle equinus.

Ref:

Herring JA (4th ed.) (2008). *Tachdjian's Pediatric Orthopaedics*, Saunders, Philadelphia.

70.  **B**

There are two classification systems commonly used to track progression with treatment in clubfeet. The Pirani classification is a numeric score based on 6 features which are scored on 3 levels as normal (0), moderately abnormal (0.5) or severely abnormal (1). The 6 features are broken down into 3 midfoot features and 3 hindfoot features:

Midfoot – medial crease, lateral border, talar head overage

Hind foot – posterior crease, heel configuration, equinus rigidity

An alternative classification was proposed by Dimeglio. Four major components of clubfoot are identified:

1.  Equinus
2.  Heel varus
3.  Medial rotation of calcaneopedal 'block'
4.  Forefoot adductus

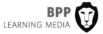

Each of these is graded clinically from 1 (most mild) to 4 (most severe). Four other parameters are also scored on points:

1.    Posterior crease
2.    Medial crease
3.    Cavus
4.    Poor muscle condition

The total numeric score is broadly stratified into 4 groups of severity from benign to very severe.

Ref:
Herring JA (4<sup>th</sup> ed.) (2008). *Tachdjian's Pediatric Orthopaedics*, Saunders, Philadelphia.

**71.    B**

The Ponseti regime has revolutionised the treatment of clubfeet and has led to initial conservative management in almost all cases. Although the likelihood of complete correction is higher if treatment is commenced within the first month of life, it can still be used in infants up to the age of 9 months. The regime involves serial casting with or without percutaneous tendo Achilles lengthening and tibialis anterior transfer. The order of deformity correction is best memorised by the mnemonic CAVE – cavus, adductus, varus then equinus. Serial, above knee casts, are applied after every manipulation. The cavus deformity is first corrected by supinating the forefoot to bring it into alignment with the hind foot. Lateral pressure over the talar head while abducting the foot corrects the forefoot adductus as well as the heel varus. The equinus component is the last element of the deformity to be addressed and may require percutaneous heel tenotomy. After the deformity is fully corrected, the child needs to wear a foot abduction orthosis consisting of two straight shoes connected by a bar and separated the distance of the child's shoulder width. The shoes are held at 70 degrees of external rotation and 5 to 10 degrees of dorsiflexion. In unilateral cases, the unaffected foot is placed in 40 degrees of external rotation. The orthosis needs to be worn full time for the first 3 to 4 months then at night time for at least 2 to 4 years.

Ref:
Herring JA (4<sup>th</sup> ed.) (2008). *Tachdjian's Paediatric Orthopedics*, Saunders, Philadelphia.

**72.    B**

Long-term studies have shown that recurrence may occur in up to one third of patients after seemingly successful treatment with the Ponseti regime. Many cases can be ascribed to early discontinuation of the abduction foot orthosis. Early recurrence can be successfully salvaged with repeat serial casting and manipulation and many would advocate this strategy even in older infants to correct as much of the deformity as possible without surgery. Untreated clubfeet with evidence of weight bearing on the outer aspect of the feet and fixed deformity is likely to require surgical correction. Contracted tissues will need to be released including tendo Achilles lengthening and posterior capsulotomy of the ankle and subtalar joints.

Ref:
Herring JA (4<sup>th</sup> ed.) (2008). *Tachdjian's Pediatric Orthopaedics*, Saunders, Philadelphia.

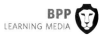

73. **E**

DDH is a very common condition in paediatric orthopaedic clinics and describes a spectrum of hip abnormalities from mildly dysplastic acetabulum to complete dislocation. Family history has shown to confer a significant risk although the condition is assumed to have polygenic inheritance. The important associations are;

- Female sex
- Breech presentation
- Family history of affected relatives
- Teratology features in other joints eg knee dislocation
- Postural moulding/Intrauterine constraint
- Torticollis
- Metatarsus adductus
- Calcaneovalgus

Ref:
Staheli LT (4th ed.) (2007). *Fundamentals of Pediatric Orthopaedics*, Lippincott Williams & Wilkins, Philadelphia.

74. **C**

The pathology in DDH affects both the acetabulum and proximal femur. The former tends to display a valgus neck with increased anteversion whereas the acetabulum is usually shallow and maldirected. If the hip is dislocated, several structures can become interposed and block reduction attempts:

- Iliopsoas/adductor longus – these cause a capsular constriction which gives rise to the hourglass appearance on contrast arthrography of the joint. These structures need to be divided if they are interposed.
- Inverted limbus – this should be extruded rather than excised during open reduction as it remodels to form the labrum
- The transverse acetabular ligament and pulvinar fat may limit the size of the acetabulum and should be removed
- The ligamentum teres is frequently hypertrophied and due to its negligible contribution to femoral head blood supply can be excised.

Ref:
Staheli LT (4th ed.) (2007). *Fundamentals of Pediatric Orthopaedics*, Lippincott Williams & Wilkins, Philadelphia.

75. **E**

Ultrasound assessment of the paediatric hip is good for screening before the ossific nucleus develops but is highly operator dependent. It is frequently used to screen the hip at risk in infants with known associations as well as evaluating the effectiveness of treatment. It can be used in the first 4–6 weeks of life but the elevated levels of circulating maternal relaxin at this time can give rise to a high number of false positive results. The Graf grading of acetabular dysplasia in DDH looks at two angles on ultrasound of the hip. The α angle is most commonly cited and is the angle between the iliac crest margin and the joint inclination. There are four grades described ranging from normal (α angle greater than 60 degrees) to severely abnormal (α angle 0 degrees).

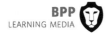

Ref:
Staheli LT (4<sup>th</sup> ed.) (2007). *Fundamentals of Pediatric Orthopaedics*, Lippincott Williams & Wilkins, Philadelphia.

76. **D**

From birth to 6 months of age, if DDH is picked up, initial management should assess if a reduction is achieved and held in a Pavlik harness. If this is the case and the hip is still reduced at 3 to 4 weeks a further period of 3–4 weeks in the harness is prescribed to make the hip more stable and then continued at night time until the radiographic findings are normal. If the hip is unreduced after 3–4 weeks of treatment, then the use of the Pavlik harness should be discontinued as ongoing splintage is likely to deform the femoral head. The hips should be examined under anaesthetic with contrast arthrography and if closed reduction is feasible this should be performed and a hip spica applied. If this is not achievable then open reduction is mandatory.

Ref:
Staheli LT (4<sup>th</sup> ed.) (2007). *Fundamentals of Pediatric Orthopaedics*, Lippincott Williams & Wilkins, Philadelphia.

77. **E**

Initial treatment in a Pavlik harness for DDH is both safe and effective if ultrasound demonstrates the hip to be concentrically reduced in this position. Treatment is usually successful in 90 to 95% of patients although parents need to be advised that if the hip is unreduced after a trial of splintage, that further treatment in the harness is unlikely to be effective. Complications are infrequent and are usually the result of mistakes in applying the harness. Avascular necrosis, skin rashes, femoral nerve palsy, brachial plexopathy, skin rashes and foot deformities have all been reported as occasional complications.

Ref:
Staheli LT (4<sup>th</sup> ed.) (2007). *Fundamentals of Pediatric Orthopaedics*, Lippincott Williams & Wilkins, Philadelphia.

78. **B**

Avascular necrosis is a devastating complication following reduction attempts in developmental hip dysplasia. The radiographic features suggesting its occurrence are

- Failure of ossific nucleus to appear in the first year of life
- Failure of ossific nucleus growth
- Fragmentation of the ossific nucleus
- Widening of the neck

The condition has been classified into different types based on severity by Kalanchi and MacEwen (1980).

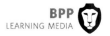

Type I – irregular ossification with no physeal bridges or deformity – usually spontaneously resolves

Type II – lateral physeal bridge occurring towards the end of growth that may cause tethering and eccentricity of the growth plate – usually treated with trochanteric transfer distally and laterally in adolescence to minimise impingement

Type III – uncommonly a medial bridge may form leading to shortening of the medial aspect of the neck and a vertical physis – treatment is to prevent abduction of the greater trochanter in abduction through transfer osteotomy

Type IV – the most severe, characterised by a central bridge with complete growth arrest and trochanteric overgrowth – trochanteric osteotomy and transfer will reduce impingement but the limb length disparity frequently requires contralateral distal femoral epiphysiodesis.

Key preventable causes of AVN are:

- Avoidance of over abducted or forced positions
- Avoidance of preliminary traction
- Care in surgical approach in open reduction
- Removal of all interposed tissues to make space to accommodate femoral head.

Ref:
Staheli LT (4th ed.) (2007). *Fundamentals of Paediatric Orthopaedics*, Lippincott Williams & Wilkins, Philadelphia.

79. **A**
Pelvic osteotomies to improve femoral head cover in DDH can be considered as two principal varieties – those which aim to reconstruct the acetabulum and utilise articular cartilage in the weight bearing surface, and those which are principally salvage procedures using fibrocartilage in the articulation (which is prone to degenerate over time).

**Reconstructive osteotomies:**

Salter – osteotomy above acetabulum which is hinged laterally and anteriorly to improve coverage and wedged open with a bone graft wedge transfixed with pins

Dega – posterior osteotomy giving posterior and lateral coverage, usually utilised in neurodysplasia

Triple – utilised in adolescence, acetabulum can be freely rotated and fixed, usually used in spherical congruity with moderate dysplasia

Pemberton – peri-acetabular osteotomy which hinges on tri-radiate cartilage, consequently alters acetabular shape and can be used in more severe dysplasia in younger patients

Ganz – technically challenging peri-acetabular osteotomy which can be done after skeletal maturity

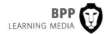

**Salvage osetotomies:**
Chiari – transverse osteotomy through ilium allowing medialisation of lateralised femoral heads
Shelf – tricortical iliac crest graft used to augment lateral acetabulum

Ref:
Staheli LT (4th ed.) (2007). *Fundamentals of Paediatric Orthopaedics*, Lippincott Williams & Wilkins, Philadelphia.

80. **B**
Juvenile idiopathic avascular necrosis (AVN) of the femoral head is known as Perthes' disease. The differentials for this condition include all other causes for femoral head AVN:

Haematological – sickle cell disease, haemophilia, lupus, protein C and S deficiencies
Infection – septic arthritis, femoral osteomyelitis
Metabolic – hypothyroidism
Trauma – slipped upper femoral epiphysis, femoral neck fracture
Tumours – lymphoma

Occasionally, a radiograph reveals bilateral synchronous AVN which can never be Perthes disease as although 10–15% of cases are bilateral the disease process is never symmetrical. In these instances, syndromes should be suspected such as:

- Gaucher's disease
- Mucopolysaccharidoses
- Multiple epiphyseal dysplasia
- Spondylo-epiphyseal dysplasia

Ref:
Staheli LT (4th ed.) (2007). *Fundamentals of Pediatric Orthopaedics*, Lippincott Williams & Wilkins, Philadelphia.

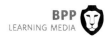

# Adult Pathology

## Hip: Question Bank

Fahad G Attar & Talal Ibrahim

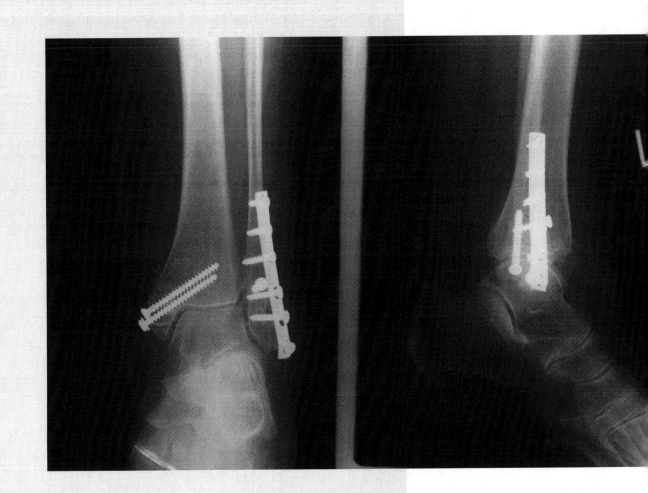

1.  The nerve most commonly injured during total hip arthroplasty is:
    A.  Femoral nerve
    B.  Obturator nerve
    C.  Sciatic nerve
    D.  Superior gluteal nerve
    E.  Lateral cutaneous nerve of thigh

2.  All of the following are recognised risk factors for the development of osteonecrosis of the hip except:
    A.  Caisson disease
    B.  Trauma
    C.  Corticosteroid use
    D.  Haemophilia A
    E.  Alcohol abuse

3.  The following factors all reduce the risk of dislocation following total hip arthroplasty except:
    A.  Elevated rim liners
    B.  Increased head to neck ratio
    C.  Cup abduction angle of 40 degrees ± 10 degrees
    D.  Constrained components
    E.  Reducing offset

4.  The following are all components of third generation cementing technique except:
    A.  Retrograde canal filling
    B.  Pressurised mixing of cement
    C.  Distal canal plug
    D.  Thorough cleaning of femoral canal
    E.  Vacuum mixing of cement

5.  A 67-year-old man presents with pyrexia of 38 degrees and 2 week history of increasing pain in the right hip. He had undergone a successful right total hip arthroplasty 2 years previously, which was functioning well. He gives a history of recent dental extraction. Blood tests reveal a CRP of 198 and WCC of 12.8. A plain radiograph shows a well fixed implant. Hip aspiration under aseptic conditions resulted in purulent material being obtained. The next step in management is:
    A.  Thorough debridement with retention of prosthesis
    B.  Two stage revision right THR
    C.  Indium-111 labelled leucocyte scan
    D.  One stage revision right THR
    E.  Parenteral antibiotic therapy

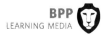

6. Risk factors for the development of heterotopic ossification following hip arthroplasty include all of the following except:
   A. Male sex
   B. Bilateral hypertrophic osteoarthritis of hips
   C. Posterior approach
   D. Ankylosing spondylitis
   E. Pagets

7. Patients presenting with meralgia paraesthetica are most likely to have:
   A. Positive straight leg test
   B. Bilateral symptoms in the majority of cases
   C. A positive Tinel's sign 1cm medial and inferior to the anterior superior iliac spine
   D. Weakness of hip abductors
   E. Symptoms are relieved by hip extension

8. The predominant cause of squeaking following ceramic on ceramic hip arthroplasty is:
   A. Edge loading with resultant stripe wear
   B. Acetabular liner fracture
   C. Excess boundary lubrication occurring
   D. Damage to the ceramic head during reduction
   E. Loosening of the implants

9. During total hip arthroplasty, excessive retroversion of the acetabular component will result in which of the following?
   A. Posterior impingement of the components
   B. Increased risk of dislocation when flexing hip
   C. Increased leg length
   D. Limitation of hip extension
   E. Cup lateralisation

10. The C-reactive protein level following total hip arthroplasty takes how long to fall back to normal pre-operative levels?
    A. 3 days
    B. 1 week
    C. 2 weeks
    D. 6 weeks
    E. 6 months

11. The anterior approach to the hip joint utilises the interval between which two muscles?
    A. Gluteus medius and tensor fascia latae
    B. Gluteus minimus and sartorius
    C. Rectus femoris and tensor fascia latae
    D. Tensor fascia latae and sartorius
    E. Rectus femoris and iliopsoas

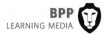

12.   The recommended optimal position for hip arthrodesis is:
    A.   20–30 degrees flexion, 5 degrees of adduction and 5–10 degrees external rotation
    B.   20–30 degrees flexion, 5 degrees abduction and neutral rotation
    C.   10 degrees flexion, 10 degrees adduction and 10 degrees internal rotation
    D.   40 degrees flexion, 10 degrees abduction and 10 degrees internal rotation
    E.   40 degrees flexion, 20 degrees adduction and 20 degrees external rotation

13.   A 19-year-old male presents with gradual onset of activity related pain in the left groin. All of the following are consistent with a diagnosis of protrusio acetabuli except:
    A.   Centre edge angle of Wiberg of 45 degrees
    B.   Medial wall of acetabulum protruding 4mm medial to ilioischial line
    C.   Reduction in hip abduction
    D.   Increased head-neck offset
    E.   Positive Trendelenburg sign

14.   Wear particle analysis from metal on polyethylene bearing surfaces in total hip arthroplasty have shown that the size of wear particle implicated in osteolysis is:
    A.   $<1\mu m$
    B.   $5–10\mu m$
    C.   $10–20\mu m$
    D.   $>20\mu m$
    E.   $>100\mu m$

15.   Which of the following bearing surfaces have been shown to have the lowest wear rate?
    A.   Ceramic on polyethylene
    B.   Cobalt chrome on polyethylene
    C.   Cobalt chrome on highly cross-linked polyethylene
    D.   Ceramic on ceramic
    E.   Cobalt chrome on cobalt chrome

16.   Which structure is most at risk during total hip arthroplasty when attempting restoration of a normal hip centre in a high dislocation following developmental dysplasia of the hip?
    A.   Rectus femoris
    B.   Femoral nerve
    C.   Femoral artery
    D.   Sciatic nerve
    E.   Iliopsoas tendon

17.   During surgical dislocation of the hip to treat femoroacetabular impingement, the preservation of which vessel is crucial to preserve the blood supply to the femoral head?
    A.   Ascending branch of lateral femoral circumflex artery
    B.   Descending branch of lateral femoral circumflex artery
    C.   Deep branch of medial femoral circumflex artery
    D.   Transverse branch of lateral femoral circumflex artery
    E.   Superficial branch of medial femoral circumflex artery

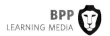

18.  A 43-year-old lady presents with a 6-month history of pain in the left groin worse after prolonged sitting and walking. She is a keen runner and is unable to run due to the pain. She is otherwise fit and well. On examination pain is reproduced on flexion of the hip to 90 degrees and adduction and internal rotation. Plain radiographs including a cross-table lateral radiograph show signs of acetabular retroversion. What is the next step in management?
     A.  Diagnostic hip injection with 0.5% bupivacaine
     B.  MRI scan
     C.  Physiotherapy
     D.  MRI arthrogram
     E.  Observation alone

19.  When performing total hip arthroplasty through a posterior approach, what is the recommended orientation of the acetabular component?
     A.  Anteverted 10–20 degrees
     B.  Abduction angle >50 degrees
     C.  Anteverted 20–40 degrees
     D.  Abduction angle <30 degrees
     E.  Retroverted 5–10 degrees

20.  The most frequent complication after fibular vascularised graft harvesting for treating osteonecrosis of femoral head is:
     A.  Sensory deficit
     B.  Motor weakness
     C.  Deep vein thrombosis
     D.  Superficial wound infection
     E.  Contracture of flexor hallucis longus

21.  During primary hip arthroplasty, fixation of the acetabular component with screws placed in the anterosuperior quadrant puts which structure at risk?
     A.  Sciatic nerve
     B.  External iliac vein
     C.  Femoral nerve
     D.  Obturator vein
     E.  Internal iliac artery

22.  Following metal on metal hip resurfacing arthroplasty, which of the following is known to lead to an increase in the serum concentration of metal ions?
     A.  Increased activity level of patient
     B.  Abduction angle of >55 degrees for the acetabular component
     C.  Larger size of components
     D.  Increased offset
     E.  Male sex

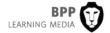

23. Hip arthroscopy is contraindicated in which of the following situations:
    A. Femoroacetabular impingement
    B. Stage 2 osteoarthritis
    C. Protrusio acetabuli
    D. Concurrent disc prolapse
    E. Inflammatory arthropathy

24. Which of the following is an absolute contraindication to simultaneous single stage bilateral total hip arthroplasty?
    A. Contralateral hip contracture
    B. Atrial septal defect
    C. Myocardial infarction 1 year prior to operation
    D. Past history of deep vein thrombosis
    E. Rheumatoid arthritis

25. A 62-year-old man undergoes an uncemented total hip arthroplasty using a porous coated femoral stem. Six months later he complains of increasing thigh pain. He has no constitutional symptoms and has a C-reactive protein level <10. Which of the following radiographic signs would indicate an unstable fixation of the femoral component?
    A. Progressive implant migration >2mm
    B. Absence of reactive lines around the porous portion of stem
    C. Presence of 'spot welds' of trabecular bone from the host to prosthesis
    D. Calcar atrophy
    E. Absence of progressive radiolucencies

26. Which of the following factors has been shown to be the single most effective method in reducing the rate of post-operative deep wound infection following total hip arthroplasty?
    A. Use of prophylactic intravenous antibiotics
    B. Limiting the number of operating room personnel
    C. Laminar air flow
    D. Use of iodophor impregnated adhesive plastic drape
    E. Whole body exhaust suits for surgeon and assistant

27. A 74-year-old man undergoes a cemented total hip arthroplasty using a metal on polyethylene bearing. The use of a high offset femoral component compared to one with a lower offset will result in which one of the following?
    A. Increased linear wear rate of the polyethylene
    B. Decreased gait efficiency
    C. Increased risk of dislocation
    D. Decreased linear wear rate of polyethylene
    E. Trendelenburg gait

28. All of the following factors can increase the femoral offset except:
    A. Increasing neck length
    B. Decreasing neck-shaft angle
    C. Trochanteric advancement
    D. Placing the femoral component in a valgus position relative to the femoral shaft
    E. Using a lateralised acetabular liner

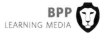

29. A 78-year-old lady presents with a 6-month history of increasing pain in her left hip. She underwent a successful total hip arthroplasty 12 years previously. She is not a diabetic and has no constitutional symptoms. Plain radiographs show progressive radiolucencies around both the acetabular and femoral components. Which of the following investigations will most reliably exclude infection as a cause of her symptoms?
   A. Technitium 99m bone scan
   B. Aspiration of hip
   C. CRP and ESR levels
   D. Indium 111 labelled white blood cell scan
   E. White cell count

30. A 62-year-old lady who has a known history of metastatic breast cancer presents with pain in her right hip. Radiographs show a lytic lesion in the femoral neck occupying 50% of the diameter of the femoral neck. The pain is described by the patient as a dull ache and is 3/10 on a visual analogue scale. What is the Mirels' score for assessing the risk of pathological fracture in this case?
   A. 5
   B. 7
   C. 9
   D. 11
   E. 12

31. A 73-year-old lady presents with a pathological fracture of the right proximal femur. She is known to have metastatic breast carcinoma. The fracture is in the basicervical region of the femoral neck and is minimally displaced. Whole length femoral radiographs do not show any other distal lesions. What is the best form of fixation for this type of fracture?
   A. Dynamic hip screw
   B. Long stem cephalomedullary nailing
   C. Standard total hip replacement
   D. Long stem total hip replacement
   E. Dynamic condylar screw

32. Which of the following structures is most likely to be injured during anterior portal placement for hip arthroscopy?
   A. Femoral artery
   B. Ascending branch of lateral femoral circumflex artery
   C. Lateral femoral cutaneous nerve
   D. Superior gluteal nerve
   E. Femoral nerve

33. The use of a constrained acetabular component for recurrent dislocation following total hip arthroplasty is indicated in which of the following cases?
   A. Impingement of femoral head against an elevated rim acetabular liner
   B. Acute avulsion of the greater trochanter
   C. Soft tissue laxity around hip
   D. Abductor muscle insufficiency
   E. Segmental acetabular bone defect

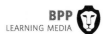

34. Which of the following is a contraindication to the use of constrained components in revision total hip arthroplasty for recurrent dislocation?
    A. Large acetabular bone defect
    B. Rheumatoid arthritis
    C. Abductor muscle insufficiency
    D. Recurrent dislocation in well positioned implants
    E. Significant leg length discrepancy

35. A 57-year-old lady presents with left groin, buttock and thigh pain of 6 months duration. The pain is worse with activity. She has some mechanical low back pain and paraesthesia in the big toe on the left side. Lumbar spine extension causes significant back pain. There is no neurological deficit in the legs, but movements of the left hip particularly rotations are restricted and painful. X-rays of the left hip show evidence of superior joint space narrowing and the presence of osteophytes. What is the next step to elucidate the cause of the pain?
    A. Plain X-rays of lumbar spine
    B. Diagnostic hip injection
    C. Root canal injection
    D. MRI scan of lumbar spine
    E. Bone scan

36. A 62-year-old man is reviewed 6 weeks following a left uncemented ceramic on polyethylene total hip replacement. On examination he has a Trendelenburg positive gait. Which of the following is least likely to explain this finding?
    A. Loss of normal femoral offset
    B. Lengthening of femoral neck
    C. Superior gluteal nerve palsy
    D. Intra-operative trochanteric fracture
    E. Detachment of hip abductors

37. Which of the following drugs has been shown to be of benefit in patients with early stage (Ficat 1 and 2) idiopathic osteonecrosis of femoral head?
    A. Statins
    B. Bisphosphonates
    C. Aspirin
    D. Non-steroidal anti-inflammatory drugs (NSAIDs)
    E. Calcium antagonists

38. What is the commonest complication after traumatic dislocation of the native hip?
    A. Sciatic nerve palsy
    B. Myositis ossificans
    C. Avascular necrosis
    D. Redislocation
    E. Osteoarthritis

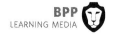

39. A 43-year-old man has sustained a traumatic posterior dislocation of the right hip after being involved in a road traffic accident. The hip has been reduced closed and CT scanning confirms fracture of the femoral head above the fovea and the presence of a large fragment of femoral head lying in the acetabulum (Pipkin type II). Open reduction and fracture fixation is planned through an anterior Smith-Peterson approach. Which of the following complications is more likely following this approach compared to a posterior approach?
    A. Inability to retrieve femoral head fragments
    B. Heterotopic ossification
    C. Avascular necrosis
    D. Redislocation
    E. Sciatic nerve injury

40. A 37-year-old man undergoes a varus osteotomy of the right hip to treat osteonecrosis of the femoral head. Which one of the following effects is seen after a varus osteotomy of the femur?
    A. Lengthening of the leg
    B. Reduced femoral offset
    C. Reduced joint reaction force
    D. Increased abductor force
    E. Displacement of joint reaction force laterally

BPP
LEARNING MEDIA

# Adult Pathology

## Hip: Answers

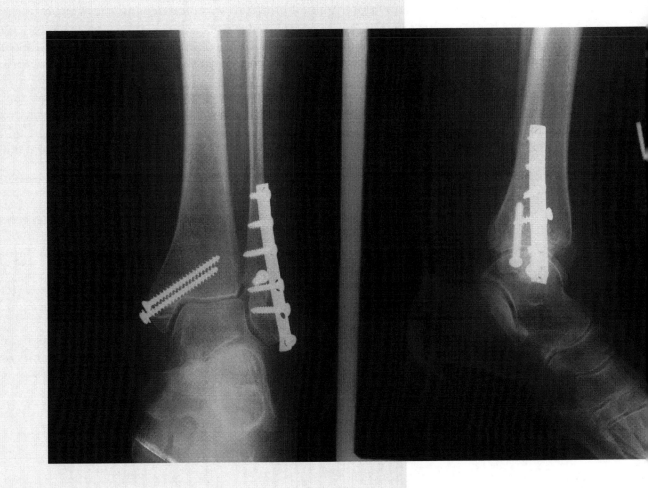

1.  **C**

    In the study by Schmalzried *et al.* 3,000 cases of total hip replacement, 53 nerve injuries occurred of which over 90% involved the sciatic nerve. Higher incidence in revisions (3–8%) possibly due to scarring and in DDH (5.8%) due to lengthening. In uncomplicated THR, the rate is quoted to be less than 1%. The peroneal division is more susceptible to injury than the tibial division.

    Ref:

    Schmalzried TP, Amstutz HC, Dorey FJ: (1991) Nerve palsy associated with total hip replacement: Risk factors and prognosis. *J Bone Joint Surg (Am)*; 73: 1074–1080.

2.  **D**

    Haemophilia A causes excess bleeding due to Factor VIII deficiency and is not linked to osteonecrosis of femoral head. Alcohol abuse and excess corticosteroids cause osteonecrosis of the femoral head by causing fat cell hypertrophy. Trauma causes loss of blood supply to the femoral head. Caisson disease also known as dysbaric osteonecrosis occurs in deep sea divers who have been exposed to hyperbaric conditions. The disorder is thought to occur secondary to nitrogen bubbles occluding blood vessels in the femoral head.

    Ref:

    Lavernia CJ, Sierra RJ, Grieco FR (1999) Osteonecrosis of the Femoral Head. *J Am Acad Orthop Surg*; 7: 250–261.

3.  **E**

    Reducing offset can have a detrimental effect on hip biomechanics leading to reduced tension in hip abductors. Decreasing offset also reduces the clearance between the femur and the pelvis, which may lead to dislocation through bony impingement. It also increases the joint reaction forces; this can increase the forces at the bone-cement or head-liner interfaces, leading to higher wear rates.

    Cup abduction of 40°±10° is also known as the safe zone of Lewinnek. The dislocation zone for implants placed outside this zone was 4 times higher than those placed within the range (6% vs. 1.5%). Increasing the head to neck ratio increases the arc to impingement and hence reduces the risk of dislocation.

    Ref:
    1.  Lewinnek GE, Lewis JL, Tarr R *et al.* (1978) Dislocations after total hip-replacement arthroplasties. *J Bone Joint Surg (Am)* 60: 217–220.
    2.  Charles MN, Bourne RB, Davey JR *et al.* (2004): Soft tissue balancing of the hip. An Instructional Course Lecture. *J Bone Joint Surg (Am)* 86: 1078–1088.

4.  **B**

    This is not a component of third generation cementing technique. The combined use of high pressure lavage, an intramedullary brush and plug, tamponade of the femoral canal, retrograde filling of the canal and proximal pressurisation and vacuum mixing of cement is the current 'third generation cementing technique'.

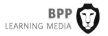

Ref:

Bulstrode C, Buckwalter J, Carr A *et al.* (2002) *Oxford textbook of Orthopaedics and Trauma,* Oxford University Press, Oxford.

5.  **A**

This case most likely represents a case of late haematogenous spread to a well functioning prosthesis. With a two-week history of pain there is a chance that the prosthesis can be retained. The chances of retaining the prosthesis are increased if the organism obtained from culture is of low virulence. These include streptococci and non-glycocalyx forming staphylococcus epidermidis and staphylococcus aureus, which are susceptible to flucloxacillin. Organisms of high virulence include gram negative bacilli and glycocalyx forming staphylococcus epidermidis and staphylococcus aureus, which are resistant to flucloxacillin.

Ref:

Fitzgerald RH (1995). Infected total hip arthroplasty: Diagnosis and Treatment. *J Am Acad Orthop Surg,* 3: 249–262.

6.  **C**

The posterior approach is associated with the lowest risk of developing heterotopic ossification (HO). The highest risk is associated with the Liverpool approach which involves taking a sliver of trochanteric bone with the gluteal flap. HO is twice as common in men as in women. Patients with a past history of HO are at particularly high risk (up to 90% without prophylaxis in some studies). Men with bilateral hypertrophic osteoarthritis have markedly higher levels of HO.

Ref:

1.  Iorio R, Healy W L (2002) Heterotopic Ossification After Hip and Knee Arthroplasty: Risk Factors, Prevention and Treatment *J Am Acad Orthop Surg,* 10: 409–416.
2.  Ritter MA, Vaughan RB (1977) Ectopic ossification after total hip arthroplasty: Predisposing factors, frequency, and effect on results. *J Bone Joint Surg (Am),* 59: 345–351.

7.  **C**

Meralgia paraesthetica involves numbness, paraesthesia and pain in the anterolateral thigh which may result from either an entrapment neuropathy or a neuroma of the lateral femoral cutaneous nerve (LFCN). The LFCN is a purely sensory nerve so compression is not associated with any motor deficits. Around 20% of patients have bilateral symptoms. Symptoms are relieved by hip flexion and aggravated by hip extension (during walking or getting into and out of a car). A positive straight leg test is a sign of a disc prolapse and is not positive in patients with meralgia paraesthetica.

Ref:

Grossman MG et al. (2001): Meralgia Paresthetica: Diagnosis and Treatment. *J Am Acad Orthop Surg* 9: 336–344.

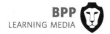

8.  **A**

    Microseparation results in edge loading and stripe wear, which is the predominant cause of squeaking following ceramic on ceramic hip arthroplasty. Microseparation can occur from acetabular malpositioning, failure to reconstruct offsets and/or leg lengths or from bony or soft tissue impingement. Clinical reports have shown that edge loading has been found at the time of revision surgery on all retrievals in patients who report squeaking.

    Ref:
    D'Antonio JA, Sutton K (Feb 2009): Ceramic materials as bearing surfaces for total hip arthroplasty. *J Am Acad Orthop Surg*, 17: 63–68.

9.  **B**

    Excessive retroversion of the acetabular component can result in hip instability when the hip is flexed and should be avoided as this will result in dislocation occurring during eg sitting. Hip flexion will also be limited and anterior impingement of components will occur.

    Ref:
    Barrack RL (2003): Dislocation after total hip arthroplasty: Implant design and orientation. *J Am Acad Orthop Surg*, 11: 89–99.

10. **C**

    This is important for monitoring possible infection after total hip arthroplasty. The C-reactive protein is an acute phase inflammatory marker which takes 2–3 days post-operative to reach peak levels and falls back to normal in around 2 weeks.

    Ref:
    Sukeik MTS, Haddad FS (2009): Management of periprosthetic infection in total hip arthroplasty. *Orthopaedics and Trauma*. 23: 342–349.

11. **D**

    The anterior approach utilises the interval between tensor fascia latae and sartorius superficially. This is a true internervous plane, tensor fascia latae (superior gluteal nerve branch of sciatic nerve) and sartorius (branch of femoral nerve). The deep layer of muscles consists of the rectus femoris and the gluteus medius.

    Ref:
    Hoppenfield S (2003) *Surgical Exposures in Orthopaedics, The Anatomic Approach*. Lippincott Williams & Wilkins, Philadelphia.

12. **A**

    This is the optimal position for hip arthrodesis. The degree of hip flexion depends on the activity of the patient. For a patient who spends a lot of time sitting at a desk 30 degrees of flexion would be appropriate, whereas 20 degrees of flexion would be more appropriate for a manual labourer who stands most of the time.

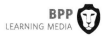

Ref:

Beaule PE, Matta JM, Mast JW (2002): Hip Arthrodesis: Current indications and techniques. *J Am Acad Orthop Surg*, 10: 249–258.

13.  **D**

Protrusio acetabuli can be primary or secondary to a number of different conditions. It results in protrusion of femoral head into the pelvis. The symptoms of protrusio develop in adolescence and patients present with activity related groin pain and stiffness. There is a reduced active and passive range of motion of hip particularly abduction. There may be a positive Trendelenburg sign due to the shortened lever arm of the mechanically disadvantaged hip abductors. Plain radiographs are diagnostic showing the medial wall of the acetabulum protruding medial to the ilioischial line (by 3mm in males and by 6mm in females). They can also be used to measure the centre edge angle of Wiberg with an angle >40 degrees said to be diagnostic of protrusio. The head neck offset is not affected by protrusio. Some of the causes of protrusio include: rheumatoid arthritis, trauma and idiopathic.

Ref:
1.   McBride MT, Muldoon MP, Santore RF *et al.* (2001): Protrusio acetabuli: Diagnosis and Treatment. *J Am Acad Orthop Surg*, 9: 79–88.
2.   Hooper JC, Jones EW: Primary protrusion of the acetabulum (1971). *J Bone Joint Surg (Br)*, 53: 23–29.

14.  **A**

Retrieval analysis of wear particle debris found in tissues surrounding total hip arthroplasty has shown that submicrometer particles induce a greater inflammatory response than larger particles, which is the mechanism responsible for osteolysis. The predominant wear mechanisms appear to involve microadhesion and microabrasion with the generation of many particles <1$\mu$m in length.

Ref:

McKellop HA, Campbell P, Park SH, *et al.* (1995): The origin of submicron polyethylene wear debris in total hip arthroplasty. *Clin Orthop*, 311: 3–20

15.  **D**

Ceramic on ceramic bearing surfaces are known to produce an extremely low rate of wear in vivo; in one study as low as 0.016mm/year, which is around one tenth of that reported for metal on polyethylene components. In order of increasing wear rates is: ceramic on ceramic (0.004mm$^3$), metal on metal (0.88mm$^3$), metal on ceramic (17.1mm$^3$) and finally metal on polyethylene (55.71mm$^3$) which produces the highest wear rates.

Ref:
1.   Jazrawi LM, Bogner E, Della Valle CJ *et al.* (Oct 1999): Wear rates of ceramic-on-ceramic bearing surfaces in total hip implants: a 12-year follow-up study. *J Arthroplasty*; 14: 781–787.
2.   Heisel C, Mauricio S, Schmalzried TP (2004): Bearing surface options for total hip replacement in young patients. *Instr Course Lect*, 53: 49–65.

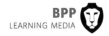

**16.    D**

During total hip arthroplasty for a high dislocated hip, bringing the hip back to a more normal centre of rotation usually requires a simultaneous femoral shortening. Although the soft tissues around the hip are at risk during the procedure, the sciatic nerve is at significant risk of injury due to the lengthening required to reduce the hip to a more normal hip centre. The direction of reduction of a dislocated hip is towards the femoral nerve and artery (ie medially) and therefore they are less at risk from lengthening. It is recommended not to lengthen a limb by more than 2–4cm as this increases the risk of injury to the sciatic nerve.

Ref:
1.    Sanchez-Sotelo J, Berry DJ, Trousdale RT, Cabanela ME (2002): Surgical Treatment of developmental dysplasia of the hip in adults: II. Arthroplasty Options: *J Am Acad Orthop Surg*, 10: 334–344.
2.    Haddad FS, Masri BA, Garbuz DS, Duncan CP (1999): Instructional Course Lectures: Primary total replacement of the dysplastic hip. *J Bone Joint Surg (Am)*; 81: 1462–1482.

**17.    C**

During surgical dislocation of the hip the critical blood supply to the femoral head from the deep branch of the medial femoral circumflex artery (MFCA) needs to be preserved. After crossing the obturator externus muscle posteriorly the MFCA runs anteriorly towards the short external rotators and crosses the femoral neck anteriorly to become the retinacular vessels penetrating the femoral neck. Preservation of the short external rotators of the hip ensures that the MFCA is not damaged during surgical dislocation of the hip.

Ref:
1.    Ganz R, Gill TJ, Gautier E *et al.* (2001) Surgical dislocation of the adult hip: A technique with full access to femoral head and acetabulum without the risk of avascular necrosis. *J Bone Joint Surg Br* 20; 83: 1119–1124.
2.    Parvizi J, Leunig M, Ganz R (2007): Femoroacetabular impingement. *J Am Acad Orthop Surg*; 15: 561–570.

**18.    D**

This is a typical presentation for femoroacetabular impingement. The examination findings of pain with flexion to 90 degrees and adduction and internal rotation is known as the impingement test. The radiographic finding of acetabular retroversion is consistent with pincer type impingement and is most common in middle-aged athletic women. Cam impingement is caused by a femoral deformity and is most common in young, athletic males in their thirties. MRI arthrogram provides visualisation of the labrum and the acetabular cartilage, which is useful to detect any associated labral tears and chondral lesions which are common associated findings in patients presenting with symptoms of impingement.

Ref:
1.    Parvizi J, Campfield A, Clohisy JC (2006): Management of arthritis of the hip in the young adult. *J Bone Joint Surg (Br)* 88: 1279–1285.
2.    Parvizi J, Leunig M, Ganz R (2007): Femoroacetabular impingement. *J Am Acad Orthop Surg* 15: 561–570.

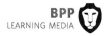

19.  **C**

Lewinnek recommended a safe zone for acetabular component positioning of 40 degrees ± 10 degrees abduction and 15 degrees ± 10 degrees anteversion. McCollum and Gray recommended cup anteversion of 20–40 degrees. It is accepted that the orientation of the acetabular component is associated with the surgical approach. With the posterior approach, greater acetabular anteversion is recommended to allow greater flexion before impingement occurs. Therefore, 20–40 degrees anteversion is preferable when using the posterior approach and 5–25 degrees for the lateral approach.

Ref:
1.    Lewinnek GE, Lewis JL, Tarr R, *et al.* (1978): Dislocations after total hip-replacement arthroplasties. *J Bone Joint Surg (Am)* 60: 217–220.
2.    McCollum DE, Gray WJ (1990): Dislocation after total hip arthroplasty: Causes and prevention. *Clin Orthop* 261: 59–170.
3.    Barrack RL (2003): Dislocation after total hip arthroplasty: Implant design and orientation. *J Am Acad Orthop Surg*, 11: 89–99.

20.  **A**

In a study of patients undergoing vascularised fibular grafting for osteonecrosis at 5 year follow-up, an abnormality was noted in 24% of lower limbs. Sensory deficit was found in 11.8% of patients, motor deficit in 2.7% and contracture of flexor hallucis longus in 2%. Deep vein thrombosis and pulmonary emboli were very rare complications.

Ref:
1.    Vail TP, Urbaniak JR (1996): Donor-site morbidity with use of vascularised autogenous fibular grafts. *J Bone Joint Surg (Am)*, 78: 204–211.
2.    Urbaniak JR, Harvey EJ (1998): Revascularisation of the femoral head in osteonecrosis. *J Am Acad Orthop Surg*, 6: 44–54.

21.  **B**

The safe zone for insertion of screws during total hip arthroplasty is the postero-superior and postero-inferior zones. The external iliac vein is most at risk from screws placed in the antero-superior quadrant.

Ref:
Illgen R, Rubash HE (2002): The Optimal Fixation of the Cementless Acetabular Component in Primary Total Hip Arthroplasty. *J Am Acad Orthop Surg*, 10: 43–56.

22.  **B**

This results in edge loading of the components, which can cause marked localised wear and increased metal ion levels. It has been shown that an abduction angle of >55 degrees causes an increase in metal ion concentrations. There is also an association of lower metal ion levels in patients implanted with larger components, which is probably due to the thicker fluid film achieved and by the greater arc of cover. Increased activity level has not been shown to be correlated to increased metal ion concentration. Increasing the offset and male sex have not been shown to have an effect on the metal ion concentration.

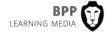

Ref:

1. De Haan R, Pattyn C, Gill HS *et al.* (2008): Correlation between inclination of the acetabular component and metal ion levels in metal-on-metal hip resurfacing replacement. *J Bone Joint Surg (Br)*, 90: 1291–1297.
2. Langton DJ, Sprowson AP, Joyce TJ (2009): Blood metal ion concentrations after hip resurfacing arthroplasty. *J Bone Joint Surg (Br)*, 91: 10–25.

**23.    C**

Hip arthroscopy is useful for treating labral tears associated with femoroacetabular impingement, debridement of the hip in early stages of osteoarthritis and synovectomy associated with inflammatory arthropathy. Contraindications to hip arthroscopy are conditions that limit traction on the leg making hip arthroscopy difficult to perform and include protrusio acetabuli, stage 4 osteoarthritis of hip and ankylosing spondylitis. Avascular necrosis of the femoral head is also considered a contraindication as there is potential for compromising the blood supply of the femoral head further due to the raised intra-articular pressure at hip arthroscopy.

Ref:

1. McCarthy JC, Day B, Busconi B (1995): Hip Arthroscopy: Applications and Techniques. *J Am Acad Orthop Surg* 3: 115–122.
2. Villar RN (1991) Arthroscopic debridement of the hip: A minimally invasive approach to osteoarthritis. *J Bone Joint Surg (Br)*, 73 (suppl 1): 170–171.

**24.    B**

Single stage bilateral total hip arthroplasty is considered as safe as unilateral hip arthroplasty in well selected patients. The ideal patient is one who has severe disabling bilateral hip arthritis and is medically fit. One of the major complications is fat embolism which can occur with increased frequency due to the reaming and subsequent insertion of a prosthesis (particularly cemented) into two femoral canals on the same day. It is contraindicated in patients who have a patent ductus arteriosus or septal defect which would allow fat emboli to access the systemic circulation and vital organs such as the brain and myocardium.

A patient with a contralateral hip contracture associated with bilateral hip arthritis may have a residual hip flexion contracture on the operated side due to their inability to stand erect during ambulation. This would make them a good candidate for bilateral procedures to increase mobility post-operatively. Rheumatoid arthritis of the hip has been shown to affect the hips bilaterally in greater than 50% of patients and in one study 17% of single stage bilateral procedures were done for rheumatoid arthritis[2].

Ref:

1. Pell ACH, Hughes D, Keating J, *et al.* (1993): Brief report: Fulminating fat embolism syndrome caused by paradoxical embolism through a patent foramen ovale. *N Engl J Med*, 329: 926–929.
2. Salvati EA, Hughes P, Lachiewicz P (1978): Bilateral total hip-replacement arthroplasty in one stage. *J Bone Joint Surg (Am)*, 60: 640–644.
3. Macaulay W, Salvati EA, Sculco TP, Pellicci PM (2002): Single stage bilateral total hip arthroplasty. *J Am Acad Orthop Surg*, 10: 217–221.

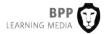

**25.    A**

One of the common causes of thigh pain in this case is aseptic loosening of the femoral component. This would be seen on radiographs as the presence of progressive radiolucencies around the stem and progressive implant migration >2mm. Engh et al[1] suggested a radiographic system to determine fixation of porous coated femoral components. They categorised fixation into osseointegration, stable fibrous ingrowth and unstable fixation. Signs of osseointegration include the absence of reactive lines around the porous portion of the stem, calcar atrophy (due to proximal stress shielding occurring after diaphyseal osseointegration of the stem) and the presence of endosteal spot welds.

Ref:

1.    Engh CA, Bobyn JD, Glassman AH: Porous-coated hip replacement (1987): The factors governing bone ingrowth, stress shielding, and clinical results. *J Bone Joint Surg (Br)*, 69: 45–55.

2.    Engh CA, Massin P, Suthers KE (1990): Roentgenographic assessment of the biologic fixation of porous-surfaced femoral components. *Clin Orthop*; 257: 107–128.

3.    Brown TE, Larson B, Shen F, Moskal JT (2002): Thigh pain after cementless total hip arthroplasty: Evaluation and management. *J Am Acad Orthop Surg*; 10: 385–392.

**26.    A**

Prophylactic antibiotic use for total joint arthroplasty has been shown to be the single most important factor in reducing post-operative deep wound infection. One study showed that the infection rate was reduced from 2.8% without prophylactic antibiotics to 0.5% with antibiotics[2]. The additional effect of laminar airflow above this reduction has not been clearly established in studies. Whole body exhaust suits and reducing the number of personnel in theatre have also been shown to reduce the bacterial counts in theatre. The use of iodophor impregnated plastic drapes to cover the operative site has also been shown to reduce the wound contamination (as measured on culture of deep wound specimens take just before closure).

Ref:

1.    Hill C, Flamant R, Mazas F, Evrard J (1981): Prophylactic cefazolin versus placebo in total hip replacement. Report of a multicentre double-blind randomised trial. *Lancet*, 1: 795–796.

2.    Marotte JH, Lord GA, Blanchard JP *et al.* (1987): Infection rate in total hip arthroplasty as a function of air cleanliness and antibiotic prophylaxis. 10-year experience with 2,384 cementless –Lord Madreporic prostheses. *J. Arthroplasty*; 2: 77–82

3.    Hanssen AD, Osmon DR, Nelson CL (March 1996): Prevention of Deep Periprosthetic Joint Infection. *J Bone Joint Surg (Am)*, 78: 458–471.

**27.    D**

Increasing the femoral offset increases the lever arm of the hip abductors, thereby reducing the abductor muscle force required for normal gait. This in turn minimises the joint reaction force across the hip and lower wear rates of polyethylene. A study comparing low offset with high offset femoral components in patients who had bilateral hip replacements has shown that the linear wear rate of polyethylene was 0.21mm/year for the low offset and 0.01mm/year for the high offset components. The risk of dislocation is reduced as the abductors maintain the hip joint under correct tension and lower risk of impingement as the femur is displaced further from the acetabulum. There is also a reduced incidence of Trendelenburg gait if femoral offset is restored to normal and increased gait efficiency.

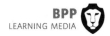
BPP
LEARNING MEDIA

Ref:
1. Sakalkale DP, Sharkey PF, Eng K, Hozack WJ *et al.* (2001): Effect of femoral component offset on polyethylene wear in total hip arthroplasty. *Clin Orthop*, 388: 125–34.
2. Charles MN, Bourne RB, Davey JR *et al.* (May 2004): Soft tissue balancing of the hip. *J Bone Joint Surg (Am)* 86: 1078–1088.

**28.    D**

This would result in a reduction in the femoral offset and medialisation of the insertion of the abductor muscles and reduction in the lever arm of the abductors. The remaining factors are all methods used to increase the femoral offset.

Ref:

Charles MN, Bourne RB, Davey JR *et al.* (May 2004): Soft tissue balancing of the hip. *J Bone Joint Surg (Am)*, 86: 1078–1088.

**29.    C**

If the C-reactive protein (CRP) and ESR are both normal and there is no suggestion of infection on clinical presentation, then infection can reliably be excluded. The ESR has been shown to have a sensitivity and specificity of 0.82 and 0.85 respectively and the CRP has a sensitivity and specificity of 0.96 and 0.92 respectively. The combined CRP and ESR have a negative predictive value of 91%. The white blood cell count is rarely elevated in patients presenting with an infection following total hip arthroplasty. A technetium 99m bone scan is non-specific and can be abnormal in aseptic loosening of the hip. Indium 111 labelled white blood cell scans can improve the accuracy of bone scans and have a sensitivity of 0.56 and specificity of 0.79.

Ref:

Spangehl MJ, Younger ASE, Masri BA, Duncan CP (Oct 1997): Diagnosis of infection following total hip arthroplasty. *J Bone Joint Surg (Am)*, 79: 1578–1588.

**30.    C**

Mirel's score is considered a useful aid to management of patients presenting with metastatic lesions and predicts the risk of pathological fracture. A score of ≥8 predicts a high risk of impending pathological fracture and prophylactic fixation is recommended.

Ref:
Mirel's H (1989): Metastatic disease in long bones. A proposed scoring system for diagnosing impending pathologic fractures. *Clin Orthop*; 249: 256–264.

**31.    D**

Pathological fractures of the femoral head and neck are best treated with a long stem total hip arthroplasty as fixation in this area is at high risk of failure. Even if no distal lesions are seen on radiographs a long stem prosthesis inserted prophylactically is recommended.

Ref:

Damron TA, Sim FH (Jan 2000): Operative treatment for metastatic disease of the pelvis and the proximal end of the femur. An Instructional Course Lecture. *J Bone Joint Surg (Am)*, 82: 114–126.

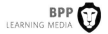

**32.  C**

Small branches of the lateral femoral cutaneous nerve lie in close proximity to the anterior portal and are damaged during portal placement. The anterior portal is placed on the intersection of a line drawn vertically down from the anterior superior iliac spine and a horizontal line across the superior margin of the greater trochanter. The femoral nerve and artery are well medial to this point. The lateral femoral cutaneous nerve has been shown to pass within an average of 0.3cm of the anterior portal.

Ref:
Byrd JWT (2006): Hip Arthroscopy. *J Am Acad Orthop Surg*, 14: 433–444.

**33.  D**

This is the main reason for using constrained acetabular components during revision THR for dislocation. If impingement is found to be the reason for dislocation then the treatment needs to be directed towards that, ie for impingement of the femoral head against an elevated rim, the femoral head, acetabular liner or shell may need to be changed. Soft tissue laxity around hip can be treated by lengthening the femoral neck or increasing the femoral offset. Segmental bone defects are a contraindication to the use of constrained components.

Ref:
Lachiewicz PF, Kelley SS (2002): The use of constrained components in total hip arthroplasty. *J Am Acad Orthop Surg*, 10: 233–238.

**34.  A**

Constrained components in revision THR lead to increased stresses being transferred to the implant-bone interface and have a high potential for loosening and failure. They are most suited to low-demand patients who lack soft tissue constraint and have a well fixed cup suitable for a constrained liner or adequate bone stock for maximal screw fixation of a constrained cup. Other contra-indications include acute dislocation, dislocation due to component loosening or malposition and the presence of acute infection.

Ref:
1. Soong M, Rubash HE, Macaulay W (2004): Dislocation after total hip arthroplasty. *J Am Acad Orthop Surg*, 12: 314–321.
2. Lachiewicz PF, Kelley SS (2002): The use of constrained components in total hip arthroplasty. *J Am Acad Orthop Surg*, 10: 233–238.
3. Goetz DD, Capello WN, Callaghan JJ *et al.* (1998): Salvage of a recurrently dislocating total hip prosthesis with use of a constrained acetabular component: A retrospective analysis of fifty-six cases. *J Bone Joint Surg (Am)*, 80: 502–509.

**35.  B**

This is an excellent technique to differentiate hip and spine pain. It has high sensitivity (97%) and specificity (91%) and can be used in cases where there is a diagnostic dilemma and a combination of hip and spine pain to determine the relative contribution of each.

Ref:
Ashok N, Sivan M, Tafazal S, Sell P (April 2009): The diagnostic value of anaesthetic hip injection in differentiating between hip and spinal pain. *Eur J Orthop Surg Traumatol*, 19: 167–171.

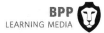

**36.** **B**

This would result in possible lengthening of the leg and is least likely to cause a Trendelenburg positive gait, which is usually seen if the femoral offset is not restored, if the hip abductors are damaged intra-operatively or they are denervated (superior gluteal nerve palsy)

Ref:

Charles MN, Bourne RB, Davey JR *et al.* (May 2004): Soft tissue balancing of the hip. An Instructional Course Lecture. *J Bone Joint Surg (Am)* 86: 1078–1088.

**37.** **B**

Recently several studies have shown that bisphosphonates may be useful in the early stages of osteonecrosis of the femoral head. They have been shown to reduce the rate of collapse of the femoral head and reduce the requirement for total hip arthroplasty. NSAIDs may be linked to an increase in risk of osteonecrosis of femoral head. Statins may be of benefit in patients with osteonecrosis secondary to steroid usage possibly be reducing the fat content in the femoral head which is increased in patients with steroid induced osteonecrosis of femoral head.

Ref:

Agarwala S, Shah S, Joshi VR (Aug 2009): The use of alendronate in the treatment of avascular necrosis of the femoral head: follow-up to eight years. *J Bone Joint Surg (Br)*, 91: 1013–1018.

**38.** **E**

This has been shown to develop in up to 20% of cases of traumatic hip dislocation. Avascular necrosis is also seen frequently, in one study, 9.6% of patients developed this complication.

Ref:
1.  Tornetta III P, Mostafavi HR (1997): Hip Dislocation: Current treatment regimens. *J Am Acad Orthop Surg*, 5: 27–36.
2.  Sahin V, Karakas ES, Aksu S, *et al.* (Mar 2003): Traumatic dislocation and fracture-dislocation of the hip: a long term follow-up study. *J Trauma*, 54: 520–529.

**39.** **B**

The preferred approach for fixation of femoral head fractures is the anterior approach which allows good visualisation of the fracture fragments. A study[1] comparing the two approaches found a comparable rate of avascular necrosis but a higher rate of heterotopic ossification possibly due to increased muscle damage during the anterior approach.

Ref:

Swiontkowski MF, Thorpe M *et al.* (1992): Operative management of displaced femoral head fractures: Case-matched comparison of anterior versus posterior approaches for Pipkin I and Pipkin II fractures. *J Orthop Trauma*, 6: 437–442.

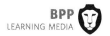

**40. C**

A varus osteotomy increases the abductor lever arm and reduces the abductor muscle force and hence reduces the joint reaction force. The joint reaction force is displaced medially and the leg is shortened. A proximal femoral varus osteotomy of 40 degrees reduces peak hip force by 25% and a valgus osteotomy increases peak hip force by approximately 25%.

Ref:

1.    Ramachandran M (2007): *Basic Orthopaedic Sciences The Stanmore Guide*. Edward Arnold, London, 164–166.
2.    Brand RA (1997): Hip osteotomies: A biomechanical consideration. *J Am Acad Orthop Surg*; 5: 282–291.

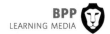

BPP
LEARNING MEDIA

# Adult Pathology

## Knee: Question Bank

Ibrar Majid, Haroon A Mann
& Fahad G Attar

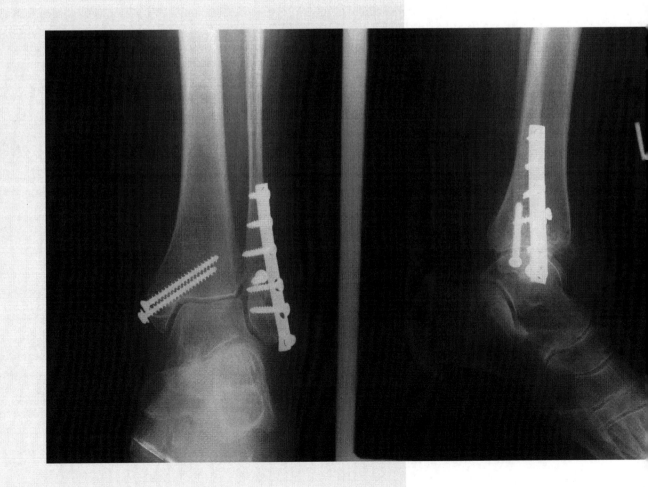

1.   In the treatment of focal knee articular defects, osteoarticular allografts most commonly fail due to
     A.   Mechanical loosening
     B.   Infection
     C.   Immune rejection
     D.   Graft collapse
     E.   Fracture

2.   A 65-year-old lady with a history of Type II diabetes presents with a sudden onset of knee pain. Clinical examination is unremarkable and blood investigations are all within normal parameters. Plain radiographs demonstrate narrowing of the tibiofemoral joint space, with flattening of the lateral femoral condyle and the presence of a 'crescent' sign. MRI scan shows a defect in the lateral femoral condyle, with collapse of the articular surface. What is the next most appropriate step in management?
     A.   Aspiration of the knee joint
     B.   Radionuclide bone scan
     C.   Arthroscopy
     D.   Total knee replacement
     E.   Conservative measures

3.   The following are all contraindications for high tibial osteotomy (HTO), except:
     A.   Varus deformity between 10–15 degrees
     B.   Inflammatory arthropathy
     C.   Lateral tibial subluxation
     D.   Multicompartment disease
     E.   Fixed flexion deformity greater than 15 degrees

4.   In total knee replacement surgery, a tight flexion gap and a normal extension gap, in the presence of a PCL sacrificing prosthesis, can be addressed by all of these except:
     A.   Increasing the amount of posterior slope on the tibial cut
     B.   Resecting more posterior femoral condyle
     C.   Releasing the posterior capsule
     D.   Downsizing the femoral component
     E.   Augmenting the posterior femoral condyle

5.   Bilateral simultaneous total knee replacements are associated with:
     A.   Increased bleeding
     B.   Less range of motion
     C.   Higher 30-day post operative mortality rates
     D.   Higher incidence of infection
     E.   Prosthesis more likely to undergo failure through loosening

6.   The most reliable diagnostic tool for diagnosing infection in a total knee replacement is:
     A.   Radionuclide scan
     B.   Serum CRP
     C.   Serum WCC
     D.   Aspiration of the knee
     E.   Plain radiographs

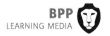

7.  Injury to the ACL is most commonly associated with a concurrent acute injury to:
    A.  MCL
    B.  LCL
    C.  PCL
    D.  Posterolateral corner
    E.  Medial femoral condyle

8.  When considering a patient for a unicompartmental knee replacement, it is essential to obtain the following radiographic view:
    A.  Horizontal beam lateral
    B.  Skyline
    C.  Merchant's view
    D.  Tunnel view
    E.  Stress view

9.  With regards autologous chondrocyte implantation (ACI):
    A.  Kissing lesions on either side of the joint can be treated simultaneously
    B.  Contained lesions around the medial femoral condyle have best outcomes
    C.  Smoking is not a contraindication
    D.  Failure is most commonly due to infection
    E.  Results seem to be better in the 25–35 age group

10. The following are all risk factors for nerve injury during TKR except:
    A.  Previous HTO
    B.  Epidural anaesthesia
    C.  Correction of varus deformity
    D.  Correction of a fixed flexion deformity
    E.  Prior lumbar laminectomy

11. The following are all **true** regarding the menisci of the knee except:
    A.  They are predominantly composed of type I collagen
    B.  The lateral meniscus is more circular than the medial
    C.  The medial meniscus receives its blood supply from the medial genicular artery
    D.  The lateral meniscus is more mobile than the medial
    E.  The lateral meniscus is more prone to tears than the medial

12. The medial parapatellar approach to the knee is associated with injury to:
    A.  Saphenous vein
    B.  Infrapatellar branch of saphenous nerve
    C.  Common peroneal nerve
    D.  Peroneal artery
    E.  Popliteus tendon

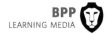

13. The posterolateral corner comprises all of the following, except:
    A. Popliteus
    B. Arcuate ligament
    C. Lateral collateral ligament
    D. The ligament of Wrisberg
    E. Posterolateral capsule

14. Regarding the medial structures of the knee, the saphenous nerve is found between:
    A. Sartorius and the superficial fascia
    B. Sartorius and semimembranosus
    C. The superficial and deep MCLs
    D. Superficial MCL and the capsule
    E. Semimembranosus and the deep MCL

15. In a young healthy adult the tensile strength of the ACL is approximately:
    A. 750 N
    B. 1000 N
    C. 2250 N
    D. 3500 N
    E. 4500 N

16. A young girl presents to the outpatient department complaining of left anterior knee pain and a sensation of her knee regularly 'popping' on physical activity. Examination reveals an increased Q angle and the presence of the J sign. The next most appropriate step in management would be:
    A. Weight bearing AP radiographs
    B. Notch view radiographs
    C. Merchant's view radiographs
    D. MRI
    E. CT

17. The most common complication of knee arthroscopy is:
    A. Articular cartilage damage
    B. Haemarthrosis
    C. Nerve injury
    D. Infection
    E. Intrarticular instrument breakage

18. All the following regarding a high riding patella are **true**, except:
    A. It is associated with patella instability
    B. Will have a Blackburne-Peel index of 1.0 or more
    C. Is often found with an abnormal trochlea
    D. Is an indication for lateral retinacular release
    E. Will have an Insall-Salvati index of 1.2 or more

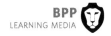

19. The Segond fracture is pathognomonic with injury to the:
    A. Posterolateral corner
    B. PCL
    C. MCL
    D. LCL
    E. Lateral mensicus

20. A 65-year-old man presents with a long history of knee pain, worse in the last six months. Examination reveals a fixed flexion deformity of 5 degrees, the presence of a small effusion and some limitation beyond 100 degrees of knee flexion. Plain radiographs reveal tricompartmental degenerative disease. MRI of the knee shows a degenerative peripheral longitudinal tear of the medial meniscus. The next most appropriate step of management would be:
    A. Intra-articular steroid
    B. Intra-articular viscosupplementation
    C. Arthroscopy plus partial menisectomy
    D. Arthroscopy plus meniscal repair
    E. Total knee replacement

21. Meniscal repair:
    A. Should be considered for all radial tears
    B. Can achieve success rates of up to 90% in acute peripheral tears in conjunction with ACL reconstruction in the young patient
    C. Has good outcomes in the ACL deficient knee
    D. Is associated with injury to the saphenous nerve during lateral repair
    E. Is best with simple vertical sutures

22. The most sensitive test for diagnosing ACL injury in the outpatient setting is:
    A. Posterior draw
    B. Lachman
    C. Anterior draw
    D. Tibial sag
    E. Pivot shift

23. A 35-year-old man who plays football three times a week presented to the Emergency Department with a painful swollen knee following a twisting injury. Examination at the time revealed a tense haemarthrosis which was aspirated. On review two weeks later he complains of his leg giving way. Examination of his knee reveals a positive Lachman test and nil else of note. KT-1000 testing reveals 4.6mm of anterior displacement of the affected knee as compared with the contralateral. The next most appropriate step in management would be
    A. A course of physiotherapy
    B. CT
    C. MRI
    D. List for arthroscopy
    E. List for arthroscopy plus ACL reconstruction

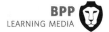

24. An elderly man is involved in an RTA and is admitted with an isolated anterior knee dislocation. His knee is reduced in the Emergency Department. The next most appropriate step in management is:
    A. Close observation
    B. Plain radiographs
    C. MRI
    D. Arteriogram
    E. External fixation

25. The following are all technical goals of knee replacement surgery, except:
    A. Restoring mechanical alignment
    B. Restoring the joint line
    C. Restoring a full range of motion
    D. Balancing ligaments
    E. Restoring a normal Q angle

26. Regarding mechanical alignment of the lower limb during knee arthroplasty surgery:
    A. The femoral anatomical and mechanical axis are coincident in the normal femur
    B. The tibial cut is perpendicular to a line which passes from the knee centre and the ankle joint centre
    C. The valgus cut angle is the angle between the femoral and tibial mechanical axis
    D. The entry point for the intramedullary rod of the femoral jig is always the intercondylar notch
    E. The valgus cut angle is often reduced in patients who are obese

27. The following are all **true** regarding ligament balancing in total knee arthroplasty, except:
    A. Balancing is required in both the coronal and sagittal planes:
    B. The peroneal nerve is at most risk in a valgus knee with a fixed flexion deformity
    C. In refractory cases, release of the PCL can be used to achieve proper balance in the varus knee
    D. Full release of the lateral collateral ligament in a valgus knee is an indication for the use of a constrained prosthesis
    E. In the medial release for varus deformity the superficial MCL is released before the deep MCL

28. Femoral rollback:
    A. Prevents hyperflexion of the knee
    B. Is closer to physiological in the PCL substituting prosthesis
    C. Refers to anterior translation of the tibia which allows the femur to flex further
    D. Reduces the effective strength of the quadriceps
    E. In the PCL substituting prosthesis is associated with more contact stresses

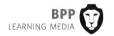

29.    A PCL substituting prosthesis would be the first choice in all of the following cases, except:
       A.    An competitive middle aged weightlifter
       B.    A patient with a history of previous PCL injury
       C.    Following a complete and extensive medial release during ligament balancing
       D.    Patients with previous patellectomy
       E.    A middle aged female with rheumatoid arthritis

30.    With regards to functional outcome following total knee replacement:
       A.    Final postoperative knee flexion is determined mostly by the level of flexion reached at discharge from hospital
       B.    Flexion contractures after surgery are always due to inadequate release at surgery
       C.    Continuous passive motion is required less often in knees closed in extension
       D.    Femoral notching is a relative contraindication to manipulation of a stiff knee replacement
       E.    Reduced quadriceps activity after total knee replacement is due to pain

31.    The Q angle is increased by all of the following except:
       A.    External rotation of the femoral component
       B.    Medialisation of the femoral component
       C.    Internal rotation of the tibial component
       D.    Valgus alignment of the leg
       E.    Lateralisation of the patella component

32.    The most common patellofemoral complication following total knee replacement surgery is:
       A.    Patella baja
       B.    Component loosening
       C.    Fracture
       D.    Patella clunk syndrome
       E.    Patella maltracking

33.    A 65-year-old man undergoes primary total knee replacement surgery with a PCL retaining prosthesis. He returns to clinic eight months after surgery, complaining of persistent pain in the knee. He does not report any preceding trauma or any other symptoms. Examination is unremarkable. Plain radiographs do not show any obvious abnormality. Blood investigations including inflammatory markers are all within normal parameters. Aspiration of the knee joint under sterile conditions does not grow any organisms. The most appropriate next step in management would be:
       A.    Radionuclide bone scan
       B.    MRI
       C.    CT
       D.    Arthroscopy
       E.    Referral to a pain specialist

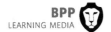

34. The minimum thickness of the polyethylene insert required to avoid catastrophic wear is:
    A. 6mm
    B. 8mm
    C. 9mm
    D. 10mm
    E. 11mm

35. Deep infections related to total knee arthroplasty are most commonly due to:
    A. Staphylococcus epidermidis
    B. Escherichia coli
    C. Pseudomonas species
    D. Klebsiella species
    E. Methicillin resistant staphylococcus aureus

36. A 40-year-old lady presents to clinic with anterior knee pain, worse on ascending stairs. She denies any previous history of trauma and is otherwise fit and well. Examination reveals tenderness over the lateral and medial facets of the patella, with no evidence of patella instability. Plain fully weight bearing AP and lateral, Merchant's and tunnel view radiographs reveal isolated patellofemoral degenerate disease. On arthroscopy there is evidence of Grade IV changes in both the patella and trochlea, with no evidence of tibiofemoral arthritis. The next most appropriate step in management would be:
    A. Intraarticular viscosupplementation
    B. Lateral retinacular release
    C. Patellofemoral replacement
    D. Total knee replacement
    E. Tibial tuberosity transfer

37. The following are all **true** regarding constrained knee prostheses, except:
    A. All have a central post that restricts opening of the knee to varus and valgus stresses
    B. In the hinged variety there is mechanical linkage between the femur and the tibia
    C. When used in revision TKR surgery, they must always be used with medullary stems in the femur and tibia
    D. The forces at the prosthesis bone interface are greater than those with unconstrained prostheses
    E. Constrained hinged prostheses are the first choice for most revision TKRs

38. In revision TKR surgery, the first step after removal of the components should be:
    A. Restoration of the femur
    B. Balancing of the ligaments
    C. Restoration of the tibia
    D. Assessing and correcting patella tracking
    E. Increasing the surgical exposure

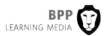

39. The following are all relative contraindications to unicompartmental knee replacement, except:
    A. ACL deficiency
    B. Significant tricompartmental disease
    C. Fixed valgus deformity
    D. Young age
    E. Knee flexion less than 90 degrees

40. The specificity of MRI in diagnosing meniscal pathology is approximately:
    A. 60%
    B. 80%
    C. 90%
    D. 95%
    E. 100%

BPP
LEARNING MEDIA

# Adult Pathology

## Knee: Answers

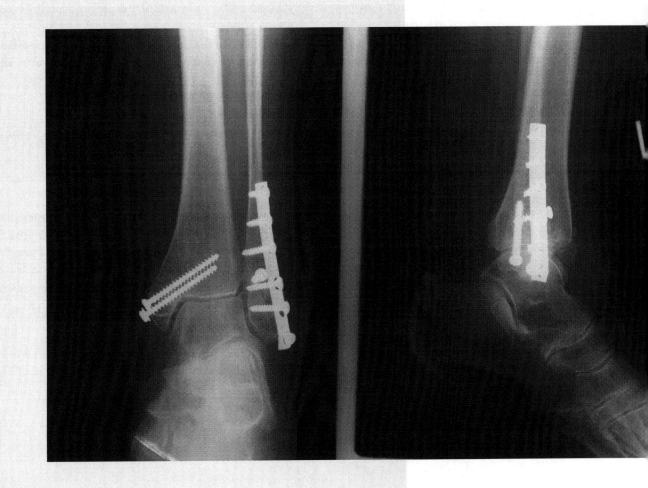

1.  **D**

    Osteoarticular allografts are an alternative to autologous chondrocyte implantation for focal knee defects. This procedure involves harvesting full-thickness fragments of articular cartilage and subchondral bone from donors. The most common mode of failure of osteoarticular allografts is by graft collapse during the revascularisation process

    Ref:

    Mandelbaum, BR. *et al.* (1998) Articular cartilage lesions of the knee, *Am J Sports Med*, 26. 6, 853–861.

2.  **D**

    Avascular necrosis of the knee can occur about either femoral condyles or tibial plateaus and most commonly occurs in women over age 60. This condition is often self-limiting and resolves with conservative management. However, in refractory, persistent cases of avascular necrosis, once there has been collapse of the articular surface, total knee replacement provides the most predictable result.

    Ref:

    Ecker, ML and Lotke, PA. (1994) Spontaneous osteonecrosis of the knee, *J Am Acad Orthop Surg*, 2, 173–178.

3.  **A**

    An HTO can be effective for treating medial compartment arthritis in the carefully selected patient. This procedure is generally considered appropriate for the younger patient with mild to moderate arthritis, preoperative ROM of 90 degrees or greater, between 10 and 15 degrees of varus deformity, and sufficient preoperative conditioning to complete the extensive rehabilitation program. It is contraindicated in inflammatory arthropathy or in those cases where more than one compartment is involved. Other contraindications include lateral tibial subluxation and a fixed flexion deformity greater than 15 degrees.

    Ref:

    Chin, K and Mehta, S. (ed.) (2007) *Orthopaedic Key Review Concepts*, Lippincott Williams & Wilkins, Philadelphia.

4.  **E**

    If the flexion gap is tight and the extension gap is normal and a PCL-sacrificing prosthesis is used several techniques can be used to address this asymmetry. These include increasing the amount of posterior slope of the tibial cut, resecting more posterior femoral condyle, downsizing the femoral component, and releasing a tight posterior capsule. Increasing the size of the femoral condyle is a useful strategy if the flexion gap is loose in the presence of a normal extension gap.

    Ref:

    Chin, K and Mehta, S. (ed.) (2007) *Orthopaedic Key Review Concepts*, Lippincott Williams & Wilkins, Philadelphia.

BPP
LEARNING MEDIA

5.  **C**

    Bilateral TKAs performed simultaneously have been shown to have a higher 30-day postoperative mortality rate. Other complications, such as bleeding, loosening, infection, and ROM, have not been shown to be significantly higher for simultaneous bilateral TKAs.

    Ref:

    Chin, K and Mehta, S. (ed.) (2007) *Orthopaedic Key Review Concepts*, Lippincott Williams & Wilkins, Philadelphia.

6.  **D**

    Studies have demonstrated that aspiration can be 100% sensitive, specific, and accurate in diagnosing infection. Serial plain X-rays can be useful adjuncts to diagnosis, particularly if they demonstrate extensive and rapid loosening or periosteal reaction. Technetium 99m bone scans and gallium scans are often not helpful because they will frequently show increased uptake for up to 3 years after the initial surgery. Serum CRP may stay elevated for up to six weeks post surgery.

    Ref:

    Chin, K and Mehta, S. (ed.) (2007) *Orthopaedic Key Review Concepts*, Lippincott Williams & Wilkins, Philadelphia.

7.  **B**

    MRI studies have shown that ACL injuries are associated with bone bruising to the lateral femoral condyle and the posterolateral tibial plateau. Concurrent ligamentous injuries are most commonly to the LCL.

    Ref:

    Miller, MD. (ed.) (2008) *Review of Orthopaedics*, Saunders Elsevier, Philadelphia. p. 257.

8.  **E**

    A relative contraindication to UKR is instability of the MCL, which presents with abnormal opening of the medial tibiofemoral joint space on valgus stressing.

    Ref:

    Miller, MD. (ed.) (2008) *Review of Orthopaedics*, Saunders Elsevier, Philadelphia. p. 251.

9.  **B**

    ACI is a good option for addressing focal articular defects in the younger patient in whom one would like to avoid arthroplasty surgery. Contraindications include kissing lesions, and patients who are smokers. Failure of the procedure is most commonly due to lack of uptake of cells, hypertrophy or the formations of abnormal fibrocartilage. Outcomes appear to be best in patients aged 18 years and younger, and in contained defects of the medial femoral condyle.

    Ref:

    Chin, K and Mehta, S. (ed.) (2007) *Orthopaedic Key Review Concepts*, Lippincott Williams & Wilkins, Philadelphia.

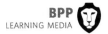

**10.  C**

Neurological injury following TKR most commonly affects the peroneal nerve. Correction of severe valgus deformities and severe flexion contractures increase the risk of peroneal nerve injury. Other risk factors for peroneal nerve palsy include prior lumbar laminectomy, epidural anesthesia, and prior HTO.

Ref:

Chin, K and Mehta, S. (ed.) (2007) *Orthopaedic Key Review Concepts*, Lippincott Williams & Wilkins, Philadelphia.

**11.  E**

The menisci are crescent shaped fibrocartilagenous structures composed mainly of type I collagen. The peripheral 20–30% of the medial meniscus and 10–25% of the lateral meniscus are vascular, receiving blood from the medial and lateral genicular arteries. The medial meniscus is C shaped, while the lateral is more circular and mobile. As a result the medial meniscus is more prone to injury, and is torn approximately three times more often than the lateral.

Ref:

Miller, MD. (ed.) (2008) *Review of Orthopaedics*, Saunders Elsevier, Philadelphia. pp. 183, 247.

**12.  B**

The infrapatellar branch of the saphenous nerve is at risk with the medial parapatellar approach to the knee joint.

Ref:

Miller, MD. (ed.) (2008) *Review of Orthopaedics*, Saunders Elsevier, Philadelphia. p. 187.

**13.  D**

The posterolateral corner (PLC) of the knee comprises of popliteus, arcuate ligament, lateral collateral ligament, posterolateral capsule and the lateral head of gastrocnemius. The ligament of Wrisberg originates from the posterolateral meniscus and lies directly behind the PCL, and is not part of the PLC

Ref:

Miller, MD. (ed.) (2008) *Review of Orthopaedics*, Saunders Elsevier, Philadelphia. p. 183.

**14.  B**

The medial structures of the knee are composed of three layers, and the saphenous nerve is found between layers I and II in the same plane as gracilis and semitendonosus. The superficial fascia and sartorius are found in layer I. The superficial part of the MCL and semimembranosus are found in layer II.

Ref:

Warren, LF. and Marshall, JL. (1979) The supporting structures and layers on the medial side of the knee: an anatomical analysis, *J Bone Joint Surg (Am)*, 61. 1, 56–62.

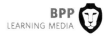

15. **C**

The tensile strengths of the ligaments in the knee of a healthy adult, in ascending order are:

| | |
|---|---|
| LCL | 750 N |
| ACL | 2250 N |
| PCL | 3000 N |
| MCL | 4500 N |

Ref:

Miller, MD. (ed.) (2008) *Review of Orthopaedics*, Saunders Elsevier, Philadelphia. p. 247.

16. **C**

Patellofemoral malalignment often presents with recurrent lateral subluxation or dislocation of the patella. Examination can reveal lateral deviation of the patella in extension (the J sign), as well as an increased Q angle. Diagnosis is aided by Merchant's views which are useful in evaluating the relationship between the patella and the trochlea surface of the femur. These are obtained with the patient supine and the knee flexed 30 degrees at the table edge and the X-ray cassette held perpendicular to the tibia. CT should be reserved for those cases in which plain radiographs are indeterminate.

Ref:

Aglietti, P. Insall, JN. Cerulli, G. (1983) Patellar Pain and Incongruence. Measurements of Incongruence, *Clin. Orthop*, 176, 217–224.

17. **A**

The most common complication of knee arthroscopy is iatrogenic articular cartilage damage. Other complications include nerve injury, haemarthrosis, infection, deep vein thrombosis and intrarticular breakage of instruments

Ref:

Miller, MD. (ed.) (2008) *Review of Orthopaedics*, Saunders Elsevier, Philadelphia. p. 253.

18. **D**

Patella alta is associated with patella instability and the presence of an abnormal trochlea. Lateral radiographs are useful in the evaluation, and the relative position of the patella can be determined by two methods. The Insall-Salvati index is a ratio of the length of the patella tendon to the diagonal length of the patella, with an index of 1.2 or more being alta. The Blackburne-Peel index is a ratio of the distance between the tibial plateau and the inferior patella articular surface, and the length of the articular surface of the patella, with an index of 1.0 or more being alta. Patella alta maybe associated with a tight lateral retinaculum, but this alone is not an indication for release

Ref:

Simmons, E Jr and Cameron, JC. (1992) Patella alta and recurrent dislocation of the patella, *Clin Orthop*, 274, 265–9.

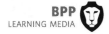

19. **A**

The Segond fracture is a small avulsion fracture of the lateral tibial condyle just below the joint line. It is recognised as being associated with ALC injury and now, more commonly injuries to the posterolateral corner.

Ref:
Campos, JC. et al. (2001) Pathogenesis of the Segond fracture: anatomic and MR imaging evidence of an iliotibial tract or anterior oblique band avulsion, *Radiology*, 219. 2, 381–6.

20. **A**

Degenerate meniscal tears in the absence of mechanical symptoms can be treated non-operatively in the first instance. Those that fail to improve with conservative measures may benefit from arthroscopy and menisectomy. The role of meniscal repair in the degenerate knee remains controversial

Ref:
Miller, MD. (ed.) (2008) *Review of Orthopaedics*, Saunders Elsevier, Philadelphia. p. 253.

21. **B**

Meniscal repair should be considered for all peripheral longitudinal tears, especially in the younger patient with an acute tear and in conjunction with ACL reconstruction. In such instances success rates of 80–90% have been reported. Repair in the ACL deficient knee has poor outcomes. The gold standard technique remains the 'inside to out' using vertical mattress sutures. Care should be taken to preserve the saphenous nerve with medial repair and the peroneal nerve with lateral repair

Ref:
Miller, MD. (ed.) (2008) *Review of Orthopaedics*, Saunders Elsevier, Philadelphia. pp. 253–255.

22. **B**

In the conscious patient the most sensitive test for ACL injury is the Lachman test (78.6%). Under anaesthesia the pivot shift is a more sensitive test (100%) and in general it is also more specific to ACL injury. Tibial sag and posterior draw are indicative of injury to the PCL.

Ref:
Jain, DK. Amaravat, R. Sharma, G. (2009) Evaluation of the clinical signs of anterior cruciate ligament and meniscal injuries, *Indian J Orthop*, 43. 4, 375–8.

23. **E**

In acute ACL injuries with a positive Lachman test and KT-1000, MRI should not be routinely employed unless there is concern regarding injury to the MCL, LCL or posterolateral corner. In the relatively active young patient such injuries should be treated with ACL reconstruction and meniscal repair if required. In the acute setting there is no role for pre-operative rehabilitation.

Ref:
Miller, MD. (ed.) (2008) *Review of Orthopaedics*, Saunders Elsevier, Philadelphia. p. 258

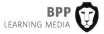

**24.    D**

The incidence of vascular injury after anterior knee dislocation is 30–50%. Therefore after reduction of the dislocation, attention should be directed to identifying and treating any associated vascular injury. Knee dislocations are also associated with multiple knee ligament injuries and these should be investigated and treated after any life or limb threatening injuries have been dealt with.

Ref:

Marks, PH. Harner, CD. (1993) The anterior cruciate ligament in the multiple ligament-injured knee, *Clin Sports Med*, 12. 4, 825–38.

**25.    C**

The technical goals of knee replacement surgery are to restore the joint line, mechanical alignment and a normal Q angle, and to balance all ligaments. Restoring a full range of motion is not from the technical goals of knee arthroplasty surgery, but rather is one of the functional goals.

Ref:

Miller, MD. (ed.) (2008) *Review of Orthopaedics*, Saunders Elsevier, Philadelphia. p. 323.

**26.    B**

The femoral anatomical axis is defined by the intramedullary canal and is distinct from the mechanical axis, which runs from the centre of the femoral head to the point of intersection with the exit point of the femoral anatomic axis. This is normally at the intercondylar notch, and is the usual entry point for the intramedullary rod of the femoral jig. In cases of distal femoral bowing, the anatomic axis may exit slightly lateral or medial to the intercondylar notch. The angle between the femoral mechanical and anatomical axis is known as the valgus cut angle, and when the distal femur is cut at this angle it ensures that the centre of the prosthesis is mechanically aligned with the centre of the femoral head. The valgus cut angle is usually between 5–7 degrees, but can be less in very tall patients. The tibial cut is perpendicular to the mechanical axis of the tibia, which runs from the centre of the knee to the centre of the ankle.

Ref:

Miller, MD. (ed.) (2008) *Review of Orthopaedics*, Saunders Elsevier, Philadelphia. p. 324.

**27.    E**

Ligament balancing is an important factor in providing optimum wear and function in total knee arthroplasty. Balancing is required in both the coronal and sagittal planes. Varus deformities require release of the medial structures, in the order: osteophytes, deep MCL, semimembranosus, superficial MCL, PCL. Valgus deformities require release of the lateral structures in the order: osteophytes, lateral capsule, iliotibial band, popliteus, LCL. Full release of the superficial MCL or the LCL is an indication for the use of a constrained device. Correction of a valgus knee with a flexion contracture is most likely to lead to a peroneal nerve palsy.

Ref:

Miller, MD. (Ed.) (2008) *Review of Orthopaedics*, Saunders Elsevier, Philadelphia. pp. 325–6.

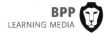

**28. B**

Femoral rollback refers to the posterior shift of the femora-tibial contact as the knee flexes and the femur rolls back on tibia. This increases the potential for further flexion by preventing posterior structures from impinging, and increases the effective strength of the quadriceps by increasing their moment arm. In the PCL substituting prosthesis this is reproduced more accurately, in the presence of a spine-cam mechanism, and there are less contact stresses on the polyethylene. In the PCL retaining prosthesis femoral rollback occurs as a consequence of roll and slide, and leads to higher contact stresses

Ref:
Fantozzi, S. Catani, F. Ensini, A. Leardini, A. Giannini, S. (2006) Femoral rollback of cruciate-retaining and posterior-stabilised total knee replacements: in vivo fluoroscopic analysis during activities of daily living, *J Orthop Res*, 24. 12, 2222–9.

**29. A**

A PCL substituting prosthesis is favoured over a PCL retaining prosthesis in patients who have or who may go on to have an abnormal PCL either due to injury or disease. This can include rupture of the PCL due to injury or an inflammatory arthropathy, as well as over release during ligament balancing. In the presence of a previous patellectomy, the PCL substituting prosthesis is preferred due to its ability to increase the extensor mechanism lever arm, and thus prevent anterior dislocation of the femur. The PCL substituting prosthesis can be problematic in the hyperflexed knee where the femur can be levered over the tibial post and dislocate. For this reason it should be avoided in cases where more than 130 degrees of knee flexion is expected.

Ref:
Miller, MD. (ed.) (2008) *Review of Orthopaedics*, Saunders Elsevier, Philadelphia. p. 328.

**30. D**

The most important determinant of final postoperative knee flexion is the preoperative flexion range, with postoperative flexion being roughly equal to preoperative +/−10 degrees. Postoperative flexion contractures are usually due to hamstring spasms and tightness, and a relative inactivity of quadriceps firing post arthrotomy. Knees closed in flexion recover quicker than those closed in extension and require less continuous passive motion. Arthrofibrosis following TKR should be treated expediently with manipulation, but care should be taken in the presence of anterior femoral notching. Reduced bending strength can lead to supracondylar fractures in these cases.

Ref:
Miller, MD. (ed.) (2008) *Review of Orthopaedics*, Saunders Elsevier, Philadelphia. p. 335.

**31. A**

The Q angle is the angle formed by the intersection of the extensor mechanism axis with the axis of the patella tendon. One of the aims of total knee replacement surgery is to maintain a normal Q angle and so prevent abnormal patella tracking. The Q angle is increased by any manoeuvre which moves the trochlea more medial (medialisation of the femoral component), externally rotates the tibial tubercle (internal rotation of the tibial component), and increases lateral tilt (internal rotation of the femoral component) or position (lateralisation of the patella component) of the patella. Valgus alignment will

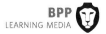

also increase the Q angle.

Ref:
Rand, JA. (1994) The patellofemoral joint in total knee arthroplasty, *J Bone Joint Surg Am*, 76. 4, 612–20.

**32.   E**
The most common patellofemoral complications following total knee replacement surgery are related to abnormal patella tracking. Patella clunk syndrome is seen with the PCL substituting prosthesis, and is due to impingement of a fibrotic nodule at the distal end of the quadriceps.

Ref:
Kelly, MA. (2001) Patellofemoral complications following total knee arthroplasty, *Instr Course Lect*, 50, 403–7.

**33.   C**
Potential causes of early failure of TKR include fracture, infection, component failure and component wear. Joint aspiration remains the most accurate investigation for diagnosing infection. Radionuclide bone scan may indicate loosening after 6–12 months, but cannot distinguish between septic and aseptic loosening so early on. The evaluation of component rotation in the context of a painful TKR is best performed with a CT scan.

Ref:
Barrack, RL. Schrader, T. Bertot, AJ. Wolfe, MW. Myers, L. (2001) Component rotation and anterior knee pain after total knee arthroplasty, *Clin Orthop Relat Res*, 392, 46–55.

**34.   B**
The polyethylene insert thickness must be at least 8mm to be able to keep the joint contact stresses below the yield strength of the UHMWPE.

Ref:
Miller, MD. (ed.) (2008) *Review of Orthopaedics*, Saunders Elsevier, Philadelphia. p. 333.

**35.   A**
Numerous studies have documented that gram-positive organisms are the most common bacteria causing infections associated with joint arthroplasty, with staphylococcus aureus and staphylococcus epidermidis causing the majority of the infections.

Ref:
Meehan, J. Jamali, AA. Nguyen, H. (2009) Prophylactic antibiotics in hip and knee arthroplasty, *J Bone Joint Surg Am*, 91. 10, 2480–90.

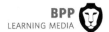

**36.** **C**

The treatment of isolated patellofemoral arthritis remains a controversial topic. However in the absence of trochlea dysplasia or patella instability it is probably best treated with patellofemoral replacement in the younger patient.

Ref:

Grelsamer, RP. Stein, DA. (2006) Patellofemoral Arthritis, *J Bone Joint Surg Am*, 88A. 8, 1849–1860.

**37.** **E**

Constrained knee prostheses are part of the armamentarium of the revision knee surgeon, and all have a large central post which can substitute for deficient collateral ligament function. In revision surgery they should always be used with both femoral and tibial medullary stems, which assist with load sharing. The first choice is usually the non hinged constrained prosthesis, but in cases of necessity, such as global ligament deficiency or tumour resections, one may consider a hinged prosthesis. The hinged prosthesis is the most constrained TKR implant and has a mechanical linkage between the femur and the tibia. Constrained implants generate greater forces at the prosthesis bone interface than unconstrained implants

Ref:

Miller, MD. (ed.) (2008) *Review of Orthopaedics*, Saunders Elsevier, Philadelphia. p. 337.

**38.** **C**

The major goals of revision TKR include extraction of knee components with minimal bone and soft tissue loss, restoration of bone defects, restoration of the original joint line and balancing of the ligaments. Once the components have been removed, it is vital to establish the joint line, and this is best done by reconstructing the tibia first.

Ref:

Miller, MD. (Ed.) (2008) *Review of Orthopaedics*, Saunders Elsevier, Philadelphia. p. 338.

**39.** **D**

Unicompartmental knee replacement in the absence of a functional ACL can lead to early failure due to increased sliding translation in the medial compartment. A rigid valgus or varus deformity cannot be adequately balanced with UKR and should thus be avoided. Significant tricompartmental disease is an indication for TKR.

Ref:

Miller, MD. (Ed.) (2008) *Review of Orthopaedics*, Saunders Elsevier, Philadelphia. p. 340.

**40.** **D**

MRI is approximately 95% specific for diagnosing meniscal pathology.

Ref:

Mackenzie, R. Palmer, CR. Lomas, DJ. Dixon, AK. (1996) Magnetic resonance imaging of the knee: diagnostic performance studies, *Clin Radiol*, 51. 4, 251–7.

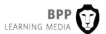

# Adult Pathology

## Spine: Question Bank

Suhayl Tafazal & Talal Ibrahim

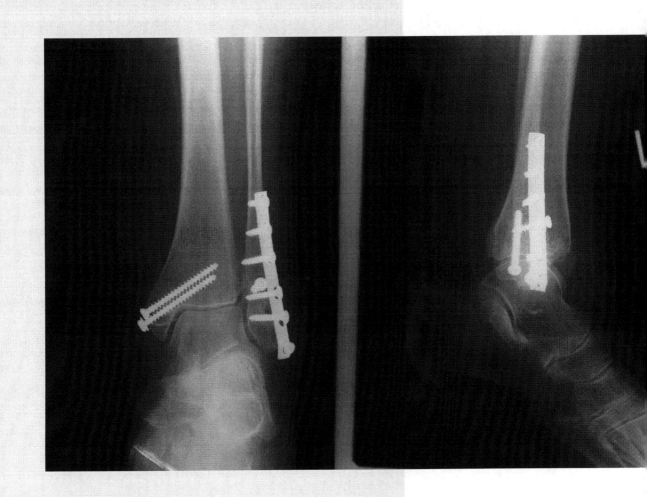

1.  Which one of the following statements regarding spinal injury syndromes is **true**?
    A.  Anterior cord syndrome is the result of extension injury in elderly patients
    B.  Brown-Sequard syndrome carries the best prognosis
    C.  Central cord syndrome affects the lower limbs greater than the upper limbs
    D.  Anterior cord syndrome carries the best prognosis
    E.  Brown-Sequard syndrome is usually due to non-penetrating trauma


2.  Which one of the following defects of vertebral body formation has the highest risk of progression in congenital scoliosis?
    A.  Block vertebra
    B.  Simple unsegmented hemivertebra
    C.  Unilateral unsegmented bar
    D.  Wedge vertebra
    E.  Unilateral unsegmented bar and contralateral hemivertebra


3.  A 16-year-old girl presents with a 3-month history of increasing mid-thoracic spine pain, with no history of trauma. The pain is worse at night, but she does not have any radicular pain. She is otherwise fit and well. On examination she is tender over T8 and plain radiographs show a mild tilting of the thoracic spine to the right, but no rotational deformity of the thoracic spine. What is the best investigation to further investigate the cause of this pain?
    A.  MRI scan
    B.  Blood tests for inflammatory markers
    C.  Bone scan
    D.  Plain radiographs of whole spine
    E.  CT myelogram


4.  A 48-year-old man presents with a 5-week history of pain in the low back radiating to the right leg along the L5 dermatome. There is some weakness of extensor hallucis longus (MRC grade 4/5) and numbness along the L5 dermatome. Clinically, this is consistent with a radiculopathy secondary to a lumbar disc prolapse. Which of the following statements is **true**?
    A.  Contained disc prolapses do well following surgery
    B.  The most likely cause of symptoms is a far lateral disc prolapse at L4/5
    C.  A plain radiograph of the lumbar spine is indicated
    D.  Discectomy will lead to a more rapid resolution of symptoms
    E.  Following surgery for a disc prolapse there is a 1520% chance of recurrent disc prolapse


5.  When performing an anterior approach to the cervical spine, which one of the following statements is **false**?
    A.  It can be used for discectomy in patients presenting with a C5 radiculopathy
    B.  There is an increased risk of injury to the recurrent laryngeal nerve with left sided approaches
    C.  Lower left sided approaches can increase the risk of injury to the thoracic duct
    D.  The platysma is retracted with the skin
    E.  Damage to the stellate ganglion can result in Horner's syndrome

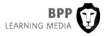

6.   All of the following statements regarding spinal stenosis are **true** except:
     A.   It is common in patients with achondroplasia
     B.   Lateral recess stenosis usually affects the exiting nerve root at that level
     C.   Central stenosis is more common in men
     D.   Surgical treatment of stenosis secondary to spondylolistheis should include a fusion procedure
     E.   L4/5 is the commonest level to be affected

7.   Which of the following statements regarding spinal tuberculosis are **true**?
     A.   It is an uncommon location for extrapulmonary tuberculosis
     B.   Skip lesions can be present in up to 50% of patients
     C.   It usually originates in the disc and spreads to the vertebral body
     D.   Vertebral collapse and progressive kyphosis is an indication for surgical intervention
     E.   Abnormalities on chest radiographs are rarely found

8.   With regards to spinal trauma, which of the following statements applies?
     A.   Widening of the interpedicular distance on antero-posterior radiographs suggests injury to the posterior column according to Denis
     B.   The thoracolumbar junction is an area not particularly susceptible to injury
     C.   A burst fracture always requires operative intervention
     D.   Lesions below L1 level have a worse prognosis
     E.   Non-contiguous injuries necessitate imaging of whole spine in patients presenting with a spinal fracture

9.   A 54-year-old diabetic man presents with mid thoracic back pain and pyrexia of 38 degrees. He has no neurological deficit. His blood tests reveal a CRP of 195 and WCC of 12.9. Blood cultures are negative. An MRI scan shows increased signal in the T8/9 disc space and a collection anterior to the vertebral bodies on both T2 and fat suppressed images. The next step in the management is:
     A.   Commence empirical intravenous antibiotics
     B.   Anterior debridement and strut grafting
     C.   Commence quadruple antituberculous chemotherapy
     D.   CT guided needle biopsy and commence empirical antibiotics
     E.   Triple phase bone scan

10.  A 38-year-old lady presents with neck pain and pain radiating down the left arm to the thumb and index fingers. She has no neurological deficit and is Hoffmann's reflex negative. The best test to further investigate this is:
     A.   CT myelogram
     B.   CT scan
     C.   MRI scan
     D.   Nerve conduction studies
     E.   Thoracic outlet views

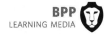

11. A 48-year-old lady has been admitted with a burst fracture at L1 with loss of anterior vertebral body height of 25 degrees and kyphosis of 15 degrees. She has no neurological deficit. The management of this is:
    A. Posterior decompression and stabilisation T12 to L2
    B. Posterior stabilisation T9 to L3
    C. 6 weeks of bed rest
    D. Analgesia and then application of an extension type orthoses/brace
    E. T12 to L2 posterior stabilisation

12. A positive Hoffmann reflex is associated with:
    A. Cervical spinal cord compression and myelopathy
    B. Cervical radiculopathy
    C. Brachial neuritis
    D. Thoracic outlet syndrome
    E. Peripheral neuropathy

13. In spinal deformity correction which of the following is associated with the highest risk of neurological damage?
    A. Anterior lumbar surgery
    B. Posterior spinal instrumentation and correction of scoliosis
    C. Posterior cervical surgery
    D Combined anterior and posterior correction of kyphosis
    E. Anterior cervical surgery

14. A 12-year-old girl presents with a right sided thoracic scoliosis with the apex at T7 measuring 18 degrees. She is Risser stage 1 and is asymptomatic with no neurological deficit. A year later the curve measures 26 degrees and she is Risser stage 2. The next step in management is:
    A. Observation alone
    B. Posterior instrumented fusion
    C. Combined anterior and posterior instrumentation
    D. Bracing
    E. Posterior instrumentation alone

15. Diffuse idiopathic skeletal hyperostosis (DISH) is associated with which of the following:
    A. Sacroilitis
    B. Thoracic kyphosis
    C. Heterotopic ossification after total hip arthroplasty
    D. Marginal syndesmophytes
    E. High risk of spinal cord compression

16. A Trendelenburg positive gait is most likely to be seen after:
    A. Paracentral disc herniation at L3/4
    B. Far lateral disc herniation at L4/5
    C. Paracentral disc herniation at L5/S1
    D. Paracentral disc herniation at L4/5
    E. Central disc herniation at L2/3

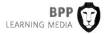

17. Which of the following factors is the key to deciding on using an anterior rather than a posterior approach to decompress the cervical spine in patients with cervical myelopathy?
    A. Significant neck pain pre-operatively
    B. Cervical kyphosis
    C. Multilevel diffuse canal stenosis
    D. High signal intensity on T2 weighted MRI scan of cervical spine
    E. Excessive cervical lordosis

18. A 36-year-old lady presents with left sided sciatica with pain radiating down to the S1 dermatome. Her past history includes a previous successful L5/S1 discectomy performed 3 years ago for similar symptoms resulting in complete relief of leg pain. Which of the following investigations are most useful to investigate the current episode of sciatica?
    A. MRI scan
    B. CT myelography
    C. Gadolinium enhanced MRI scan
    D. CT scan
    E. Bone scan

19. The preferred approach to the L4/5 level during an anterior transperitoneal approach is:
    A. Left
    B. Midline
    C. Right
    D. Directly anterior to L4 vertebral body
    E. Directed to the right side of the aorta

20. Which of the following factors do **not** influence the risk of development of a pseudoarthrosis after lumbar spinal fusion?
    A. Steroid use
    B. Smoking
    C. NSAID use
    D. Radiation therapy
    E. Hyperthyroidism

21. A 45-year-old man presents with a 1-week history of severe mechanical low back pain with no radicular symptoms. He does not report any weight loss and there is no history of trauma. On examination the pain is made worse by lumbar flexion and extension, but he has no neurological deficit in his legs. The best course of action is:
    A. Lumbar MRI scan
    B. Facet joint injections
    C. Analgesia, limited bed rest and return to normal activities as pain allows
    D. Epidural steroid injections
    E. Oral corticosteroids

22. A 52-year-old man presents with a 2-week history of low back pain and pain radiating down the left leg to the L5 dermatome. Which of the following would reassure the surgeon to continue non-operative management?
    A. Weight loss

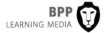

B. Fever
C. Straight leg raise restricted to 30 degrees
D. Loss of perianal sensation
E. History of trauma

23. Which structure is most at risk of damage during harvesting of bone graft from the posterior iliac crest during posterior lumbar decompression and fusion procedures?
   A. Genitofemoral nerve
   B. Ilioinguinal nerve
   C. Lateral femoral cutaneous nerve
   D. Iliohypogastric nerve
   E. Superior cluneal nerves

24. A 38-year-old man undergoes anterior cervical decompression and fusion at C4/5 for a large disc herniation. At 2 weeks post-operatively he complains of dysphagia. Which of the following is the least likely explanation for this complication?
   A. Damage to recurrent laryngeal nerve
   B. Post-operative soft tissue swelling
   C. Haematoma formation
   D. Damage to hypoglossal nerve
   E. Injury to the pharyngeal plexus

25. Risk factors for bone graft extrusion after anterior cervical surgery include all of the following except:
   A. Three level corpectomy
   B. Osteoporosis
   C. Combined anterior and posterior spinal instrumented fusion
   D. Graft overtensioning
   E. Previous cervical laminectomy

26. Which of the following is the commonest region of the spine to have neurologic compromise due to spinal metastases?
   A. Upper cervical
   B. Upper lumbar
   C. Thoracic
   D. Lower cervical
   E. Lumbosacral junction

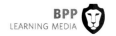
BPP
LEARNING MEDIA

27. A 78-year-old lady presents with a 3-week history of mid to lower thoracic spine pain. There is no preceding history of trauma. She has no constitutional symptoms and no neurologic compromise. Her past history includes breast carcinoma 10 years ago treated with mastectomy. A plain X-ray of the thoracic spine shows a compression fracture of T9. Which of the following investigations would help best to determine if the fracture is due to osteoporosis or metastatic disease?
    A. DEXA scan
    B. MRI scan
    C. CT scan
    D. Bone scan
    E. CT myelogram

28. Which of the following is a contraindication to the use of percutaneous vertebral augmentation by kyphoplasty or vertebroplasty for the treatment of vertebral compression fractures?
    A. Interruption of posterior vertebral cortex
    B. Pain for 4 months
    C. Metastatic compression fracture
    D. Kyphosis of 25 degrees
    E. Previous compression fracture

29. Which of the following carries the highest risk of post-operative wound infection?
    A. Posterior L4/5 decompression and fusion without instrumentation
    B. L5/S1 discectomy
    C. Posterior instrumentation for T12 burst fracture
    D. Anterior cervical decompression and fusion for disc herniation
    E. Lumbar decompression for L4/5 stenosis

30. Which of the following is the commonest level for symptomatic thoracic disc herniations?
    A. C7/T1
    B. T1/2
    C. T4/5
    D. T7/8
    E. T12/L1

31. A 15-year-old boy presents with a thoracic kyphotic deformity and pain made worse with activity and eased by rest. Which of the following radiographic findings would most support the diagnosis of Scheuermann's kyphosis?
    A. Thoracic kyphosis of 30 degrees
    B. Wedging of 5 degrees of 3 successive vertebra
    C. Hyperextension radiographs showing correction of the deformity
    D. Presence of an anterior bar
    E. Presence of marginal syndesmophytes

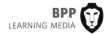

32.  A 68-year-old man presents with symptoms of neurogenic claudication. He has back and bilateral leg pain made worse on walking 400 yards. He is considered suitable for a lumbar decompression procedure. Which one of the following factors would be an indication for concomitant spinal fusion?
     A.  Pre-operative symptoms of bladder dysfunction
     B.  Black disc on MRI scanning
     C.  Presence of degenerative spondylolisthesis
     D.  Multilevel spinal stenosis
     E.  Loss of sagittal balance


33.  A 32-year-old lady is admitted as an emergency following a road traffic accident. Initial assessment according to ATLS principles is performed. The patient is noted to have neck pain and paraesthesia and numbness in the right C6 dermatome and power MRC grade 4/5 for elbow flexion. A lateral radiograph of the cervical spine and a CT scan confirm a bifacet dislocation at C5/6. The next step in management is:
     A.  Immediate closed reduction with Halo traction
     B.  Urgent anterior cervical decompression and plating
     C.  Posterior reduction and fusion
     D.  MRI scan
     E.  Flexion-extension views


34.  Which of the following non-operative treatments have been shown to be of benefit in patients with lumbar spinal stenosis?
     A.  Facet joint injections
     B.  Periradicular steroid injections
     C.  Salmon calcitonin
     D.  Spinal manipulation
     E.  Ultrasound therapy


35.  Which of the following factors in a patient presenting with isthmic spondylolisthesis is related to a low risk of progression of the slip?
     A.  Female sex
     B.  >50% slip
     C.  Pre-menarche
     D.  Unilateral pars defect
     E.  Risser stage 4


36   A 14-year-old male athlete presents with increasing low back pain. He recalls no history of trauma and he has to curtail his activities due to the pain. On examination he has some tenderness over the paraspinal muscles but no neurological deficit. Plain radiographs including an oblique view are normal. What is the next step in management?
     A.  6 weeks of restricted activities
     B.  TLSO brace
     C.  MRI scan
     D.  Physiotherapy
     E.  Single photon emission computed tomography (SPECT) scanning

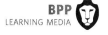

37. Which of the following is unlikely to be a cause of infantile torticollis?
    A. Trauma
    B. Spinal cord tumour
    C. Sternocleidomastoid tumour
    D. Occipitocervical synostosis
    E. Atlantoaxial rotatory displacement

38. Atlantoaxial subluxation can occur in all of the following conditions except:
    A. Spina bifida occulta
    B. Rheumatoid arthritis
    C. Marfan's syndrome
    D. Psoriatic arthropathy
    E. Down's syndrome

39. A 45-year-old man presents with back and right leg pain of 6 months' duration. On neurological testing he has some weakness of the right extensor hallucis longus with power grade 4/5. He reports reduced sensation along the lateral aspect of the lower leg. Which of the following pathologies would best explain his symptoms?
    A. L5/S1 postero-lateral disc protrusion
    B. Far lateral L4/5 disc protrusion
    C. L4/5 foraminal stenosis
    D. L5/S1 foraminal stenosis
    E. L3/4 posterolateral disc protrusion

40. A 48-year-old man with a long history of low back pain undergoes L4-S1 posterior stabilisation and posterior lumbar interbody fusion using polyetheretherketone (PEEK) cages at L4/5 and L5/S1. On day 1 post-operatively, he reports severe dyaesthesia and pain in the left L5 dermatome. This is best explained by:
    A. Penetration of the anterior longitudinal ligament
    B. Unrecognised dural tear
    C. Superior breach of L5 pedicle during pedicle screw insertion
    D. Inferior breach of L5 pedicle during pedicle screw insertion
    E. Epidural haematoma

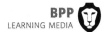

BPP
LEARNING MEDIA

# Adult Pathology

## Spine: Answers

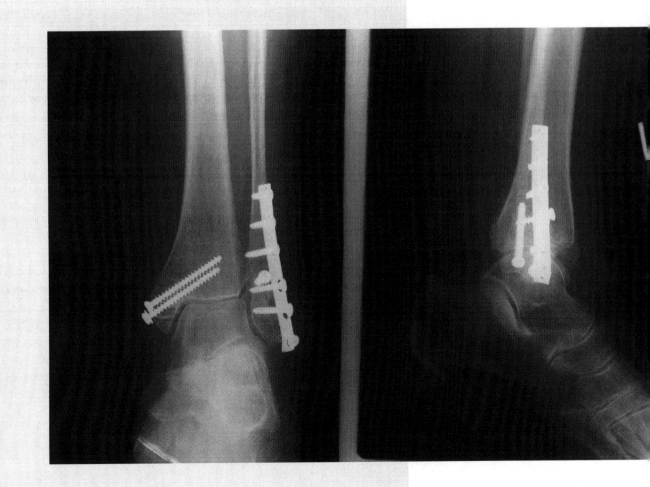

1.  **B**

    Brown-Sequard is caused by penetrating trauma, results in ipsilateral loss of motor function and vibration and position sense, contralateral loss of pain and temperature. This syndrome has the best prognosis.

    Central cord syndrome occurs due to an extension injury in elderly patients. It affects the upper limbs greater than the lower limbs resulting in motor and sensory loss.

    Anterior cord syndrome is caused by a flexion compression injury resulting in motor loss, but the dorsal columns are spared. This syndrome carries the worst prognosis.

    Ref:
    Miller MD (2008) *Review of Orthopaedics*. Saunders Elsevier, Philadelphia.

2.  **E**

    These anomalies are usually located in the thoracic spine and are the most aggressive of all congenital scoliotic deformities. There is potential for rapid progression as one side of the vertebra continues to grow (hemivertebra) and the other (bar) restricts growth.

    Block vertebra and simple unsegmented vertebrae have little growth potential and progress at a slow rate.

    Ref:
    Marks DS, Qaimkhani SA (2009). The natural history of Congenital Scoliosis and Kyphosis. *Spine*; 34: 1751–1755.

3.  **C**

    The most likely diagnosis here is an osteoid osteoma of the thoracic spine. A bone scan will show increased uptake in the region of the lesion and is an excellent screening tool for the diagnosis of back pain in children. An osteoid osteoma is a benign tumour, 10% of them occur in spine (posterior elements) and may cause a scoliosis. The usual age group is 5–25 years.

    Ref:
    Garg S, Dormans JP (2005): Tumors and tumor-like conditions of the spine in children. *J Am Acad Orthop Surg*; 13: 372–381.

4.  **D**

    Peul *et al.* showed that early surgery achieved more rapid relief of sciatica than conservative care, but outcomes were similar by one year and these did not change during the second year.

    Contained disc prolapses have the worst prognosis when operated on – in one study 37.5% rate of recurrent sciatica (Carragee E *et al.* (2003) Clinical outcomes after lumbar discectomy for sciatica. *J Bone Joint Surg (Am)*, 85: 102–108.) There is no place for plain radiography in the investigation of sciatica. There is a 5% risk of recurrent disc prolapse after surgery.

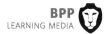

Ref:

Peul WC, van den Hout WB, Brand R *et al.* (2008): Prolonged conservative care versus early surgery in patients with sciatica caused by lumbar disc herniation: two year results of a randomised controlled trial. *BMJ*; 336: 1355–1358.


5.  **B**

This is **false** as the recurrent laryngeal nerve is more likely to be injured with a right sided approach and hence left sided approaches are preferred. During the approach the platysma is retracted with the skin and the interval between the carotid sheath and trachea is developed. There is risk of injuring the thoracic duct particularly with low left sided approaches.

Ref:

Miller MD (2008) *Review of Orthopaedics*. Saunders Elsevier, Philadelphia.


6.  **B**

This is **false** as lateral recess stenosis (also known as subarticular compression) occurs when there is compression between the medial aspect of a hypertrophic superior articular facet and the posterior aspect of the vertebral body and disc. This affects the traversing root (L5 at the L4/5 level). Foraminal stenosis affects the exiting nerve root (L4 at L4/5 level). It is commoner in men as they have a smaller spinal canal at L3-L5 level. Patients with achondroplasia have an increased risk of developing spinal stenosis due to short pedicles.

Ref:

Miller MD (2008) *Review of Orthopaedics*. Saunders Elsevier, Philadelphia.


7.  **D**

The spine is the commonest site for extrapulmonary tuberculosis. It originates in the metaphysis of the vertebral body and spreads under the anterior longitudinal ligament. Anterior vertebral body destruction with preservation of the disc, distinguishes tuberculosis from pyogenic infection. Skip lesions occur in up to 15% of patients. About two-thirds of patients have abnormal chest radiographs.

Ref:

Miller MD (2008) *Review of Orthopaedics*. Saunders Elsevier, Philadelphia.


8.  **E**

The entire spine must be imaged to rule out non-contiguous injuries as these can occur in up to 10% of patients. In the study by Vaccaro *et al.*, 31% of patients had a secondary injury initially missed with an average delay in diagnosis of 7.1 days. In 25% of these missed injuries, a neurologic deficit developed or progressed due to improper initial immobilisation. As the spinal cord ends at L1, lesions below L1 have a better prognosis as roots rather than cord are involved.

Widening of the interpedicular distance on AP radiographs and a change in the height of the posterior cortex of the vertebral body on a lateral radiograph of the spine indicates injury to the middle column according to Denis. This represents a potentially unstable injury.

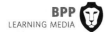

Stable burst fractures can be managed non-operatively. At the thoracolumbar junction there is a fulcrum of increased motion and this area is more commonly affected by spinal trauma.

Ref:
Vaccaro AR, An HS, Lin S *et al.* (1992) Noncontiguous injuries of the spine. *J Spinal Disord;* 5: 320–329.

9. **D**

The most likely diagnosis here is disc space infection. The next step would involve obtaining tissue diagnosis either by blood cultures or by obtaining tissue from CT guided or open biopsy and then commencing empirical antibiotics while awaiting microbiology results. Anterior debridement and strut grafting is only indicated if there is neurological deterioration, failure to respond to antibiotics, extensive bony destruction or marked deformity. A bone scan is useful to show the site of infection and possible skip lesions.

Ref:
Miller MD (2008) *Review of Orthopaedics.* Saunders Elsevier, Philadelphia.

10. **C**

The most likely diagnosis here is a cervical radiculopathy. MRI is a non-invasive modality used to provide excellent imaging of the spine and soft tissues. MRI scan is useful to demonstrate herniated discs as well as central and foraminal stenosis. A CT scan would not provide as much definition of the soft tissues around the spine, but is very useful to image the bony structures. A cervical myelogram is an invasive test and has been superceded by MRI scan.

Ref:
Rhee JM, Yoon T, Riew KD (2007) Cervical Radiculopathy, *J Am Acad Orthop Surg;* 15: 486–494.

11. **D**

This is a stable spinal fracture as described by McAfee. Factors that indicate instability include loss of anterior vertebral body height of >50% and initial kyphosis >20 degrees and progressive neurological deficit.

Ref:
Miller MD (2008) *Review of Orthopaedics.* Saunders Elsevier, Philadelphia.

12. **A**

A positive Hoffmann reflex is a highly sensitive test for cervical myelopathy due to cervical spinal cord compression. In one study, 94.5% of asymptomatic individuals had cord compression due to disc protrusion.

Ref:
Sung RD, Wang JC (Jan 2001) Correlation between a positive Hoffmann's reflex and cervical pathology in asymptomatic individuals. *Spine;* 26: 67–70.

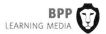

**13. D**

Possible mechanisms of spinal cord damage include hyperkyphosis and combined anterior and posterior surgery. The majority of injuries reflect vascular insufficiency due to disturbance of blood supply during exposure, reduced blood pressure and perfusion pressure during the peri- and post-operative periods and overzealous correction. Direct damage to the cord is a rare cause of paraplegia.

Ref:

Bulstrode C, Buckwalter J, Carr A *et al.* (2002) *Oxford textbook of Orthopaedics and Trauma.* Oxford University Press, Oxford. pp. 577–578.

**14. D**

There is a risk of progression especially as the child is Risser stage 2 so bracing may be effective here. 68% of curves of 20–29 degrees will progress in children that are Risser stages 0 or 1. A meta-analysis of bracing vs. natural history came out in favour of bracing.

Ref:

1. Bulstrode C, Buckwalter J, Carr A *et al.* (2002) *Oxford textbook of Orthopaedics and Trauma,* Oxford University Press, Oxford. pp. 577–578.
2. Rowe D, Berbstein S, Riddick M *et al.* (1997): A meta-analysis of the efficacy of non-operative treatment for idiopathic scoliosis. *J Bone Joint Surg (Am)*; 79: 664–74.

**15. C**

Patients with diffuse idiopathic skeletal hyperostosis (DISH) are at increased risk of heterotopic ossification after total hip arthroplasty. In one study by Fahrer *et al.*, heterotopic ossification developed in 30% of patients with DISH vs. 10% of those without DISH.

Ref:

1. Belanger TA, Rowe DE (2001) Diffuse Idiopathic Skeletal Hyperostosis: Musculoskeletal manifestations. *J Am Acad Orthop Surg*; 9: 258–267.
2. Fahrer H, Koch P, Ballmer P, Enzler P, Gerber N (1988) Ectopic ossification following total hip arthroplasty: Is diffuse idiopathic skeletal hyperostosis a risk factor? *Br J Rheumatol*; 27: 187–190.

**16. D**

A trendelenburg positive gait is due to weakness of gluteus medius which is innervated by the L5 nerve root. This nerve root is compressed after a paracentral disc herniation at L4/5. A far lateral disc herniation at L4/5 and a paracentral disc herniation at L3/4 affects the L4 nerve root. A paracentral disc herniation at L5/S1 results in compression of the S1 nerve root. Another possible cause of L5 root compression would be a far lateral disc herniation at L5/S1.

Ref:

Bulstrode C, Buckwalter J, Carr A *et al.* (2002) *Oxford textbook of Orthopaedics and Trauma.* Oxford University Press, Oxford.

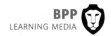

17. **B**

This is the key to deciding on using an anterior over a posterior approach. Most patients with cervical spondylosis have predominately anterior compression. Any posterior decompressive procedure is an indirect technique that requires posterior shifting of the cord in the thecal sac to diminish the effect of the anterior compression. For this to occur, the preoperative sagittal alignment of the cervical spine must be at least straight or preferably lordotic. A kyphotic spine is less likely to allow sufficient posterior translation of the spinal cord to diminish symptoms. The posterior approach is still preferred for patients with diffuse multilevel canal stenosis and congenitally narrow canals as these patients require decompression of virtually the entire cervical spine. This is more readily achieved with posterior laminoplasty techniques. Some authors prefer the anterior approach for patients with two level disease and posterior surgery for those with involvement at three or more levels.

Ref:
1. Emery SE: Cervical Spondylotic Myelopathy (2001): Diagnosis and Treatment. *J Am Acad Orthop Surg*; 9: 376–388.
2. Yonenobu K, Fuji T, Ono K *et al.* (1985) Choice of surgical treatment for multisegmental cervical spondylotic myelopathy. *Spine*; 10: 710–716.

18. **C**

The likely diagnosis is a recurrent disc prolapse and this is best diagnosed using a gadolinium enhanced MRI scan which will also distinguish between scar tissue from the previous discectomy and recurrent disc. The other investigations will not be able to distinguish between scar and recurrent disc.

Ref:
1. Sotiropoulos S, Chafetz NI, Lang P *et al.* (1989) Differentiation between postoperative scar and recurrent disk herniation: Prospective comparison of MR, CT, and contrast-enhanced CT. *AJNR Am J Neuroradiol*; 10: 639–643.
2. Boden SD, Wiesel SW (1996): Lumbar Spine Imaging: Role in clinical decision making. *J Am Acad Orthop Surg*; 4: 238–248.

19. **A**

The aorta and vena cava are held firmly onto the anterior parts of the lower lumbar vertebrae by the lumbar vessels. These segmental vessels must be mobilised to permit the aorta and vena cava to be moved. Because the arterial structures are easier to dissect and more muscular than are the thin walled venous structures, the preferred approach to the L4–5 disc space is from the left, the more arterial side.

Ref:
Hoppenfield S (2003) (3rd ed.) *Surgical Exposures in Orthopaedics. The Anatomic Approach.* Lippincott Williams & Wilkins, Philadelphia.

20. **E**

All of the other risk factors inhibit spinal fusion. Thyroid hormone is known to have a positive effect on bone healing. Prior to any spinal fusion procedure, patients should be advised to stop smoking and discontinue NSAID use.

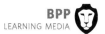

Ref:
1. Larsen JM, Capen DA (1997) Pseudoarthrosis of the lumbar spine. *J Am Acad Orthop Surg*; 5: 153–162.
2. Brown CW, Orme TJ, Richardson HD (1986) The rate of pseudarthrosis (surgical non-union) in patients who are smokers and patients who are non-smokers: A comparison study. *Spine*; 11: 942–943.

**21.    C**

Facet joint injections, epidural steroid injections and oral corticosteroids have shown no benefit in patients with acute mechanical low back pain. An MRI scan is not indicated as there are no radicular symptoms.

Ref:

Shen FH, Samartzis D, Andersson GBJ (2006): Nonsurgical management of acute and chronic low back pain. *J Am Acad Orthop Surg*; 14: 477–487.

**22.    C**

The remaining factors are all considered red flag signs indicating signs of serious spine pathology and require urgent further investigation and management.

Ref:
1. Shen FH, Samartzis D, Andersson GBJ (2006)Nonsurgical management of acute and chronic low back pain. *J Am Acad Orthop Surg*; 14: 477–487.
2. Samanta J, Kendall J, Samanta A (March 2003) Chronic low back pain. *BMJ*; 326: 535.

**23.    E**

These nerves are at risk when harvesting bone graft from the posterior iliac crest. These nerves cross the iliac crest and can be avoided by placing the incision no more than 8cm anterolateral to the posterior superior iliac spine. The nerves supply sensation to the skin over the cluneal (gluteal area) and are composed of the posterior primary rami of L1, L2 and L3. Damage to these nerves can result in numbness over the buttock area and occasionally a painful neuroma can form. The lateral femoral cutaneous nerve most commonly passes 1cm medial to the anterior superior iliac spine and so is not at risk with harvesting bone graft from the posterior iliac crest. The ilioinguinal, iliohypogastric and genitofemoral nerves are again more at risk during anterior approaches to the iliac crest with overzealous retraction of the abdominal muscles.

Ref:

Hoppenfield S. *Surgical Exposures in Orthopaedics. The Anatomic Approach.* 3rd edition. p. 346.

**24.    D**

Dysphagiais one of the commonest complications of anterior cervical surgery. It is reported to occur in 28–57% patients and usually occurs in the intermediate post-operative period between 1–6 weeks post-op. Its causes are multifactorial, potential causes are denervation of the oesophagus, post-op haematoma formation and soft tissue swelling and damage to specific nerves involved in swallowing. The hypoglossal nerve which is involved in both the oral and pharyngeal phases of swallowing is most at risk of damage during

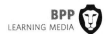

surgical procedures above the level of C3. Anterior cervical spine surgery between C2–5 risks injury to the nerves of the pharyngeal plexus, which arise from the vagus nerve. Irritation or injury to these nerves can occur as a result of traction and can cause significant pharyngeal dysphagia. The superior laryngeal nerve is at risk during surgery at C3–4 level and damage to this nerve can lead to laryngeal sensory impairment and dysphagia. Surgery to the lower cervical spine C5–T1 can place the recurrent laryngeal nerve at risk of injury, which can cause mild dysphagia, mainly during swallowing of liquids.

Ref:
1. Daniels AH, Riew DK, Yoo JU *et al.* (2008) Adverse events associated with anterior cervical spine surgery. *J Am Acad Orthop Surg*; 16: 729–738.
2. Frempong-Boadu A, Houten JK, Osborn B *et al.* (2002) Swallowing and speech dysfunction in patients undergoing anterior cervical discectomy and fusion: A prospective, objective preoperative and postoperative assessment. *J Spinal Disord Tech*; 15: 362–368.

25. **C**

Bone graft extrusion after anterior cervical surgery is a potentially serious complication with a reported incidence of 6.4% in one study. It can lead to acute airway compromise if the bone graft is displaced anteriorly and spinal cord compression if displaced posteriorly. Three level corpectomy is known to increase the risk of graft extrusion. Sasso *et al.*[3] reported a 6% failure rate after two level corpectomy and 71% failure rate after three level corpectomy, despite use of a locking plate. Osteoporosis, graft overtensioning and previous cervical laminectomy are all risk factors for graft extrusion due to vertebral body fracture and secondary graft displacement. Combined anterior and posterior surgery is not known to increase the risk of graft extrusion; in general a patient requiring corpectomy of two or more levels should be considered for simultaneous posterior instrumented spine fusion.

Ref:
1. Daniels AH, Riew DK, Yoo JU *et al.* (2008) Adverse events associated with anterior cervical spine surgery. *J Am Acad Orthop Surg*; 16: 729–738.
2. Emery SE, Bohlman HH, Bolesta MJ, Jones PK (1998): Anterior cervical decompression and arthrodesis for the treatment of cervical spondylotic myelopathy: Two to seventeen-year follow-up. *J Bone Joint Surg (Am)* 80: 941–951.
3. Sasso RC, Ruggiero RA, Reilly TM, Hall PV (2003) Early reconstruction failures after multilevel cervical corpectomy. *Spine*; 28: 140–142.

26. **C**

Although the lumbar region is the commonest site for vertebral metastases based on autopsy studies (due to the larger size of the vertebral bodies here), most metastatic lesions of the spine causing neurologic compromise are known to occur in the thoracic spine. This is due to the smaller ratio between the diameter of the spinal canal and the traversing spinal cord within the thoracic spine. In a study of 1585 cases of metastatic spinal tumours that caused neurologic compromise, 70% of lesions were found in the thoracic spine, 22% in the lumbosacral spine and 8% in the cervical spine.

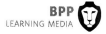

Ref:
1.  White AP, Kwon BK, Lindskog DM (2006) Metastatic disease of the spine. *J Am Acad Orthop Surg;* 14: 587–598.
2.  Schaberg J, Gainor BJ (1985) A profile of metastatic carcinoma of the spine. *Spine;* 10: 19–20.
3.  Brihaye J, Ectors P, Lemort M, Van Houtte P (1988) The management of spinal epidural metastases. *Adv Tech Stand Neurosurg;* 16: 121–176.

27. **B**

In the elderly patient it can be difficult to determine the underlying cause of a compression fracture. MRI scan can be particularly useful in these situations. In both situations T2 sequences will show increased signal intensity, whereas on T1 sequences metastatic disease shows diminished signal intensity compared to osteoporotic fractures which appear isointense. Metastatic pathologic fractures show involvement of the pedicle and posterior elements as well as an associated epidural or paraspinal mass, which can also be assessed on MRI scan. In patients with metastatic spine disease, MRI evaluation of the entire spine is necessary to determine if there are any skip lesions present.

Ref:
1.  White AP, Kwon BK, Lindskog DM (2006) Metastatic disease of the spine. *J Am Acad Orthop Surg;* 14: 587–598.
2.  Chan JHM, Peh WCG, Tsui EYK *et al.* (2002): Acute vertebral body compression fractures: Discrimination between benign and malignant causes using apparent diffusion coefficients. *Br J Radiol;* 75: 207–214.

28. **A**

Both kyphoplasty and vertebroplasty are percutaneous techniques used to treat vertebral compression fractures due to osteoporosis or metastatic disease. An acute compression fracture with ≥ 20 degrees kyphosis or ≥ 40% collapse are indications for these techniques. Kyphoplasty more reliably corrects kyphotic deformity although both techniques are known to provide good pain relief following acute compression fractures. Interruption of the posterior vertebral cortex is a contraindication as both techniques involve injecting cement into the vertebral body and without a posterior cortex there is no posterior barrier to cement extrusion into the spinal canal. The presence of pain for 4 months and a previous compression fracture and are not contraindications to treatment. Other contraindications include vertebra plana and fractures or neoplasms with spinal canal compromise.

Ref:
Spivak JM, Johnson MG (2005) Percutaneous treatment of vertebral body pathology. *J Am Acad Orthop Surg;* 13: 6–17.

29. **C**

Post-operative wound infection following spinal surgery varies depending on the type of procedure performed. Anterior spinal surgery carries the lowest risk of infection. Lumbar discectomy is reported to have a 0.7% post-op infection rate. Spinal fusion without instrumentation seems to have a lower rate of infection than instrumented cases. In elective surgical instrumented cases the incidence of infection has been reported to be 2.8% to 6%. Spinal surgery for trauma has an increased infection rate of up to 10%. The higher infection risk may be the result of greater localised tissue hypoxia resulting from soft tissue injury.

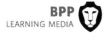

Ref:

Sasso RC, Garrido BJ (2008) Post-operative spinal wound infections. *J Am Acad Orthop Surg*; 16: 330–337.


**30.  E**

Herniations are extremely rare in the upper thoracic spine, T1/2 to T4/5 herniations account for approximately 1–3% of all thoracic disc herniations. Approximately 50–75% of thoracic disc herniations occur between the T8 and L1 levels. The T11/12 and T12/L1 interspaces are the most frequent sites of **symptomatic** thoracic disc herniations. This is thought to be due to the increased mobility at these levels and potential for developing degenerative disease.

Ref:
1.  Vanichkachorn JS, Vaccaro AR (2000) Thoracic Disk Disease: Diagnosis and Treatment. *J Am Acad Orthop Surg*; 8: 159–169.
2.  Rogers MA, Crockard HA (1994) Surgical treatment of the symptomatic herniated thoracic disk. *Clin Orthop*; 300: 70–78.


**31.  B**

The main criteria for diagnosing Scheuermann's kyphosis is wedging of 5 degrees of 3 successive vertebra on plain radiographs. The Scoliosis Research Society has stated that the accepted range of normal thoracic kyphosis is 20–40 degrees for a growing adolescent. Correction of the kyphosis on hyperextension radiographs suggests a diagnosis of postural kyphosis. The presence of an anterior bar would be consistent with a congenital kyphosis and marginal syndesmophytes are seen in ankylosing spondylitis.

Ref:

Tribus CB: Scheuermann's kyphosis in adolescents and adults (1998) Diagnosis and Management. *J Am Acad Orthop Surg*; 6: 36–43.


**32.  C**

This factor indicates instability and therefore concomitant fusion is recommended. In one study[1] comparing decompression alone and decompression with intertransverse fusion, 96% of patients had satisfactory results after decompression and fusion compared with 44% of those who did not undergo fusion. Progression of the slip occurred in 28% of the group who underwent fusion compared to 96% of patients who had decompression alone. A meta-analysis[2] has also shown that a satisfactory outcome was reported in 69% of patients with degenerative spondylolisthesis undergoing decompression alone , compared with 90% of patients having a concomitant fusion.

Ref:
1.  Herkowitz HN, Kurz LT (1991) Degenerative lumbar spondylolisthesis with spinal stenosis: A prospective study comparing decompression with decompression and intertransverse process arthrodesis. *J Bone Joint Surg (Am)*; 73: 802–808.
2.  Mardjetko SM, Connolly PJ, Shott S (1994) Degenerative lumbar spondylolisthesis: A meta-analysis of literature, 1970–1993. *Spine*; 19 (suppl 20): 2256S–2265S.
3.  Herkowitz HN, Sidhu KS (1995) Lumbar spine fusion in the treatment of degenerative conditions: current indications and recommendations. *J Am Acad Orthop Surg*; 3: 123–135.

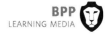

33. **D**

A bifacet dislocation is a highly unstable injury and can be associated with significant spinal cord injury. The definitive treatment includes a combination of posterior reduction with fusion and anterior decompression and fusion. Prior to this an MRI scan is essential as there is a risk of an associated cervical disc extrusion and attempts at closed reduction can result in displacement of the disc material into the spinal cord and conversion of an incomplete neurological deficit to a complete deficit. If a significant disc extrusion is seen on MRI scanning, then anterior cervical discectomy and plating is perfomed, however if the dislocation cannot be reduced anteriorly then after anterior discectomy, the patient will require a posterior reduction and fusion and then turned to the supine position for completion of the procedure by anterior plating.

Ref:
1. Timothy J, Towns G, Girn HS (2004) Cervical spine injuries. *Current Orthopaedics*; 18: 1–16.
2. Slucky AV, Potter HG (1998) Use of magnetic resonance imaging in spinal trauma: Indications, techniques and utility. *J Am Acad Orthop Surg*; 6: 134–145.
3. Kwon BK, Vaccaro AR, Grauer JN *et al.* (2006) Subaxial cervical spine trauma. *J Am Acad Orthop Surg*; 14: 78–89.

34. **B**

These have been shown to produce some benefit in patients with lumbar spinal stenosis but the effect is only moderate improvement compared to patients having similar injections for sciatica due to lumbar disc herniation. In a study[2] by Ng *et al.*, 37% of patients with spinal stenosis had a 10% reduction in the Oswestry Disability Index at 3 months post-injection.

Ref:
1. S Tafazal, L Ng, N Chaudhary, P Sell (2009) Corticosteroids in Peri-radicular Infiltration for Radicular Pain- a Randomised Double Blind Controlled Trial. One year results and subgroup analysis. *Eur Spine J*; 18: 1220–1225.
2. Ng L, Sell P (2004) Outcomes of a prospective cohort study on peri-radicular infiltration for radicular pain in patients with lumbar disc herniation and spinal stenosis. *Eur Spine J*; 13: 325–329.

35. **D**

Children presenting pre-menarche, girls and those with >50% slip at presentation are most likely to progress. In one study with a 45 year follow-up of patients with spondylolysis and spondylolistheis no patient with a unilateral pars defect progressed to slippage over the course of follow up.

Ref:
1. Beutler WJ, Fredrickson BE, Murtland A (2003) The natural history of spondylolysis and spondylolisthesis: 45-year follow up evaluation. *Spine*; 28: 1027–1035.
2. Boxall D, Bradford DS, Winter RB, Moe JH (1979) Management of severe spondylolisthesis in children and adolescents. *J Bone Joint Surg Am*; 61: 479–495.

**36.   E**

The most likely diagnosis here is an acute spondylolysis and SPECT scanning of the lumbosacral spine is the most effective method of detecting this. MRI has a high false-positive rate and is not routinely used in adolescents presenting with spondylolysis and spondylolisthesis.

Ref:

Bodner RJ, Heyman S, Drummond DS, Gregg JR (1988) The use of single photon emission computed tomography (SPECT) in the diagnosis of low-back pain in young patients. *Spine*; 13: 1155–1160.

**37.   D**

Occipitocervical synostosis condition is associated with a short neck, low posterior hair line and limited range of motion of the neck and is not known to cause infantile torticollis. The other rare causes need to be ruled out in an infant presenting with torticollis before a diagnosis of muscular torticollis is made.

Ref:

Copley LA, Dormans JP (1998) Cervical spine disorders in infants and children. *J Am Acad Orthop Surg*; 6: 204–214.

**38.   A**

Atlantoaxial subluxation can occur in all the other conditions. It occurs due to either a bony or ligamentous abnormality resulting in excessive mobility of C1 on C2. The most common abnormalities involve the transverse ligament or odontoid process. Atlantoaxial subluxation is defined as an atlantodens interval of greater than 3mm in adults and greater than 5mm in children.

Ref:

Frymoyer JW, Wiesel SW, An HS *et al.* (2004) *The Adult and Paediatric Spine*; Lippincott Williams & Wilkins, Philadelphia.

**39.   D**

The symptoms are consistent with L5 root compression which would occur with L5/S1 foraminal stenosis. Posterolateral disc protrusions usually affect the more distal nerve root at a particular level; therefore a L5/S1 posterolateral disc protrusion would affect the S1 root. The more proximal root is affected in far lateral disc protrusions or foraminal pathology, so foraminal stenosis at L5/S1 would affect the L5 nerve root.

Ref:

Frymoyer JW, Wiesel SW, An HS *et al.* (2004) *The Adult and Paediatric Spine*. Lippincott Williams & Wilkins, Philadelphia.

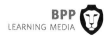

**40.  D**

The lumbar nerve roots exit below their corresponding pedicle and tend to hug the medial and inferior aspect of the pedicle. The lumbar nerve roots tend to fill the superior third of the foramen. Therefore, an inferior pedicle breach is much more likely to cause nerve root injury compared to a superior breach of the pedicle.

Ref:

Frymoyer JW, Wiesel SW, An HS *et al.* (2004) *The Adult and Paediatric Spine*. Lippincott Williams & Wilkins, Philadelphia.

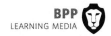

BPP
LEARNING MEDIA

# Adult Pathology

## Foot & Ankle: Question Bank

Haroon A Mann & Fahad G Attar

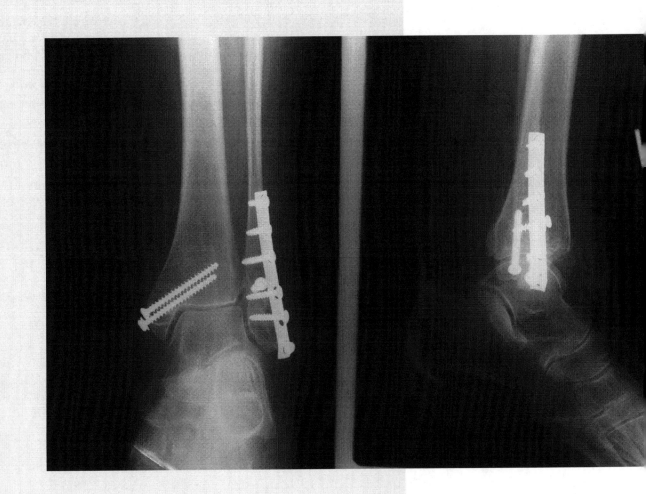

1.  Chronic instability of the peroneal tendons can best be demonstrated by positioning the ankle in:
    A.  Dorsiflexion against resisted inversion
    B.  Dorsiflexion against no resistance
    C.  Plantar flexion against resisted inversion
    D.  Dorsiflexion against resisted eversion
    E.  Plantar flexion against resisted eversion

2.  Which of the following tendons is considered the functional antagonist of the peroneus longus tendon?
    A.  Peroneus brevis
    B.  Posterior tibial tendon
    C.  Flexor digitorum longus
    D.  Extensor hallucis longus
    E.  Tibialis anterior

3.  A 42-year-old manual labourer has significant pain around the Hallux metatarsophalangeal joint. Three years ago he underwent removal of a bone spur, with some relief. Radiographs demonstrated arthritis in the Hallux MPJ joint. The appropriate treatment would be:
    A.  Resection of the first metatarsal head
    B.  Keller's procedure
    C.  Proximal phalangeal closing wedge osteotomy and interpositional arthroplasty
    D.  Arthrodesis of the first metatarsophalangeal joint
    E.  Silastic implant arthroplasty

4.  Examination of a 24-year-old man with hereditary motor sensory neuropathy reveals a correctable cavovarus. Recommended treatment would consist of:
    A.  Split anterior tibial tendon transfer
    B.  First metatarsophalangeal arthrodesis and achilles tendon lengthening
    C.  Dwyer calcaneal osteotomy and posterior tibial tendon transfer
    D.  Triple arthrodesis
    E.  Plantar fascial release, dorsal closing wedge osteotomy of the first metatarsal, and peroneus longus to peroneus brevis tendon transfer

5.  Blood supply to the talar body is mainly provided by the:
    A.  Dorsalis pedis artery
    B.  Deltoid branch of the posterior tibial artery
    C.  Perforating peroneal artery
    D.  Artery of the tarsal sinus
    E.  Artery of the tarsal canal

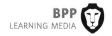

Foot & Ankle: Question Bank

6.  A 55–year-old woman has a flexible adult-acquired flatfoot deformity characterised by a positive too-many toes sign and medial foot and ankle swelling. She is unable to perform a single leg heel raise. These findings are classified as what stage of posterior tibial tendon dysfunction?
    A.  I
    B.  II
    C.  III
    D.  IV
    E.  V

7.  An active 46-year-old woman has had an 18-month history of progressive hindfoot pain that has failed to respond to nonsurgical therapy. She has unilateral collapse of her arch and an equinus contracture of the Achilles tendon. The foot remains flexible. Recommended treatment should include:
    A.  Triple arthrodesis
    B.  Isolated flexor digitorum longus (FDL) transfer to the navicular
    C.  Medialising calcaneal osteotomy, FDL transfer to the navicular and a gastroc recession
    D.  Lateralising calcaneal osteotomy, FDL transfer to the navicular, and gastroc recession
    E.  Plantar flexion first tarsometatarsal fusion (lapidus) and lateralising calcaneal osteotomy

8.  During the normal gait cycle, at push off phase of stance, the hindfoot:
    A.  Inverts and the transverse tarsal joints lock
    B.  Pronates and the transverse tarsal joints lock
    C.  Everts and the transverse tarsal joints unlock
    D.  Supinates and the transverse tarsal joints lock
    E.  Remains neutral and the transverse tarsal joints lock

9.  Plantar heel pain may be associated with a compression neuropathy of:
    A.  First branch of the lateral plantar nerve
    B.  First branch of the calcaneal nerve
    C.  Deep branch of the peroneal nerve
    D.  Superficial branch of the peroneal nerve
    E.  Sural nerve

10. Which of the following is less likely to predispose to hallux rigidus?
    A.  Long first metatarsal
    B.  Hyperlaxity
    C.  Flat or chevron-shaped metatarsophalangeal joint
    D.  Osteochondral fracture
    E.  Hallux valgus interphalangeus

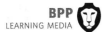

231

11. The Sanders classification of calcaneal fractures is based upon:
    A. Position of secondary fracture line on a broadens view radiograph
    B. Position of secondary fracture line on Harris axial radiograph
    C. Number and location of articular fragments on saggittal CT scan
    D. Position of primary fracture line on a Canale view
    E. Number and location of articular fragments on coronal CT scan

12. Retrocalcaneal bursitis is often associated with:
    A. Plantar fasciitis
    B. Rheumatoid arthritis
    C. Haglund's deformity
    D. Non-inflammatory arthropathy
    E. Tibialis posterior tenosynovitis

13. Adult-acquired flatfoot deformity secondary to posterior tibial tendon dysfunction is associated with which of the following physical findings?
    A. Hindfoot varus
    B. Forefoot adduction
    C. Achilles tendon contracture
    D. Plantar fascial rupture
    E. Hallux varus

14. A common cause of heel pain in athletes is caused by entrapment of which nerve?
    A. Sural nerve
    B. Lateral plantar nerve
    C. Superficial peroneal nerve
    D. Medial plantar nerve
    E. Interdigital nerve

15. The plantar plate of the Hallux MTPJ does not:
    A. Stabilise the digit along with collateral ligaments
    B. Stabilise intrinsic and extrinsic muscles
    C. Attach to the sesamoids
    D. Form part of the Windlass mechanism
    E. Help to guide the line of pull of various muscles attaching to the digits

16. What complication is frequently associated with a lesser metatarsal distal, oblique osteotomy (Weil) in treating a lesser toe deformity?
    A. Excessive shortening
    B. Dorsal displacement of the metatarsal head
    C. Osteonecrosis of the metatarsal head
    D. Nonunion
    E. Extension of the toe leading to stiffness

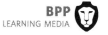

17.  A 22-year-old medical student sustains a bimalleolar ankle fracture during a rugby tackle. Which of the following is considered the most reliable means of predicting a tear of the intraosseous membrane?
     A.  The level of the fibular fracture
     B.  The Weber fracture type
     C.  The Lauge-Hansen fracture type
     D.  The results of an intra-operative stress test
     E.  Widening of the medial clear space

18.  A 19-year-old netball player who sustained an ankle sprain 6 weeks ago while playing netball has been unable to return to play. She reported a painful popping sensation behind the lateral malleolus. Which best clinical test will be diagnostic for her problem?
     A.  Anterior draw
     B.  Posterior draw
     C.  External rotation stress test
     D.  Resisted inversion
     E.  Resisted eversion

19.  Surgical treatment of the Achilles tendon ruptures offers what advantage over non-surgical management?
     A.  Improved pain relief
     B.  Earlier return to running
     C.  Lower re-rupture rate
     D.  Fewer complications
     E.  Faster return to work

20.  A displaced calcaneal fracture is treated with an ORIF. Postoperative radiographs reveal that one of the medially directed screws beneath the posterior facet is 5mm too long. What structure is most at risk?
     A.  Posterior tibial tendon
     B.  Posterior tibial neurovascular bundle
     C.  Abductor hallucis muscle
     D.  Flexor digitorum longus tendon
     E.  Flexor hallucis longus tendon

21.  Which of the following statements about ankle ligaments is **true**?
     A.  Dorsiflexion tightens the ATFL
     B.  Eversion with neutral flexion tightens the CFL
     C.  The CFL is the weakest of all the ankle ligaments
     D.  The ATFL is the weakest of all the ankle ligaments
     E.  The deltoid ligament comprises of 3 layers

22.  In muscles of the foot:
     A.  Fourth plantar layer contains flexor digiti minimi brevis
     B.  Plantar interosseous are contained in the third plantar layer
     C.  FDL and FHL are in the first plantar layer
     D.  Dorsal interosseous are in the fourth plantar layer
     E.  Quadrates plantae is in the third plantar layer

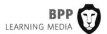

23. In ankle arthroscopy, all of these are **true** except:
    A. Anterolateral portal is routinely placed just lateral to peroneus tertius
    B. Posterolateral portal is routinely placed just lateral to Achilles tendon
    C. Anterocentral portal is routinely placed just lateral to EDC
    D. Saphenous nerve can be damaged while inserting an anteromedial portal
    E. Small saphenous vein can be injured while inserting a posterolateral portal

24. While considering the normal physiological angles in the foot, the angle that is not within the normal physiological limits is:
    A. Hallux valgus angle is usually <15 degrees
    B. First and second intermetatarsal angle is usually <9 degrees
    C. Hallux valgus interphalangeal angle is usually <15 degrees
    D. Hallux valgus angle is usually <10 degrees
    E. Hallux valgus interphalangeal angle is usually <10 degrees

25. Which of these is **false** in osteochondral lesions of the talus?
    A. Osteochondral lesions are commonly observed anterolaterally on the talar dome
    B. There is an increased risk of developing diffuse osteoarthritis following a focal osteochondral lesion
    C. MRI is the favoured screening tool
    D. Arthroscopic evaluation is more accurate than MRI or CT
    E. Autologous chondrocyte transplantation has proven effective while considering follow up results

26. Arch height is maintained during the stance phase of gait primarily by?
    A. Achilles tendon contraction
    B. Posterior tibial tendon contraction
    C. Bony and ligamentous structures
    D. Unlocking of the transverse tarsal joints
    E. Balanced contraction of the peroneus longus and anterior tibialis

27. A 42-year-old man has had a 10-year history of intermittent but recurrent ankle sprains. Examination reveals a varus heel position that corrects with a Coleman block test. On lateral stress testing there is no lateral ligament instability. What type of orthotic should be prescribed?
    A. Medial arch support
    B. Arizona brace
    C. Rigid orthotic with a medial arch support and 5 degrees of medial heel posting
    D. Semi-rigid orthotic with a recessed first metatarsal, a lateral forefoot post, a reduced medial arch, and a 5 degrees of lateral heel post
    E. Carbon fibre insole

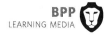

28. A 47-year-old man has had plantar heel pain for the past 5 months. The pain is most severe when he arises out of bed in the morning and when he stands after being seated for a period of time. Treatment should consist of:
    A. Surgical lengthening of the Achilles tendon
    B. Surgical release of the plantar fascia
    C. A custom orthotic
    D. Night splints, a stretching programme and a cushioned insert
    E. A corticosteroid injection

29. A 32-year-old woman who previously underwent excision of the lateral (fibular) sesamoid for a painful intractable plantar keratosis now has a painful hypertrophic callus under the medial (tibial) sesamoid. Conservative treatment has failed to provide relief. What is the most common surgical complication of which the patient should be made aware?
    A. Claw toe deformity
    B. Painful neuroma
    C. Painful scar
    D. Hallux varus
    E. Hallux valgus

BPP
LEARNING MEDIA

# Adult Pathology

## Foot & Ankle:
## Answers

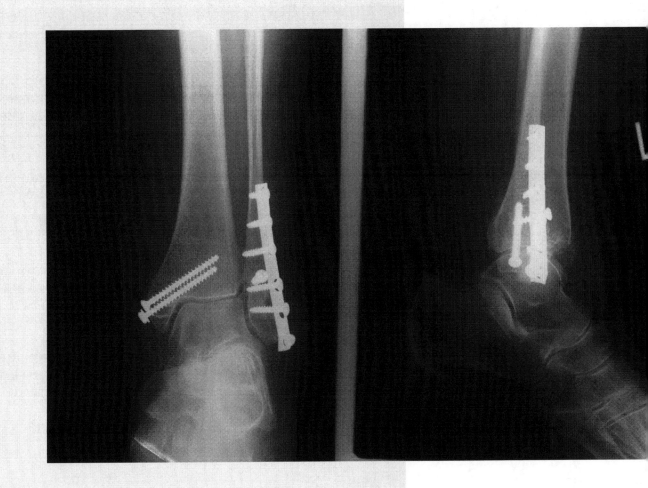

1. **D**

   Function of peroneal tendons:

   - The peroneus longus serves to plantar flex the first ray, evert the foot, and plantar flex the ankle
   - The peroneus brevis everts and plantar flexes the foot.

   Test for peroneal tendon instability:

   The patient's relaxed foot is examined hanging in a relaxed position with the knee flexed 90 degrees. Slight pressure is applied to the peroneal tendons posterior to the fibula. The patient then is asked to forcibly dorsiflex and evert the foot. Pain may be elicited, or the tendons may be felt to sublux.

   Ref:
   Greer E and Richardson MD (2003) *Orthopaedic Knowledge Update: Foot and Ankle 3*. American Academy of Orthopaedic Surgeons.

2. **E**

   This question relates to the treatment of HMSN: Charcot Marie Tooth disease. The peroneus longus muscle (remains strong) which is opposed by a weak anterior tibialis muscle resulting in plantar flexion of the first ray.

   Ref:
   Greer E and Richardson MD (2003) *Orthopaedic Knowledge Update: Foot and Ankle 3*. American Academy of Orthopaedic Surgeons. p. 135.

3. **D**

   Hallux rigidus can be managed surgically by many different means. Options include synovectomy, cheilectomy with or without dorsiflexion osteotomy, resection arthroplasty, arthrodesis and interpositional arthroplasty. The patient has already had a cheilectomy. Arthrodesis remains the gold standard procedure for pain relief.

   Ref:
   Greer E and Richardson MD (2003) *Orthopaedic Knowledge Update: Foot and Ankle 3*. American Academy of Orthopaedic Surgeons.

4. **E**

   The cavovarus foot in HSMN or CMT is caused by muscle imbalance in which the peroneus longus, relatively unopposed by a weak tibialis anterior, causes plantar flexion of the first ray and a compensatory hindfoot varus. A weak peroneus brevis also contributes to the foot and ankle inversion.

   In patients with a flexible foot who have no degenerative arthritic changes in the midfoot, release of the plantar fascia, dorsal closing wedge osteotomy of the first metatarsal, and transfer of the peroneus longus muscle to the peroneus brevis muscle are indicated.

   In older patients with fixed deformity and/or degenerative changes, a triple arthrodesis is recommended.

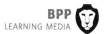

A calcaneal slide is preferred to a lateral closing wedge calcaneal osteotomy (Dwyer). Theoretically, the sliding osteotomy may be preferable, as the Dwyer osteotomy effectively lengthens the Achilles tendon and may impact push-off force with gait.

Ref:
Lee MC, Sucato DJ. Paediatric Issues with Cavovarus Foot Deformities. *Foot Ankle Clin N Am* 2008; 13: 199–219.

5.   **B**
Arterial blood supplies to the talus, in order of importance, are the posterior tibial, anterior tibial, and peroneal. Artery of the tarsal canal (from posterior tibial artery) provides most of the blood supply to the talar body. Artery of the tarsal sinus (from anterior tibial and peroneal arteries) provides most of the blood supply to the talar head.

Ref:
Brinker MR (2000) *Review of Orthopaedic Trauma.* Saunders, Philadelphia.

6.   **B**
Johnson and Strom describe posterior tibial tendon dysfunction in 3 clinical stages:

- Stage I:
    - pain and swelling of medial aspect of foot and ankle
    - Length of tendon normal
    - Tendinitis may be associated with mild degeneration
    - Mild weakness, minimal deformity

Initial management is non-operative and includes immobilisation, medial longitudinal arch support using an orthotic device, and NSAIDS.

- Stage II:
    - Tendon torn, limb weak
    - Unable to stand on tiptoes on affected side
    - Secondary deformity present as midfoot pronates and forefoot abducts at transverse tarsal joint
    - Subtalar joint stays flexible

Management is a possible lateral column lengthening, medial calcaneal osteotomy, and FDL transfer.

- Stage III:
    - Degeneration of tendon
    - Deformity more severe
    - Hindfoot rigid

Management is triple arthrodesis.

- Stage IV (described by Myerson MS 1997):
    - Valgus angulation of talus
    - Early degeneration of ankle joint

Management includes pantalar arthrodesis, ankle replacement and triple arthrodesis.

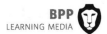

Ref:

Myerson MS: Adult acquired flatfoot deformity: Treatment of dysfunction of the posterior tibial tendon. *Instr Course Lect* 1997; 46: 393–405.

7.   **C**
Ref:

Bluman EM, Title CI, Myerson MS. Posterior Tibial Tendon Rupture: A Refined Classification System. *Foot Ankle Clin 2007;* 12(2): 233–249.

8.   **A**
Ref:

Gage JR. Gait Analysis: Principles and Applications. *J Bone Joint Surg Am* Oct 1995; 77: 1607–1623.

9.   **A**
Ref:

Thordarson DB (ed.) (2004) *Foot and Ankle: Orthopaedic Surgery Essentials.* Lippincott Williams & Wilkins, Philadelphia.

10.   **A**
Ref:

Coughlin *et al.* Hallux rigidus: demographics, aetiology, and radiographic assessment. *Foot Ankle Int* 2003 October; 24(10): 731–43

11.   **E**
The Sanders classification is based on the number and location of articular fragments on Coronal CT scan. There are 4 types, based on the number of fragments of the posterior facet, with displacement of 2mm considered significant.

Ref:

Eastwood DM, Gregg PJ, Atkins RM. Intra-articular fractures of the calcaneum. Part I: Pathological anatomy and classification. *J Bone Joint Surg [Br]* 1993; 75-B: 183–8.

12.   **C**
Ref:

Thordarson DB (2004) *Foot and Ankle Surgery: Orthopaedic Surgery Essentials.* Lippincott Willians & Wilkins, Philadelphia.

13.   **C**
Because posterior tibial tendon dysfunction often is associated with an equinus contracture, correction of deformity requires Achilles tendon lengthening. Clinical evaluation is characterised by pain and tenderness along the posterior tibial tendon and inability to perform a single limb heel rise. In the early stages of the disease, single limb heel rise may be possible but painful; eventually, the heel fails to turn into physiologic varus, and ultimately unsupported single limb heel rise is no longer possible. With advancing

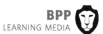

disease, subfibular (calcaneofibular) impingement develops with tenderness over the compressed peroneal tendons. The initial medial pain subsides and subfibular lateral foot pain produces the greatest symptoms. Loss of the longitudinal arch, hindfoot valgus, and forefoot abduction ('too many toes' sign) are evident with progressive posterior tibial tendon attenuation.

Ref:

Greer E and Richardson MD (2003) *Orthopaedic Knowledge Update: Foot and Ankle 8.* American Academy of Orthopaedic Surgeons.

**14.  B**

Ref:

Schon LC, Baxter DE. Neuropathies of the foot and ankle in athletes. *Clin Sports Med.* 1990 Apr; 9(2): 489–509.

**15.  C**

The plantar plate has a variety of roles in foot function. It is a fibrocartilaginous structure that aids in stabilising the digit along with collateral ligaments, intrinsic and extrinsic muscles. It acts as an attachment for the plantar fascia and has a role in the windlass mechanism. Its cartilaginous structure helps to reduce compressive loads on the metatarsal heads. Combined with other adjacent structures it also helps to guide the line of pull of various muscles attaching to the digits, specifically the lumbricals and flexor digitorum longus

Ref:

David B *et al.* (2004) Hallux Valgus, Hallux Varus, and Sesamoid Disorders. In Thordarson DB (ed.) *Foot and Ankle Surgery: Orthopaedic Surgery Essentials.* Lippincott Williams & Wilkins, Philadelphia.

**16.  E**

Depression of the plantar fragment always occurs after a Weil osteotomy. This depression changes the center of rotation of the MTP joint, and the interosseous muscles then act more as dorsiflexors than as plantarflexors.

Ref:

Trnka HJ, Nyska M, Parks BG *et al.* Dorsiflexion contracture after the Weil osteotomy: Results of cadaver study and three-dimensional analysis. *Foot Ankle Int* 2001; 22: 47–50.

**17.  D**

Adequate reduction of the syndesmosis is necessary to achieve optimal long term results after bimalleolar and trimalleolar ankle fracture. The literature states correlations between:

• The adequacy of reduction of the syndesmosis and late arthritis
• Adequacy of the initial reduction of the syndesmosis and late stability of the syndesmosis
• Late stability of the syndesmosis and final outcome

Identification of a syndesmotic injury is of great importance and different potential markers of syndesmotic injury have been investigated, including the level of fibular fracture which does not correlate with the integrity or extent of interosseous membrane tears.

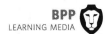

Intra-operative stress test is direct radiographic evidence of a syndesmotic injury.

Ref:

Herscovici *et al.*, Avoiding Complications in the Treatment of Pronation-External Rotation Ankle Fractures, Syndesmotic Injuries, and Talar Neck Fractures. *J Bone Joint Surg Am* 2008; 90 (4): 898.

18. **E**

The most reliable method to reproduce this condition can be with resisted eversion of the foot.

Recurrent peroneal tendon subluxation is an uncommon sports-related injury. Peroneal tendon subluxation is commonly associated with longitudinal splits in the peroneus brevis tendon and lateral ankle instability. Disruption of the lateral collateral ankle ligaments places considerable strain on the superior peroneal retinaculum. This explains why the two conditions commonly coexist. In recurrent subluxation, patients usually give a history of previous ankle injury, which may have been misdiagnosed as a sprain. An unstable ankle that gives way or is associated with a popping or snapping sensation is another common complaint. The peroneal tendons may actually be seen subluxing anteriorly on the distal fibula during ambulation.

Ref:
1.  Garrick JG. (2004) *Orthopaedic Knowledge Update: Sports Medicine 3*. American Academy of Orthopaedic Surgeons. pp. 233–248.
2.  Maffulli N, Ferran NA, Oliva F *et al.* Recurrent subluxation of the peroneal tendons. *Am J Sports Med* 2006; 34: 986–992.

19. **C**

The outcomes of open repair of Achilles tendon rupture demonstrate a lower re-rupture rate, however a higher risk of compilations is reported, such as infection, adhesions, and altered skin sensation.

Ref:

Khan RJK *et al.* Treatment of Acute Achilles Tendon Ruptures: A Meta-Analysis of Randomized, Controlled Trial. *J Bone and Joint Surgery (Am)* 2005; 87: 2202–2210.

20. **E**
Ref:

Hoppenfield S, Deboer P. (2003) (3rd ed.) *Surgical Exposures in Orthopaedics: The Anatomic Approach*. Lippincott Williams & Wilkins, Philadelphia.

21. **D**

Deltoid ligament comprises 2 layers – superficial (tibionavicular and tibiocalcaneal) and deep (anterior and posterior tibiotalar). The lateral fibular ligaments are: ATFL, CFL and PTFL. The ATFL is the weakest and is intracapsular.

Ref:

Miller MD (2008) *Review of Orthopaedics*. Saunders Elsevier, Philadelphia.

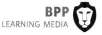

**22.  D**

Muscles and tendons in the plantar layers in the foot:

First plantar layer – abductor hallucis, flexor digitorum brevis, abductor digiti minimi

Second plantar layer – quadrates plantae, lumbricals, FDL & FHL

Third plantar layer – flexor hallucis brevis, adductor hallucis, flexor digiti minimi brevis

Fourth plantar layer – dorsal interosseous, plantar interosseous (peroneous longus and tibialis posterior)

Ref:
Miller MD (2008) *Review of Orthopaedics*. Saunders Elsevier, Philadelphia.

**23.  C**

The location of the anterocentral portal is medial to EDC, lateral to EHL.

Ref:
Miller MD (2008) *Review of Orthopaedics*. Saunders Elsevier, Philadelphia.

**24.  C**

Ref:
Coughlin MJ. Hallux Valgus in men: effect of the distal metatarsal articular angle in the hallux valgus correction. *Foot and Ankle Int* 1997; 18: 463–470.

**25.  B**

No clear association between focal osteochondral lesions of the talus and development of diffuse ankle osteoarthritis has been identified.

Ref:
Greer E and Richardson MD. (2003) *Orthopaedic Knowledge Update: Foot and Ankle 8*. American Academy of Orthopaedic Surgeons.

**26.  C**

Ref:
1.  Erdemir *et al*. Dynamic loading of the plantar aponeurosis in walking. *JBJS Am* 2004; 86: 546–552.
2.  Nyska *et al*. The contribution of the medial calcaneal osteotomy to the correction of flatfoot deformities. *Foot Ankle Int* 2001; 22:278–282.
3.  Deland *et al*. Posterior tibial tendon insufficiency. *Foot Ankle Int* 2005; 26: 427–435.
4.  Canale T. (2003) (10<sup>th</sup> ed.) *Campbell's Operative Orthopaedics*. Elsevier, St Louis.

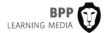

27.   **D**

Coleman block testing is used to determine if the subtalar joint complex is fixed, cannot be passively corrected, or flexible (supple), passively correctable.

This question refers to the subtle cavus foot. The deformity corrects with the Coleman block indicates that the orthotic described in d would correct his deformity.

Ref:
1.   Manoli A II, Graham B. The subtle cavus foot, 'the underpronator'. *Foot Ankle Int* 2005; 26: 256–263.
2.   Miller MD (2008) *Review of Orthopaedics*. Saunders Elsevier, Philadelphia.

28.   **D**

Plantar fasciitis is caused by repetitive strain of the plantar fascia causing inflammation of the fascia at its origin on the calcaneus. Ultrasound and histologic examination confirms the inflammatory nature of the process, but the biomechanical stress causing the inflammation is not completely understood.

Ref:
1.   Pfeffer G *et al.* Comparison of custom and prefabricated orthoses in the initial treatment of proximal plantar fasciitis. *Foot Ankle Int* 1999 Apr; 20(4): 214–21.
2.   Coughlin MJ, Mann RA, Saltzman CL (1999) *Surgery of the Foot and Ankle* (7th ed.) St Louis, Mosby. pp. 1090–1209.

29.   **A**

The sesamoids play a vital role in the function of the great toe by absorbing weight-bearing pressure, reducing friction, and protecting tendons. Excision of both sesamoids should be avoided if possible as a claw toe deformity (MTP dorsiflexed, PIP plantarflexed, DIP plantarflexed) will develop.

Ref:
1.   Richardson EG. Hallucal sesamoid pain: causes and surgical treatment. *J Am Acad Orthop Surg* 1999 Jul–Aug; 7(4): 270–8.
2.   Dedmond BT, Cory JW, McBryde A Jr. The hallucal sesamoid complex. *J Am Acad Orthop Surg* 2006 Dec; 14(13): 745–53.

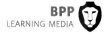

# Tumour & Metabolic Bone Diseases

## Question Bank

Haroon A Mann &
Fahad G Attar

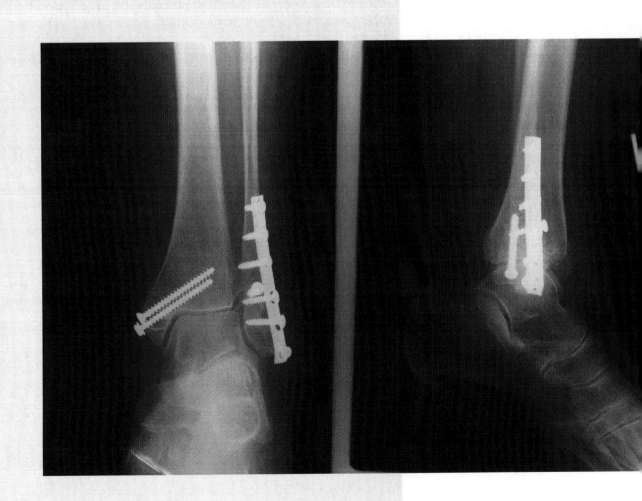

1.  Which one of the following statements is **false** for osteosarcoma?
    A.  Is a malignant spindle cell sarcoma of bone
    B.  Is composed of small round cells in a sparse intracellular stroma
    C.  Has a chondroid matrix surrounding malignant chondrocytes with a characteristic clear cytoplasm
    D.  Is usually responsive to neo-adjuvant chemotherapy
    E.  Patients with pulmonary metastasis have a 5 year survival rate of 20–40%

2.  Radio frequency ablation can be used as the primary treatment of:
    A.  Chondroblastoma
    B.  Aneurysmal bone cyst
    C.  Giant cell tumour
    D.  Osteoid osteoma
    E.  Enchondroma

3.  Pre-operative embolisation to decrease blood loss intra-operatively is commonly used in:
    A.  Metastatic renal cell carcinoma
    B.  Osteosarcoma
    C.  Osteoid osteoma
    D.  Enchondroma
    E.  Osteoblastoma

4.  Hereditary multiple exostosis is an autosomal dominant inherited disorder associated with mutations of EXT1 and EXT2 genes. What part of the growth plate is affected?
    A.  Proliferating chondrocytes
    B.  Prehypertrophic chondrocytes
    C.  Hypertrophic chondrocytes
    D.  Periosteum
    E.  Synovium

5.  The following are benign tumours except:
    A.  Adamantinoma
    B.  GCT
    C.  Chondroblastoma
    D.  Aneurysmal bone cyst
    E.  Osteochondroma

6.  Which of the following is considered a critical step in the pathological process of metastasis for a malignant cell?
    A.  Loss of cell motility
    B.  Intravasation
    C.  Loss of extravasation
    D.  Prevention of angiogenesis
    E.  Increased apoptosis

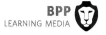

7.  For which of the following skeletal tumour is radiation therapy routinely used for definitive local control?
    A.  Osteogenic sarcoma
    B.  Ewing's sarcoma
    C.  Chondrosarcoma
    D.  Pleomorphic sarcoma
    E.  Paget's sarcoma

8.  For patients with metastatic carcinoma to bone, which of the following primary cancers are associated with the the greatest morbidity following pathologic fracture?
    A.  Thyroid
    B.  Breast
    C.  Prostate
    D.  Lung
    E.  Renal

9.  Aneurysmal bone cyst of the spine is most common in which of the following region?
    A.  Lumbar
    B.  Lower
    C.  Thoracic
    D.  Upper thoracic
    E.  Sacral

10. What process most closely resembles the radiographic and histologic presentations of mulicentric giant cell tumour?
    A.  Paget's disease
    B.  Campanacci's disease (osteofibrous dysplasia)
    C.  Ollier's disease (enchondromatosis)
    D.  Transient osteoporosis
    E.  Hyperparathyroidism

11. Which of the following soft tissue sarcomas is most common in children?
    A.  Epithelioid sarcoma
    B.  Rhabdomyosarcoma
    C.  Synovial sarcoma
    D.  Liposarcoma
    E.  Extraskeletal Ewing's sarcoma

12. Factors that decrease renal calcium absorption are:
    A.  PTH
    B.  Calcitonin
    C.  Glucocorticoids
    D.  Chronic thiazide diuretic use
    E.  1, 25 dihydroxyvitamin D

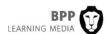

13. Regarding Osteopetrosis:
    A. Associated with cranial nerve deficits
    B. Associated with hyposplenism
    C. Disorder of bone remodelling
    D. All patients are symptomatic
    E. Iatrogenic suppression of osteoblast activity is another potential aetiology

14. Which statement is **false** in fibrous dysplasia?
    A. Developmental abnormality that can be mono or polyostotic
    B. Ground glass appearance is seen on X-ray
    C. Associated with Gs-alpha protein
    D. Associated with café au lait spots – coast of California
    E. Fibrous dysplasia heals with fibrous dysplasia

15. The following chromosomal translocation and association is **not true**:
    A. Ewing's sarcoma (11; 22)
    B. Synovial sarcoma (X; 18)
    C. Clear cell sarcoma (12; 22)
    D. Myxoid liposarcoma (12; 18)
    E. Chondrosarcoma (9; 22)

16. Regarding parosteal osteosarcoma:
    A. Most common site is posterior aspect of distal humerus
    B. Grade of lesion is intermediate
    C. Prognosis is excellent
    D. Histologically the lesion is predominantly chondroblastic
    E. Occurs most commonly in the diaphysis of long bones

17. All statements are **true** about chordomas except:
    A. Malignant neoplasm
    B. Predominantly occurs at the ends of the vertebral column
    C. About 10% occur in the vertebral bodies
    D. Chordomas rarely metastasise
    E. Cells of origin are from primitive notochordal tissue

18. The most common tumours that metastasise to bone in decreasing order of incidence are:
    A. Breast, lung, prostate, kidney, thyroid
    B. Breast, prostate, lung, kidney, thyroid
    C. Breast, prostate, kidney, lung, thyroid
    D. Prostate, breast, lung, kidney, thyroid
    E. Prostate, lung, breast, kidney, thyroid

19. Which of the following statements is **not true** regarding non-ossifying fibroma?
    A. Common lesion that rarely requires surgical intervention
    B. Are incidental findings
    C. Histologically show benign spindle cells and benign giant cells
    D. Histologically show multinucleate giant cells and mononuclear stromal cells
    E. Can cause mechanical pain

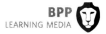

20. Histology of a lesion shows low grade spindle cell sarcoma with islands of epithelial cells that may resemble cutaneous basal cells, this same lesion could also show islands of neoplastic cells surrounded by columnar cells in a palisading fashion. The lesion most likely is a:
    A. Giant cell tumour
    B. Adamantinoma
    C. Liposarcoma
    D. Haemangioma
    E. Round cell tumours

21. What is the most common site of skeletal metastases?
    A. Pelvis
    B. Humerus
    C. Tibia
    D. Skull
    E. Spine

22. Which of these is the second most common site for metastatic disease?
    A. Pulmonary
    B. Hepatic
    C. Bone
    D. Brain
    E. Retro-peritoneum

23. A chordoma is most likely to be found in:
    A. Cervical spine
    B. Thoracic spine
    C. Lumbar spine
    D. Sacrum
    E. Pelvis

24. Regarding chondromyxoid fibroma:
    A. Occurs from first through third decades of life
    B. Is a relatively common tumour
    C. Is often located in the humerus
    D. Presents as a sclerotic diaphyseal lesion
    E. Presents with a periosteal reaction

25. Which of the following is **false** about Vitamin D?
    A. It is a steroid hormone
    B. Undergoes hydroxylation in liver and kidney
    C. It decreases insulin secretion
    D. It down regulates the rennin-angiotensin system
    E. Production of vitamin D is severely impaired by the use of sunscreens

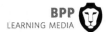

26. The following is associated with osteopetrosis:
    A. Characterised by increased bone mass
    B. Characterised by abnormal bone remodeling
    C. Characterised by decreased bone mineralisation
    D. Characterised by reduced bone mass
    E. All of the above to varying degrees

BPP
LEARNING MEDIA

# Tumour & Metabolic Bone Diseases

## Answers

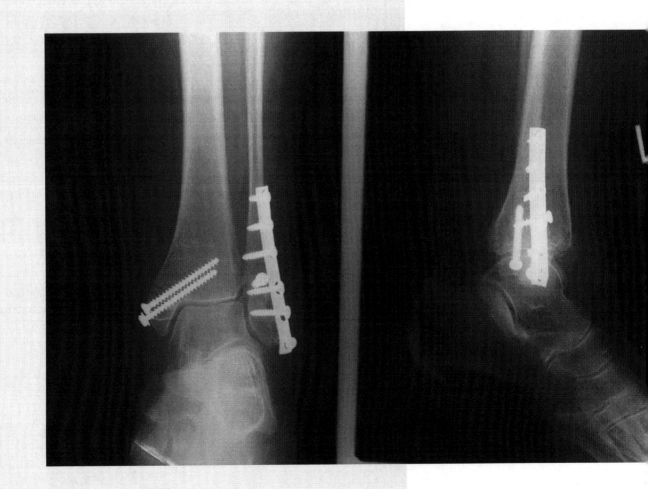

1.  **B**

    Ewing's sarcoma is characterised by small round cells in a sparse intracellular stroma.

    Ref:

    Miller, M (2004) (4<sup>th</sup> ed.) *Review of Orthopaedics*. Saunders, Philadelphia.

2.  **D**

    Ref:

    Rosenthal DI *et al.* Osteoid osteona: percutaneous radio-frequency ablation. *Radiology* 1995 Nov; 197(2): 451–4.

3.  **A**

    Ref:

    Munro NP *et al.* The role of transarterial embolisation in the treatment of renal cell carcinoma: *BJU International* 2003; vol. 92, no. 3: 240–244.

4.  **B**

    Hereditary multiple exostosis is an autosomal dominant disorder with full penetrance. Linkage analysis has identified two mutations in the EXT gene family (EXT1 and EXT2), which account for 50% of cases.

    Ref:

    Steiber JR, Dormans JP. Manifestations of hereditary multiple exostoses. *JAAOS* 2005; 13: 110–120.

5.  **A**

    Ref:

    Miller, M (2004) (4<sup>th</sup> ed.) *Review of Orthopaedics*. Saunders, Philadelphia.

6.  **B**

    The sequence of events of for distant metastasis is

    1.  Growth of tumour
    2.  Neovascularisation of the tumour
    3.  Erosion of the basement membrane with matrix metalloproteinase
    4.  Entry of tumour cells into blood vessels (Intravasation)
    5.  Detachment
    6.  Embolisation
    7.  Attachment and intravasation from the blood vasculature into tissue parenchyma

    Ref:

    Miller, M (2004) (4<sup>th</sup> ed.) *Review of Orthopaedics*. Saunders, Philadelphia.

7.  **B**

    Ewing's sarcoma has a high propensity to metastasise to the lungs and bone. Without intensive chemotherapy, the five-year survival is less than 25%. Patients are treated with systemic chemotherapy to control micro metastases and either external beam irradiation

BPP
LEARNING MEDIA

to the local site or wide surgical resection. Wide surgical resection is often utilised for the sites which will not result in major morbidity. If the surgical margins are positive, the patient then undergoes external beam radiation.

Radiation therapy is only effective for:

- Ewing's
- Multiple myeloma
- Lymphoma
- Metastatic bone disease
- Hemangioendothelioma

Ref:
McCarthy EF, Frassica FJ (1989) *Pathology of Bone and Joint Disorders*. Saunders, Philadelphia.

8.  **B**
The skeleton is the most common organ to be affected by metastatic cancer, and tumours arising from the breast, prostate, thyroid, lung, lymphoma and kidney possess a special propensity to spread to bone. Breast carcinoma, the most prevalent malignancy, causes the greatest morbidity.

Ref:
Coleman RE. Skeletal complications of malignancy. *Cancer* 1997; 80: 1588–1594.

9.  **A**
Ref:
Miller, M (2004) (4th ed.) *Review of Orthopaedics*, Saunders, Philadelphia.

10.  **E**
Multicentric giant cell tumour is a rare subset, comprising one percent of giant cell tumours. Other diseases such as brown tumour of hyperparathyroidism, Paget's disease, multiple myeloma, adamantinoma, angiosarcoma, fibrous dysplasia, fibrosarcoma, osteosarcoma, metastasis and multifocal infection can all present with multicentric lesions. Not only do brown tumours present with similar radiographic findings of an eccentric radiolucent lesion, giant cells can also be present in biopsy specimens of brown tumours. All patients suspected of having multicentric giant cell tumours should have a hyperparathyroid work-up.

Ref:
Cummins CA, Scarborough MT, Enneking WF. Multicentric giant cell tumor of bone. *Clin Orthop* 1996; 322: 245–52.

11.  **B**
Rhambdomysarcoma is the most common soft tissue tumour in children. Synovial sarcoma and neural tumours are most frequent in children than in adults. MFH, which is the common soft tissue sarcoma in adults, is rare in children.

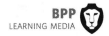

Ref:

Pappa A Parham D *et al*. Soft tissue sarcomas in children. *Seminars in Surg Onc 1999;* 16: 121–43.

**12.    C**

Factors that increase renal calcium resorption are: PTH, PTH-related peptide, 1, 25 dihydroxyvitamin D, calcitonin, increased phosphate intake, chronic thiazide diuretic use.

Factors that decrease renal calcium resorption are: increased sodium intake, increased calcium intake, metabolic acidosis, phosphate depletion, glucocorticoids, frusemide, cyclosporine A.

Ref:

Greer E, Richardson MD (2003) *Orthopaedic Knowledge Update: Foot and Ankle 8.* American Academy of Orthopaedic Surgeons.

**13.    A**

Osteopetrosis is a disorder characterised by increased bone mass. Infantile osteopetrosis is rapidly fatal and is associated with cranial nerve deficits, delayed dental eruption, hypersplenism and haemolysis.

Intermediate osteopetrosis causes short stature, recurrent fractures and possible cranial nerve deficits.

Some individuals with adult osteopetrosis are asymptomatic.

Ref:

Greer E, Richardson MD (2003) *Orthopaedic Knowledge Update: Foot and Ankle 8.* American Academy of Orthopaedic Surgeons.

**14.    D**

Fibrous dysplasia is associated with café au lait spots ie coast of Maine (coast of California is seen with neurofibromatosis). Common location is in the proximal femur.

Ref:

Malinzak RA, Albritton MJ (2006) (International ed.) *First Aid for the Orthopaedic Boards.* McGraw-Hill.

**15.    D**

Myxoid liposarcoma (12; 16)

Alveolar rhabdomyosarcoma (2; 13)

Ref:

Malinzak RA, Albritton MJ (2006) (International ed.) *First Aid for the Orthopaedic Boards.* McGraw-Hill.

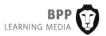

16. **C**

Low grade osteosarcoma, occurring on the surface of the metaphysis of long bones. Common sites are posterior aspect of distal femur, proximal tibia and proximal humerus. More common in females than males.

Ref:
Miller, M (2004) (4<sup>th</sup> ed.) *Review of Orthopaedics*, Saunders, Philadelphia.

17. **D**

Chordomas metastasise in 30–50% of cases and they often take the patient's life because of local extension.

Ref:
Miller, M (2004) (4<sup>th</sup> ed.) *Review of Orthopaedics*, Saunders, Philadelphia.

18. **B**

Ref:
Miller, M (2004) (4<sup>th</sup> ed.) *Review of Orthopaedics*, Saunders, Philadelphia.

19. **D**

Giant cell tumours histologically show multinucleate giant cells and mononuclear stromal cells. All others are true for non-ossifying fibromas. When the diagnosis remains elusive, open biopsy with curettage and some form of bone grafting is reasonable. After surgical excision and grafting, these lesions usually completely heal by 8 weeks, whereas such healing would commonly take 2 years or more without surgical intervention.

Ref:
Greer E, Richardson MD (2003) *Orthopaedic Knowledge Update: Foot and Ankle 8*. American Academy of Orthopaedic Surgeons.

20. **B**

Adamantinoma is a characteristic lesion usually found in the anterior cortex of the midshaft of the tibia. It usually appears as a 'soap bubble' sclerotic lesion and can mimic fibrous cortical dysplasia. Cortical fibrous dysplasia commonly occurs predominantly in males in the first and second decade of life, whereas adamantinoma occurs in both genders and in all age groups occurring from the first through to the fourth decade.

Ref:
Greer E, Richardson MD (2003) *Orthopaedic Knowledge Update: Foot and Ankle 8*. American Academy of Orthopaedic Surgeons.

21. **E**

The high incidence of metastasis to the spine has been attributed to presence of Batson's plexus.

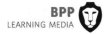

Ref:

Batson OV. Role of the vertebral veins in metastatic processes. *Ann Intern Med* 1942; 16: 38–45.

**22.  B**

Hepatic metastases is the second most common site for metastatic disease, first being pulmonary and third most common being bone.

Ref:

Harrington KD. Metastatic disease of the spine. *J Bone Joint Surg Am* 1986; 68: 1110–1115.

**23.  D**

Ref:

Greer E, Richardson MD (2003) *Orthopaedic Knowledge Update: Foot and Ankle 8.* American Academy of Orthopaedic Surgeons.

**24.  A**

Chondromyxoid fibroma is a rare tumour usually presenting as a lytic metaphyseal lesion with cortical thinning but no periosteal reaction. This tumour usually occurs from the first through to the third decades of life and is most often located in the proximal tibia. It frequently has the appearance of a very large non-ossifying fibroma.

Ref:

Greer E, Richardson MD (2003) *Orthopaedic Knowledge Update: Foot and Ankle 8.* American Academy of Orthopaedic Surgeons.

**25.  C**

Vitamin D is a steroid hormone derived from cholesterol and undergoes hydroxylation in the liver and the kidney. Its primary role is to maintain Calcium levels within the normal range by increasing intestinal absorption of calcium and by increasing maturation of osteoclasts to mobilise calcium from the bone when needed. It enhances insulin secretion and down regulates the rennin-angiotensin system. It is produced in the skin by exposure to sunlight and is also absorbed from dietary intake.

Ref:

Greer E, Richardson MD (2003) *Orthopaedic Knowledge Update: Foot and Ankle 8.* American Academy of Orthopaedic Surgeons.

**26.  A**

Ref:

Greer E, Richardson MD (2003) *Orthopaedic Knowledge Update: Foot and Ankle 8.* American Academy of Orthopaedic Surgeons.

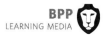

# MCQ Paper 1

## Question Bank

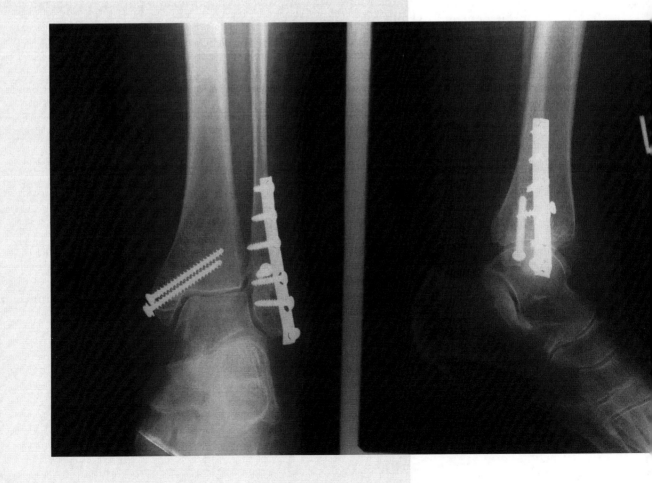

1.  What type of loading procedure produces a spiral fracture?
    A.  Shear
    B.  Bending
    C.  Compression
    D.  Tension
    E.  Torsion

2.  Loosening of an external fixator pin can be reduced by drilling the bone hole of what size?
    A.  Bone hole of the same size as the pin
    B.  Oversize the bone hole by 0.1mm
    C.  Undersize the bone hole by 0.1mm
    D.  Oversize the bone hole by 0.3mm
    E.  Undersize the bone hole by 0.3mm

3.  Best treatment for a fractured radial head with a coronoid process fracture following a fracture dislocation of elbow is:
    A.  Stabilisation in an above elbow cast for 3 weeks and then mobilisation
    B.  Excision of radial head and coronoid process
    C.  Excision of radial head and ORIF of coronoid process
    D.  ORIF radial head and coronoid process
    E.  Replacement of radial head and ORIF coronoid process

4.  In a polytrauma patient, the following parameter in a borderline patient is associated with poor outcome and risk of rapid deterioration, except:
    A.  Injury severity score <40
    B.  Core temperature <35 degrees
    C.  Systolic BP <90mm of hg
    D.  Chest trauma (AIS >2)
    E.  Bilateral femoral fractures

5.  Management of a minimally displaced radial head fracture after a fall will include:
    A.  Broad arm sling for 1 week and active ROM exercise
    B.  Broad arm sling for 3 weeks and active ROM exercise
    C.  Above elbow backslab for 1 week
    D.  Use of hinged elbow orthosis for 3 weeks
    E.  Active mobilisation after radiological union

6.  The Mangled Extremity Severity Score (MESS) includes all of the following components except:
    A.  Age of the patient
    B.  Glasgow coma score of the patient
    C.  Systolic blood pressure of the patient
    D.  Capillary refill time
    E.  Type of the fracture

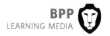

7. Following an operative treatment of radius and ulna, the most important action to achieve a maximal forearm rotation is.
    A. Early mobilisation
    B. Compression fixation of the radius and ulna
    C. Restoration of radial bow
    D. End to end reduction of the ulna fracture
    E. Less than 5mm shortening of the radius following fixation

8. The following fractures and displacement of the pelvis can be easily visualised on an inlet film, except in:
    A. Subtle fractures of the sacrum
    B. Antero-posterior displacement of injured hemipelvis
    C. Rotational displacement of injured hemipelvis
    D. Widening of sacroiliac joint or symphysis pubis
    E. Cephalad and caudad displacement of injured hemipelvis

9. All of the following statements are **true** regarding type I lateral compression fractures of the pelvis except:
    A. Most common type of pelvic ring disruption
    B. Fractures often pass through the sacral foramina
    C. Associated with disruption of sacrotuberous and sacrospinous ligaments
    D. Fracture is vertically stable and rotationally unstable
    E. Associated with a pubic rami fracture

10. The force used in the reduction manoeuvre to counteract the typical sacroiliac displacement following an APC III fracture is described as:
    A. Anterior and caudal
    B. Posterior and caudal
    C. Anterior and cephalad
    D. Posterior and cephalad
    E. Pure anterior

11. A 64-year-old lady with rheumatoid arthritis with symptoms of cervical myelopathy secondary to atlantoaxial subluxation undergoes posterior decompression and fusion. The strongest predictor of post-operative neurological recovery is:
    A. Age
    B. Duration of paralysis
    C. Degree of pre-operative neurologic deficit
    D. Pre-operative anterior atlanto-dental interval
    E. Sex

12. During placement of anterior pins for a halo fixator, which structure is at risk if the pin is placed medial to the safe zone?
    A. Supraorbital nerve
    B. Superficial temporal artery
    C. Infraorbital nerve
    D. Oculomotor nerve
    E. Infratrochlear nerve

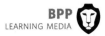

13. The most common complication associated with halo fixation following cervical spine trauma is:
    A. Dural tear
    B. Pin site bleeding
    C. Pin loosening
    D. Dysphagia
    E. Nerve injury

14. A 28-year-old man has been involved in a road traffic accident in which he was the driver of a vehicle and was seat belted. He is complaining of severe low thoracic spine pain and has tenderness and bruising posteriorly. He is neurologically intact. Plain radiographs of the spine reveal a compression fracture of T12 with 50% loss of anterior height. An MRI scan is performed which shows increased signal posteriorly on STIR images. The posterior column is most likely to have failed by which mode?
    A. Compression
    B. Tension
    C. Shear
    D. Rotation
    E. Translation

15. Which of the following factors has been shown to decrease the pullout strength of pedicle screws used during spinal stabilisation?
    A. Use of supplemental PMMA cement
    B. Reduced bone mineral density
    C. Increased screw diameter
    D. Bicortical purchase
    E. Use of converging screws

16. In the management of Legg-Calve-Perthes' disease, the most important prognostic factor is:
    A. The duration of symptoms during the acute phase
    B. The extent of synovitis
    C. The extent of femoral head involvement as classified by Catterall
    D. The sphericity of the femoral head at maturity
    E. The integrity of the medial pillar on plain radiography during the active stages of the disease

17. A 4-year-old child is diagnosed with Legg-Calve-Perthes' disease. The plain anteroposterior and lateral pelvic radiographs show late fragmentation with a Catterall grade 4 and Herring grade B. The child is currently symptomatic with knee pain on the affected side and has been limping for several months. The next most appropriate step in management would be:
    A. Obtain plain radiographs of the knee
    B. Request an MRI scan of the affected hip
    C. Prescribe analgesia for symptomatic relief, direct activity into less physical tasks and review the patient again in 3 months
    D. Abduction splintage of the affected hip
    E. Discuss with the parents and the child the need for containment surgery in the near future to preserve femoral head sphericity

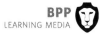

18. In Legg-Calve-Perthes' disease, how long does the fragmentation phase last?
    A. 4–6 weeks
    B. 1–3 months
    C. 6–12 months
    D. 1–2 years
    E. 3–4 years

19. Which of the following conditions is not associated with pes cavus deformity?
    A. Hereditary sensorimotor neuropathy
    B. Friedriech's ataxia
    C. Diastematomyelia
    D. Arthrogryposis
    E. Cerebral palsy

20. Which of the following statements regarding the Herring classification of Legg-Calve-Perthes' disease is **false**?
    A. The classification is based on the radiographic appearances of the integrity of the lateral pillar
    B. There are three discrete grades
    C. Herring grade A is defined as 100% preservation of the pillar
    D. The classification is best applied during the synovitis stage of the disease
    E. Herring grade B is defined as less than 100% but greater than 50% preservation of the pillar

21. With regards to autologous chondrocyte implantation, better outcomes are associated with lesions at:
    A. Supero-medial trochlea
    B. Lateral femoral condyle
    C. Medial patella facet
    D. Supero-lateral trochlea
    E. Medial tibial plateau

22. The number of bursae around the knee joint is:
    A. 12
    B. 10
    C. 9
    D. 8
    E. 7

23. The main advantage of the Southern approach to the knee is:
    A. Can be used in all knees
    B. Less likely to require lateral release
    C. It provides better exposure
    D. Less pain
    E. Spares the extensor mechanism

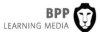

24.  The most common complication following knee arthrodesis is:
    A.  Bony fracture
    B.  Pin track infection
    C.  Nonunion
    D.  Failure of metalwork
    E.  Thrombophlebitis

25.  An active 55-year-old man presents to your clinic with knee pain and instability, two years following re-revision TKR for infection. Investigations confirm the presence of further infection. The next best step in management would be:
    A.  Above knee amputation
    B.  One stage revision arthroplasty
    C.  Two stage revision arthroplasty
    D.  Arthrodesis
    E.  Long term antibiotics

26.  Regarding the morphology and arrangement of chondrocytes in the various layers of articular cartilage, which of these statements is **true**?
    A.  In the calcified zone, the chondrocytes are small and randomly arranged
    B.  In the deep zone, the chondrocytes are small and randomly arranged
    C.  In the deep zone, chondrocytes have a flat parallel array
    D.  In the middle zone, chondrocytes have a flat parallel array
    E.  In the superficial zone, chondrocytes are spherical in shape

27.  With regards to meniscal healing and repair, which of these statements is **false**?
    A.  Meniscal repairs have a success rate of about 95% when associated with a concomitant ACL reconstruction
    B.  Meniscal repairs have a success rate of about 50% when associated with an ACL deficient knee
    C.  Healing rates of meniscal repairs are lower in ACL intact knees when compared with healing rates in ACL reconstructed knees
    D.  Healing rates of meniscal repairs are lower in ACL reconstructed knees when compared with healing rates in ACL intact knees
    E.  Healing rates of meniscal repairs are lower in ACL deficient knees when compared with healing rates in ACL reconstructed knees

28.  With regards to muscle contractions:
    A.  Concentric – joint moves with a load and the muscle contracts
    B.  Eccentric – variable load with constant velocity
    C.  Isokinetic – fixed load with no joint motion
    D.  Concentric – results in muscle lengthening while controlling a load during joint motion
    E.  Isometric – variable load with constant velocity

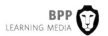

29. Which of the statements is **true** for the characteristics of human skeletal muscle fibres:
    A. Type 1 fibres are white, fast twitch fast, have a high strength of contraction, a low aerobic capacity and a larger motor unit size
    B. Type 2A fibres are white, fast twitch fast, have a low strength of contraction, a high aerobic capacity and the largest motor unit size
    C. Type 2B fibres are white, fast twitch fast, have a low strength of contraction, a small motor unit size and a high aerobic capacity
    D. Type 2B fibres are fast, have a high strength of contraction, are the most fatigable, have a low aerobic capacity and high anaerobic capacity with the largest motor unit size
    E. Type 2B fibres are fast, glycolytic, have a fast speed of contraction, have a low strength of contraction, are fatigue resistant, have a low aerobic capacity and a small motor unit size

30. With regards to increasing age related changes in articular cartilage, which following statement is **false**?
    A. With increasing age, there is a decrease in the ratio of chondroitin sulphate to total glycosaminoglycans
    B. An increase in the production of chondroitin 6 sulphate
    C. A decrease in the production of chondroitin 4 sulphate
    D. A decreasing response to TGF-β
    E. A decrease in the production of chondroitin 6 sulphate

31. Which one of the following is **not** a structure in the posterolateral corner?
    A. Popliteus
    B. Arcuate ligament
    C. Fibular collateral ligament
    D. Posterior cruciate ligament
    E. Lateral head of the gastrocnemius

32. With respect to unicompartmental knee replacements (UKR), which one of the following statements is **false**?
    A. 10-year survival results of unicondylar knee replacement (UKR) are better than High tibial osteotomy
    B. Revision of a UKR to another UKR has been shown to be associated with poor results
    C. Rheumatoid arthritis is not a contraindication to UKR
    D. Chondrocalcinosis is a relative contraindication to UKR
    E. Patello-femoral pain is a relative contraindication to UKR

33. The knee joint receives nerve fibres from:
    A. Sciatic and femoral nerves
    B. Obturator, femoral, tibial and common peroneal
    C. Sciatic nerve only
    D. Femoral and obturator nerves
    E. Femoral nerve only

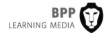

34. In osteotomy for the management of osteoarthritis of the knee, the following statement is **true**:
    A. Results of high tibial osteotomy are similar at 5 and 10 year follow up
    B. High tibial osteotomies are indicated for patients over 60 years of age
    C. The complication of nonunion is common
    D. A varus tibial osteotomy is performed for a valgus knee
    E. The principle of high tibial osteotomy (HTO) is to over-correct the deformity by just under degrees

35. During a knee replacement procedure, if the knee is well balanced for collaterals but flexion gap is smaller than extension gap, you should:
    A. Cut more distal femur
    B. Cut more proximal tibia
    C. Downsize the femur
    D. Release posteromedial corner and semimembranosus
    E. Release deep menisco-tibial ligament

36. Physical therapy in patients with isolated posterior cruciate ligament tears should most focus on strengthening which muscle group?
    A. Knee extensors
    B. Knee flexors
    C. Hip flexors
    D. Hip abductors
    E. Hip extensors

37. A 78-year-old lady is admitted after sustaining a periprosthetic fracture around the stem of a left total hip arthroplasty. The fracture is a long oblique fracture centred over the middle of the stem. The stem appears loose but there is reasonable bone stock in the femur (Vancouver type B2). The most appropriate method of management is:
    A. A Extensively porous coated uncemented long stem revision total hip arthroplasty
    B. Proximally porous coated uncemented long stem revision total hip arthroplasty
    C. Open reduction and internal fixation using a long locking plate
    D. Open reduction and internal fixation using a locking plate and cortical strut graft
    E. Proximal femoral replacement

38. During surgical hip dislocation to treat femoroacetabular impingement which muscle must not be damaged to preserve the blood supply to the femoral head?
    A. Gluteus minimus
    B. Rectus femoris
    C. Vastus lateralis
    D. Gluteus medius
    E. Obturator externus

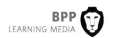

39. Which of the following radiographic findings is consistent with femoroacetabular impingement?
    A. Centre edge angle <25 degrees
    B. Positive cross over sign
    C. Femoral head lateral to ilioischial line
    D. Decreased neck-shaft angle
    E. Increased head-neck offset

40. Which one of the following factors is most important to achieve maximal fluid film lubrication with metal on metal bearing surfaces in total hip arthroplasty?
    A. Increased radial clearance
    B. Reduced radial clearance
    C. Using smaller diameter heads
    D. Increasing surface roughness
    E. Increasing carbide content of the cobalt chromium alloy

41. The reported rate of avascular necrosis following surgical hip dislocation is:
    A. <1%
    B. 10–20%
    C. 20–30%
    D. 30–40%
    E. >50%

42. In total elbow arthroplasty:
    A. Patient operated on for post-traumatic arthritis tend to have a greater range of movement compared to rheumatoid patients
    B. Linked prosthesis restores better range of movement than unlinked prosthesis
    C. Linked implants have a lower rate of loosening compared to unlinked implants
    D. Overall revision rate is around 13%
    E. All of the above

43. With regards to osteosarcomas of the proximal humerus:
    A. Second most common site for this tumour
    B. Have a better prognosis than those around the knee
    C. On presentation most will have a significant extra osseous component
    D. A raised alkaline phosphatase is diagnostic
    E. Chemotherapy has a minimal role in treatment

44. Which of the following statements regarding brachial plexus injuries is **false**?
    A. Scapuloplexy is an established form of treating longstanding scapula winging
    B. CT myelogram is helpful in identifying root avulsions
    C. Potential for return of intrinsic hand function is poorer for lower trunk lesions
    D. Postganglionic reconstruction or repair of nerves should be delayed for at least 6 months
    E. Intercostal nerves can be used for grafting

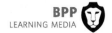

45.  The following are potential sites of compression for the median nerve except:
     A.  Ligament of Struthers
     B.  Lacertus fibrosus
     C.  Gantzer's muscle
     D.  Arcade of Froche
     E.  Flexor digitorum superficialis


46.  Regarding the brachial plexus:
     A.  Long thoracic nerve supplies latissimus dorsi
     B.  Dorsal scapular nerve supplies the levator scapulae
     C.  Musculocutaneous nerve terminates as the medial cutaneous nerve of forearm
     D.  Thoracodorsal nerve supplies serratus anterior
     E.  Subclavius nerve supplies infraspinatus


47.  Regarding shoulder arthrodesis, choose the **false** statement:
     A.  Indicated in post traumatic brachial plexus injuries
     B.  Indicated in paralysis of deltoid and rotator cuff muscle
     C.  Ideal position of arm in arthrodesis should have minimal internal rotation
     D.  Ideal position should have less flexion and abduction
     E.  Patient satisfaction after procedure has found to be 80%


48.  Regarding elbow instability, which statement is **false**?
     A.  Ulnohumeral articulation is a primary static stabiliser
     B.  Medial collateral ligament is a primary static stabiliser (anterior portion)
     C.  Radial head is a primary static stabiliser
     D.  Flexor and extensor origins are secondary stabilisers
     E.  Anconeus is a dynamic stabiliser


49.  Regarding elbow instability:
     A.  A stage I dislocation involves disruption of the anterior and posterior capsule
     B.  A stage II dislocation involves disruption of lateral collateral ligament
     C.  A stage III dislocation may have a partially intact medial collateral ligament
     D.  The coronoid process fractures are most commonly approached from a medial approach
     E.  Terrible triad of Hotckiss involves the olecranon


50.  Regarding the intracapsular ligaments of the wrist:
     A.  Scapholunate is an extrinsic
     B.  lunotriquetral is an extrinsic
     C.  Radioscaphocapitate is an intrinsic
     D.  Triquetrum is pivotal for rotational movements
     E.  Space of Poireur is an area of thickening in the capsule

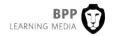

51.  In diagnostic procedures for carpal pathology, which of the following is **true**?
     A.  MRI with gadolidium enhancement is gold standard
     B.  The triangular fibrocartilage complex is poorly defined by arthrography
     C.  Arthrography is more accurate and specific than arthroscopy
     D.  Plain radiographs – 4 views are taken
     E.  Triple phase injection arthrography is particularly helpful for intrinsic ligament pathology

52.  A 22-year-old professional volleyball player complains of pain in the shoulder, exacerbated by overhead activities. On examination there is tenderness around the spinoglenoid notch and the cross-adduction test causes pain. The most likely diagnosis is:
     A.  Frozen shoulder
     B.  Cuff tear
     C.  Brachial plexopathy
     D.  Suprascapular nerve entrapment
     E.  Amyotropic neuralgia

53.  With regards the anatomy of the suprascapular nerve:
     A.  Mixed motor and sensory peripheral nerve
     B.  Passes through posterior triangle of neck
     C.  Variable contribution from fourth cervical root
     D.  At suprascapular notch passes over the superior transverse scapular ligament
     E.  Can be injured in middle and distal third clavicle fractures

54.  Regarding quadrilateral space syndrome, which statement is **not true**?
     A.  Rare cause of axillary nerve compression
     B.  Symptoms are not related to motion
     C.  Point tenderness localised to area of quadrilateral space
     D.  Subclavian arteriogram aids diagnosis
     E.  Neurology examination is usually normal

55.  Regarding elbow biomechanics, choose the **false** statement:
     A.  Resisted flexion at the elbow can transmit forces up to 4 times the body weight
     B.  Radiocapitellar joint takes 60% of the load in the elbow joint
     C.  Axis of forearm rotation passes through capitellum and radial head
     D.  The functional arc of the elbow is 0–130 degrees
     E.  Range of pronation-supination is from 70 degrees of pronation to 80 degrees of supination

56.  In re-plantation surgery in the upper limb, re-plantation is generally contraindicated or relatively contraindicated for all the following except:
     A.  Localised crush amputation of thumb
     B.  Through elbow amputation
     C.  Very high arm amputation
     D.  Warm ischaemia time > 12 hours in a hand amputation
     E.  Patient with serious injuries or illness

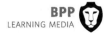

57. Which of the following statements best describes the production of collagen at the fracture site in the first two weeks of fracture healing?
    A. Type I collagen production high, type II collagen production low
    B. Type I collagen production high, type II collagen production high
    C. Type I collagen production low, type II collagen production high
    D. Type I collagen production absent, type II collagen production low
    E. Type I collagen production high, type II collagen absent

58. Which of the following principally occurs by a process of intramembranous ossification?
    A. Embryonic long bone formation
    B. Bone transport
    C. Callus formation during fracture healing
    D. Spinal fusion through use of demineralised bone matrix
    E. Bone formation by epiphyseal secondary centres of ossification

59. Which of the following materials can be considered as being the least isotropic?
    A. Highly cross linked polyethylene
    B. Alumina
    C. Stainless steel
    D. Cortical bone
    E. Trabecular bone

60. Teicoplanin belongs to which of the below groups of antibiotics?
    A. Cephalosporins
    B. Carbapenems
    C. Aminoglycosides
    D. Macrolides
    E. Glycopeptides

61. Which of the following statements describes the transition in the centre of rotation of the glenohumeral joint after reverse shoulder arthroplasty?
    A. The centre of rotation moves laterally
    B. The centre of rotation moves medially
    C. The centre of rotation is lowered and moves medially
    D. The centre of rotation is raised and moves medially
    E. The centre of rotation is lowered and moves laterally

62. Which of the following statements regarding the actions and uses of bisphosphonates is **false**?
    A. They are characterised chemically by having a POP region
    B. They act by stabilising the hydroxyapatite crystal
    C. They act by inhibiting osteoclastic activity
    D. Uses include treatment of malignant hypercalcaemia, osteoporosis and Paget's disease
    E. Gut absorption is affected by ingestion with milk

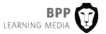

63. With respect to magnetic resonance imaging, T2 is defined as:
    A. Time taken for the longitudinal magnetisation vector to fall to 63% of its maximal value
    B. Time taken for the longitudinal magnetisation vector to fall to 37% of its maximal value
    C. Time taken for the transverse magnetisation vector to fall to 63% of its maximal value
    D. Time taken for the transverse magnetisation vector to fall to 37% of its maximal value
    E. Time taken between successive radiofrequency pulses

64. Which of the following is not a common site for bone densitometry using dual energy X-ray absorptiometry?
    A. Proximal femur
    B. Forearm
    C. Lumbar spine
    D. Proximal humerus
    E. Calcaneum

65. Which of the following statements regarding tuberculosis is **false**?
    A. They are aerobic bacilli
    B. The most common skeletal area affected is the lumbar spine
    C. Culture is usually done in Lowenstein-Jensen medium and can take weeks
    D. They exhibit resistance to decolorisation with mineral acids after Ziehl-Nielsen staining
    E. The characteristic finding on histology is one of caseating granulomas with central necrosis

66. In a triple phase bone scan, how long after injection are images taken for the blood pool phase?
    A. Less than 1 minute
    B. 1–2 minutes
    C. 2–5 minutes
    D. 10–15 minutes
    E. 1 hour

67. A 5-year-old boy presents with a bilateral hindfoot equinus and mid foot cavus deformity. Muscle function testing shows MRC grade 5 posterior tibial function, MRC grade 3 tibialis anterior and weak peroneal function. Further assessment reveals a correctable hindfoot. The most appropriate treatment would be?
    A. Subtalar fusion
    B. Posteromedial release
    C. Calcaneal osteotomy and tendo-achilles lengthening
    D. Custom orthotics
    E. Plantar fascia release, posterior tibial tendon transfer via interoseus membrane to the dorsum, and tendo-achilles lengthening

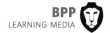

68. A 36-month-old boy has a rigid 30-degree lumbar scoliosis. MRI confirms a partially segmented L4 hemivertebra at the apex of the deformity. The examining doctor notes a single café au lait on his torso. Treatment may consist of:
    A. Posterior fusion.
    B. Conservative with follow-up in 3 months
    C. Convex hemiepiphyseodesis
    D. Hemivertebral resection and fusion
    E. Thoracolumbosacral (TLS) orthotic bracing

69. The primary goal of serial manipulation and casting in a newborn infant with bilateral clubfeet is:
    A. Simultaneous adduction of the metatarsals and dorsiflexion of the talus
    B. Lateral translation of the subtalar joint
    C. Rotation of the foot laterally around the fixed talus
    D. Translation of the navicular in an anterolateral direction
    E. Plantarflexion of the calcaneus

70. An 9-year-old African-Carribean girl has had a fever, pain and swelling over the lateral aspect of her right elbow for the past 7 days. Examination reveals warmth, swelling, and tenderness over the lateral epicondyly. Blood tests show a elevated white cell count, an erythocyte sedimentation rate of 124 and a C-Reactive Protein of 19. Aspiration yields 2ml of purulent fluid. Management should now consist of:
    A. Oral antibiotics and a follow up in clinic in 48 hours
    B. Incision and drainage of the distal humeral metaphysis.
    C. Indium-labelled WBC scan.
    D. Antituberculous medication for 3 months.
    E. Three-phase technetium 99m bone scan

71. A 12-year-old girl with hallux valgus reports pain after playing basketball. Radiographs show a hallux valgus (HV) angle of 19 degrees, an intermetatarsal (IM) angle of 10 degrees, a distal metatarsal articular angle (DMAA) of 10 degrees. The recommended treatment should consist of:
    A. Scarf osteotomy
    B. Proximal crescentic osteotomy with distal soft tissue realignment
    C. Mitchell osteotomy
    D. Chevron osteotomy
    E. Shoe wear modification

72. A histological specimen of a physis in a paediatric renal patient with slipped capital femoral epiphysis (SCFE) would reveal:
    A. A dense perichondral ring
    B. An abnormality at the metaphyseal primary and secondary spongiosa
    C. Increased undulations of the growth plate
    D. Granulation tissue in the hypertrophic zone
    E. Abnormal proliferative zone

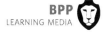

73. Criteria for diagnosis of neurofibromatosis include all the clinical signs below, except:
    A. An osseous lesion
    B. Neurological deficit
    C. Iris pigmentation
    D. Café au lait spots
    E. Axillary or inguinal freckling

74. Which of the following is **not** a feature of the foot deformity in hereditary motor sensory neuropathy?
    A. Plantar flexed first ray
    B. Interphalangeal (IP) joint flexion
    C. Forefoot pronation
    D. Metatarsophalangeal (MTP) joint hyperextension
    E. Hindfoot valgus

75. The COMP gene Chromosome 19 defect is responsible for the following disorder:
    A. Marfan syndrome
    B. Cleidocranial dysplasia
    C. Achondroplasia
    D. Fibrous dysplasia
    E. Pseudochondroplasia

76. Features of Klippel-Feil syndrome include all following except:
    A. Hypoplasia of the scapulae
    B. Cervical instability
    C. Hearing impairment
    D. A low posterior hairline congenital cervical fusion
    E. Cervical stenosis

77. Rickets affects which zone of the growth plate?
    A. Maturation zone
    B. Secondary bony epiphysis
    C. Primary spongiosa
    D. Zone of provisional calcification
    E. Proliferative zone

78. Acute haematogenous osteomyelitis affects the growth plate at which level?
    A. Zona reticularis
    B. Reserve zone
    C. Secondary spongiosa
    D. Proliferative zone
    E. Primary spongiosa

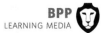

79.   Duchenne muscular dystrophy is associated with a mutation in the gene coding for:
   A.   Tropomyosin
   B.   Myosin
   C.   Actin
   D.   Dystrophin
   E.   Calcitonin

80.   The following statement is true with respect to lateral condyle fractures of the distal humerus in children:
   A.   The most common mechanism of injury is forearm supination and a valgus stress on the extended elbow
   B.   The Milch type 1 injury is a Salter Harris type II injury
   C.   The most commonly affected age group is 10–12 years
   D.   The Milch type 1 injury is most common type of injury
   E.   Reduction manoeuvres for displaced fractures include flexion and supination

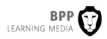

# MCQ Paper 1

## Answers

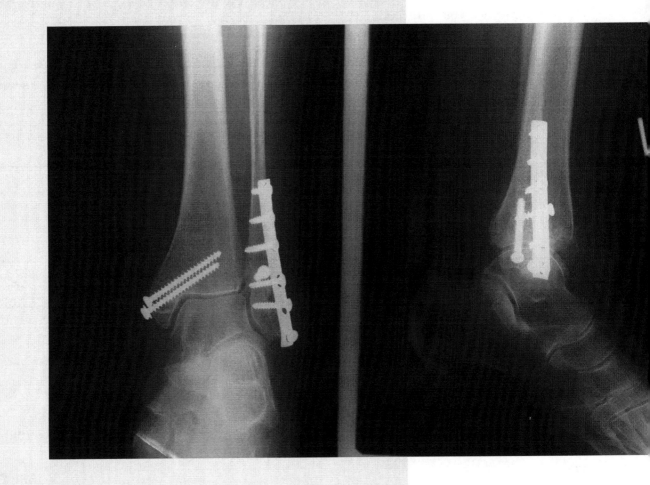

1. **E**
   Application of torsional load to bone results in appearance of the crack perpendicular to the elongating collagen fibrils that progresses through the perimeter of bone resulting in a spiral fracture.

   Ref:
   Tencer AF. Biomechanics of fixation and fracture. In Rockwood & Greens (2006) (6th ed.) *Fracture in Adults* Lippincott Williams & Wilkins, Philadelphia.

2. **C**
   A bone hole of the same size as the pin diameter causes loosening of the pins by micro motion leading to bone resorption, under sizing the bone hole by 0.3 mm leads to micro fractures and hence under sizing the bone hole by approximately 0.1 reduces the loosening of the external fixator pins.

   Ref:
   Huiskes R, Chao EYS, Cripen TE. Parametric analysis of pin-bone stress in external fracture fixation. *J Ortho Res* 1985; 3: 341–349

3. **D**
   Dislocation of the elbow (poster lateral) with fracture of the radial head and coronoid process forms the terrible triad of instability for the elbow. The treatment rationale is stabilisation of the elbow achieved by ORIF radial head, coronoid process and LCL. Replacement of the radial head with metal prosthesis provides good results but replacement should be sought if the radial head fracture is more than 3 fragments, there is loss of fragments or metaphyseal comminution.

   Ref:
   1. Regan W, Morrey B. Fracture of coronoid process of ulna. *JBJS Am* 1989; 71: 1348–54.
   2. Ring D. Fracture and dislocation of elbow. In Rockwood & Greens (2006) (6th ed.) *Fracture in Adults* (2006) (Lippincott Williams & Wilkins, Philadelphia.

4. **A**
   Borderline patients are patients who have responded to initial stabilisation but have clinical parameters associated with poor outcome and risk of rapid deterioration. These parameters include:

   a. ISS>40
   b. Hypothermia (temp<35)
   c. Mean pulmonary arterial pressure of >24mm of hg (Initial)
   d. Systolic BP<90 mm of hg
   e. Chest trauma, AIS>2
   f. Bilateral femoral fractures
   g. Moderate to severe head injury
   h. Radiographic evidence of pulmonary contusion

   Ref:
   Pape H, Giannoudis P. Management of the multiply injured patient. In Rockwood & Greens (2006) (6th ed.) *Fracture in Adults* Lippincott Williams & Wilkins, Philadelphia.

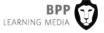

5. **A**

Broad arm sling provides adequate support with early active ROM exercises and physiotherapy helps regain early function in minimally displaced radial head fracture. Longer immobilisation increases the risk of elbow stiffness and loss of ROM. Backslab immobilisation is hardly required as these fractures are stable in nature.

Ref:

Morrey BF (1985) *The elbow and its disorders.* Saunders, Philadelphia.

6. **B**

The Mangled Extremity Severity Score is one the scoring systems used in evaluation of patients with trauma. The score is divided into 4 categories based on the soft tissue/skeletal injury or energy of trauma (scored 1–4); limb ischaemia (scored 1–3); shock (scored 0–2); and age (scored 0–2). The maximum score achieved is 11 and the minimum score achieved is 2.

An arbitrary cut off point of 7 is used to evaluate survivorship of the limb and considering reconstruction versus amputation.

Ref:

Helfet D, Howey T, Sanders R, Johansen K. Limb salvage versus amputation. Preliminary results of mangled extremity severity score. *Clin Ortho Relt Res* 1990; 256: 80–86.

7. **C**

80% of the normal rotational function of the forearm is achieved by maintaining the radial bow in closed or open treatment of the forearm fractures.

Ref:

Schemitsch EH, Richards RR. The effect of malunion on functional outcome after plate fixation of fractures of both bones of the forearm in adults. *JBJS Am* 1992; 74; 1068–78.

8. **E**

The initial radiographic evaluation of pelvic fracture includes pelvis AP radiograph assisted with an inlet and out let view. The inlet film is obtained by tilting the beam approximately 40 degrees cephalad. The X-ray demonstrates subtle fractures of sacrum, antero-posterior displacement of injured hemipelvis, degree and severity of rotational displacement of the injured hemipelvis. Widening of the scaroiliac joint or symphysis pubis joint is clearly visible on inlet view. Fractures of the pubic rami are also usually well visualised. The outlet view visualises the cephalad and caudal displacement of the injured hemipelvis.

Ref:

Starr AJ, Malekzadeh AS. Fractures of the Pelvic Ring. In Rockwood & Greens (2006) (6th ed.) *Fracture in Adults* Lippincott Williams & Wilkins, Philadelphia.

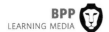

9.  **C**

    A laterally applied force that acts to compress the affected side of the pelvis causes lateral compression fractures. These fractures are divided into 3 types, however the most common type of pelvic ring disruption is the type I lateral compression fracture. This type of fracture often passes through the sacral foramina or there is a sacral 'buckle' fracture. These injuries are not associated with disruption of the posterior ligament or the sacro-tuberous or sacro-spinous ligament and hence are vertically stable. There is some degree of rotational instability. The anterior ring injury usually involves a pubic rami fracture.

    The type II lateral compression fractures are associated with greater force and is associated with iliac wing fractures. This commonly leaves crescent-shaped portions of the iliac wing attached to the sacrum and are also known as 'crescent fractures'. The posterior ligaments and the sacro-tuberous and sacro-spinous ligaments are intact. There is vertical stability and rotational instability. The type III fractures may be associated with rupture of the posterior ligaments making these fractures not only rotationally unstable but also vertically unstable.

    Ref:
    Starr AJ, Malekzadeh AS. Fractures of the Pelvic Ring. In Rockwood & Greens (2006) (6th ed.) *Fracture in Adults* Lippincott Williams & Wilkins, Philadelphia.

10. **A**

    The antero-posterior compression fractures (APC) occurs from an anteriorly directed force to the pelvis. This typically creates and 'open-book' fracture. APC fractures are divided into 3 types: The type 1 fracture has >2cm widening of the pubic symphysis with no disruption of the SI joint. Type 2 has anterior disruption of the SI joint while the type 3 is associated with disruption of both anterior and posterior ring. These injuries have a very high association with neurovascular injury, hemorrhage and mortality. The sacroiliac joint is typically displaced posterior and cephalad and hence the reduction maneuver should counteract this displacement.

    Ref:
    Starr AJ, Malekzadeh AS. Fractures of the Pelvic Ring. In Rockwood & Greens (2006) (6th ed.) *Fracture in Adults* Lippincott Williams & Wilkins, Philadelphia.

11. **C**

    This has been shown to be the strongest predictor of post-operative neurologic recovery in patients with cervical myelopathy secondary to rheumatoid arthritis.

    Ref:
    Peppelman WC *et al*. Cervical spine surgery in rheumatoid arthritis: Improvement of neurologic deficit after cervical spine fusion. *Spine* 1993; 18: 2375–2379.

12. **A**

    The supraorbital nerve and supratrochlear nerve are both at risk of injury if the anterior pins are placed too medially (medial to the safe zone). The safe zone for anterior pin placement is 1cm above the orbital rim below the equator of the skull and cephalad to the lateral two-thirds of the orbit.

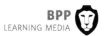

Ref:
Botte MJ, Byrne TP, Abrams RA, Garfin SR. Halo Skeletal Fixation: Techniques of application and prevention of complications. *J Am Acad Orthop Surg* 1996; 4: 44–53.

13. **C**

Pin loosening has been shown to occur in 36–60% of patients. In the absence of infection, the pin can usually be retightened or moved to an adjacent site. Dural tear is very rare and usually due to a fall with the fixator in position. Pin site bleeding is more common in patients on anticoagulation and is said to occur in 1% of cases. Nerve injury and dysphagia (due to hyperextension of neck) were shown in one study to occur in 2% of cases.

Ref:
Garfin SR, Botte MJ, Waters RL *et al.* Complications in the use of the halo fixation device. *J Bone Joint Surg (Am)* 1986; 68: 320–325.

14. **B**

The most likely mechanism of failure here is a flexion-compression injury with the anterior column failing under compression and the posterior column fails under tension. The mechanistic method of describing thoracolumbar spine injuries was proposed by Ferguson and Allen.

Ref:
Ferguson RL, Allen BL Jr. A mechanistic classification of thoracolumbar spine fractures. *Clin Orthop* 1984; 189: 77–88.

15. **B**

This factor has been shown to reduce the pullout strength of pedicle screws. It has been shown that patients with osteoporotic compression fractures are not good candidates for surgery using pedicle screw based internal fixation systems.

Ref:
Gaines RW. The use of pedicle screw internal fixation for the operative treatment of spinal disorders. *J Bone Joint Surg (Am)* 2000; 82: 1458–1476.

16. **D**

The natural history of Legg-Calve Perthes' disease (LCP) is one of repeated bouts of infarction with subsequent necrosis and collapse followed by healing and remodelling. The disease process only affects the femoral head although secondary changes in the acetabulum may occur in severe cases. Indirectly, the age of onset is important as this dictates the amount of available time for remodelling to occur and for normal femoral head anatomy to be restored. The most important prognostic factor for later life and the risk of hip osteoarthritis is the sphericity of the femoral head at maturation and research has been directed at determining which cases require intervention and at what stage in the disease intervention is likely to produce the best results in this regard. The current evidence base would suggest that the age of onset and the integrity of the lateral pillar as assessed by the Herring classification during the fragmentation phase are important guides in determining when and in which cases surgical intervention is required to contain the femoral head.

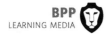

Ref:
Staheli LT (2007) (4<sup>th</sup> ed.). *Fundamentals of Paediatric Orthopaedics*. Lippincott Williams & Wilkins, Philadelphia.

17.  **C**

The important management principle of LCP disease is to avoid treating patients who are likely to do well without intervention. Generally patients under the age of 5 years are likely to do well and treatment should be aimed at symptomatic relief. There is no proven role for abduction splints. Physiotherapy can help to preserve range of motion. It must be borne in mind that occasionally a poor result is seen in young patients due to the development of metaphyseal cysts and physeal bridges and therefore future follow up is essential. The patients where surgical intervention may be required to contain the femoral head and promote sphericity are patients older than 8 years with severe disease as classified by Herring. This may take the form of a varus femoral osteotomy or more rarely a pelvic osteotomy in late cases where the head has begun to extrude.

Ref:
Staheli LT (2007) (4<sup>th</sup> ed.). *Fundamentals of Paediatric Orthopaedics*. Lippincott Williams & Wilkins, Philadelphia.

18.  **D**

The temporal classification of LCP disease usually involves four sequential stages in which the time spent in each stage is independent of the extent of epiphyseal involvement. The stages are:

Synovitis – characterised by synovitis, effusion and cartilaginous hypertrophy and typically lasts a few weeks

Necrosis/collapse – 6–12 months
Fragmentation – 1–2 years
Remodelling – several years

Ref:
Staheli LT (2007) (4<sup>th</sup> ed.). *Fundamentals of Paediatric Orthopaedics*. Lippincott Williams & Wilkins, Philadelphia.

19.  **D**

Bilateral pes cavus deformity may arise as a benign condition existing at the extreme end of the normal spectrum of arch height. However, it may arise as a result of specific pathology within the central nervous system or a systemic neuromuscular disorder. The important underlying causes to be aware of are:

- Neuromuscular disorders
    - Muscular dystrophy
    - Charcot Marie Tooth disease
    - Friedriech's ataxia
    - Roussy-Levy syndrome
- Central nervous system disorders
    - Cerebral palsy
    - Poliomyelitis

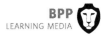

- Spinal pathology
  - Spinal dysraphism
  - Diastematomyelia
  - Spina bifida
  - Myelomeningocele
  - Syringomyelia
  - Spinal cord tumour
- Muscle pathology
  - Crush injury
  - Burns
  - Compartment syndrome

Depending on the underlying cause, the condition may be unilateral or bilateral. Unilateral cases cannot be ascribed to a benign physiological origin without further investigation.

Ref:

Staheli LT (2007) (4<sup>th</sup> ed.). *Fundamentals of Paediatric Orthopaedics.* Lippincott Williams & Wilkins, Philadelphia.

**20.** **D**

The Herring classification has three grades of increasing collapse with respect to the lateral pillar of the femoral head on an antero-posterior radiograph. Grade A has 100% preservation, grade B has greater than 50% but less than 100% preservation and grade C is defined as greater than 50% collapse of the lateral pillar. The Herring grade should be judged during the late necrosis/early fragmentation phase of the disease to be a useful tool in directing management.

Ref:

Staheli LT (2007) (4<sup>th</sup> ed.). *Fundamentals of Paediatric Orthopaedics.* Lippincott Williams & Wilkins, Philadelphia.

**21.** **B**

Lesions at the medial femoral condyle seem to have best outcomes following autologous chondrocyte implantation, followed by those at the lateral femoral condyle. Lesions in the patellofemoral joint seem to have the worst outcomes.

Ref:

Smith GD, Knutsen G, Richardson BJ A clinical review of cartilage repair techniques. *J Bone Joint Surg Br* 2005; 87-B: 445–449.

**22.** **A**

There are a total of twelve bursae around the knee, four anterior, four posterior, and two on either side. Anteriorly, they are the suprapatellar, prepatellar, and the superficial and deep infrapatellar. Laterally there are bursae between the lateral collateral ligament and the biceps femoris and the popliteus tendons. Medially, a bursa separates the medial collateral ligament from the tendons of the muscles forming the pes anserinus, and deeper to the ligament a bursa separates it from the tibia. Posteriorly, two bursae separate the joint capsule from the medial and lateral heads of the gastrocnemius, the semimembranosus bursa separates the muscle from the medial head of gastrocnemius, and there is a burse between the popliteus tendon and the back of the tibia and fibula.

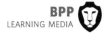

Ref:
Sinnatamby CS (ed.) (2001) *Last's Anatomy Regional and Applied*. Churchill Livingstone, London. p. 134.

23.  **E**

The Southern approach to the knee (also known as the subvastus approach) preserves the integrity of the extensor mechanism by sparing the quadriceps tendon. However, it is less versatile than other exposures.

Ref:
Hofmann AA, Plaster RL, Murdock LE Subvastus (Southern) approach for primary total knee arthroplasty. *Clin Orthop Relat Res*, 1991; 269: 70–7.

24.  **C**

The most common complication after arthrodesis of the knee is non union. Other complications include pin track infection, failure of metalwork, bony fracture, hip pain and thrombophlebitis

Ref:
Conway JD, Mont MA, Bezwada HP. Arthrodesis of the knee. *J Bone Joint Surg Am* 2004; 86-A 4: 835–48

25.  **D**

The rate of failure following re-revision of a revision total knee replacement complicated by infection is significantly high enough to warrant consideration of other surgical options. In the presence of pain and instability long term antibiotic therapy in not sufficient to address the underlying cause of the symptoms. In such instances knee arthrodesis should be considered, and although controversial, the available evidence does suggest that it may be preferable to an above knee amputation.

Ref:
Conway JD, Mont MA, Bezwada HP. Arthrodesis of the knee. *J Bone Joint Surg Am* 2004; 86-A 4: 835–48.

26.  **A**

Articular cartilage can be divided into 4 distinct layers: superficial, middle, deep and calcified. These layers differ in cellular morphology, biomechanical composition and structural properties. In the superficial layer the collagen orientation is parallel to the surface. It changes to a more random, less densely packed array in the middle zone. The collagen bundles are perpendicular to the joint surface and subchondral bone in the deep and calcified layers. The deep zone has the largest collagen fibres, highest concentration of proteoglycans and the lowest concentration of water. In the calcified zone, the chondrocytes are small and randomly arranged. The chondrocytes transition to a columnar arrangement and spherical shape in the deep zone, to a more random array of cells in the middle zone, and to a flat parallel array of cells in the superficial zone.

Ref:
Buckwalter JA, Mankin HJ. Articular cartilage: Degeneration and osteoarthritis, repair, regeneration, and transplantation. *Instr Course Lect* 1994; 43: 137–148.

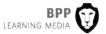

27. **D**

The increased rates of healing in ACL reconstructed knees is possibly a result of drilling, which provide an exogenous source of blood to promote healing of the repair.

Ref:
1. Arnoczky SP, Warren RF, Spivak JM. Meniscal repair using an exogenous fibrin clot: An experimental study in dogs. *J Bone Joint Surg Am* 1988; 70: 1209–1217.
2. Vaccaro AR (ed.) (2005) *Orthopaedic Knowledge Update: Home study syllabus 8*. American Academy of Surgeons.

28. **A**

Isometric – Fixed load with no joint motion

Concentric – Joint moves with a load and the muscle contracts

Eccentric – Results in muscle lengthening while controlling a load during joint motion

Isokinetic – Variable load with constant velocity

Ref:
Woo SL-Y, Debski RE, Withrow JD, Janqueshek MA: Bio-mechanics of knee ligaments. *Am J Sports Med* 1999; 27: 533–543.

29. **D**

|  | Type 1 | Type 2A | Type 2B |
|---|---|---|---|
| Other names | Red, slow-twitch slow, oxidative | White, fast-twitch fast, oxidative, glycolytic | Fast, glycolytic |
| Speed of contraction | Slow | Fast | Fast |
| Strength of contraction | Low | High | High |
| Fatigability | Fatigue-resistant | Fatigable | Most fatigable |
| Aerobic capacity | High | Medium | Low |
| Anaerobic capacity | Low | Medium | High |
| Motor unit size | Small | Larger | Largest |
| Capillary density | High | High | Low |

Ref:
Garrett WE Fr, Best TM. Anatomy, physiology, and mechanics of skeletal muscle. In Simon SR (ed) (1994) *Orthopaedic Basic Science*. American Academy of Orthopaedic Surgeons.

30. **E**

With increasing age: decrease in the ratio of chndroitin sulphate to total glycosaminglycans, an increase in chondroitin 6 sulphate, a decrease in chondroitin 4 sulphate, decreased response to growth factors, especially TGF-β, decrease in the water content of cartilage, increase in decorin concentration, increase in collagen cross-linking, increase in collagen fibril diameter

Ref:
Vaccaro AR (ed.) (2005) *Orthopaedic Knowledge Update: Home study syllabus 8*. American Academy of Surgeons.

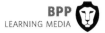

**31.** **D**

The posterolateral corner is made up of three layers. Layer 1 comprises a fascial layer made up of iliotibial band and biceps femoris. Layer 2 comprises the lateral quadriceps retinaculum, the lateral (fibular) collateral ligament and the 2 patellofemoral ligaments. Layer 3 comprises the joint capsule, popliteus tendon, the coronary, fabellofibular, arcuate and popliteofibular ligaments.

Ref:

Hoppenfeld S, Deboer P (2007) (3rd ed.) *Surgical Exposures in Orthopaedics: The Anatomic Approach*. Lippincott Williams & Wilkins, Philadelphia.

**32.** **C**

Ref:

Price AJ, Waite JC, Svard U. Long-term clinical results of the medial Oxford unicompartmental knee arthroplasty. *Clin Orthop Relat Res* 2005; 435: 171–180.

**33.** **B**

Ref:

Gray H. *Gray's Anatomy* (1980) (36th ed.) Churchill-Livingstone. p. 488.

**34.** **E**

Ref:

Coventry MB. Upper tibial osteotomy for osteoarthritis. *J Bone Joint Surg [Am]* 1985; 67: 1136–1140.

**35.** **C**

The posterior slope of tibia may be incorrect.

Ref:

Whiteside LA *et al.* Selective Ligament release in total knee asthroplasty of the knee in valgus. *CORR* 1999; 367: 141–148.

**36.** **A**

The main function of the PCL complex is to resist posterior tibial translation. Studies have shown that isolated sectioning of the PCL complex results in increased posterior translation, most pronounced at 90 degrees of flexion. Quadriceps strengthening acts to counteracts the posterior tibial subluxation caused by the PCL tear. Moreover, in acute PCL injuries, LE is immobilised in full extension to maintain tibial reduction and minimise posterior tibial sag. In doing so, it counteracts the effect of hamstring muscles on posterior tibial translation

Ref:

Harner CD, Hoher J. Evaluation and treatment of posterior cruciate ligament injuries. *Am J Sports Med* 1998; 26:471–482.

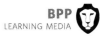

37.   **A**

In this situation where the stem is loose, but there is good bone stock the best option is revision to a long stem uncemented total hip arthroplasty which is extensively porous coated to provide adequate distal fixation for the prosthesis. In one study, proximally porous coated stems were associated with the poorest results. Fixation of the fracture is only appropriate for Vancouver type B1 (fracture around a well fixed prosthesis) and C fractures (fracture well distal to prosthesis). Proximal femoral replacement is used to treat type B3 fractures where there is associated severe segmental bone loss.

Ref:
1.   Patil S, Masri BA, Duncan CP (2006). Periprosthetic fractures of the hip. *Current Orthopaedics*; 20: 179–91.
2.   Lewallen DG, Berry DJ (Dec 1997). Periprosthetic fracture of the femur after total hip arthroplasty. *J Bone Joint Surg (Am)*; 79: 1881–1890.

38.   **E**

This muscle is one of the short external rotators and the critical blood supply to the femoral head (deep branch of the medial femoral circumflex artery) runs on top of it. In order from superior to inferior posteriorly lie the piriformis, superior gamellus, obturator internus, inferior gamellus and then the obturator externus which lies on the piriformis fossa of the femoral neck. During surgical hip dislocation the short external rotators of the hip need to be protected to prevent damage to the blood supply to the femoral head.

Ref:
1.   Parvizi J, Leunig M, Ganz R (2007). Femoroacetabular impingement. *J Am Acad Orthop Surg*; 15: 561–570.
2.   Moore KL (1992) (3rd ed.) *Clinically orientated anatomy*, Lippincott Williams & Wilkins, Baltimore.

39.   **B**

This is a radiographic sign seen on a true AP radiograph of the pelvis which indicates acetabular retroversion, which can cause pincer impingement due to excessive anterior overhang of the acetabulum.

Ref:
Schilders E, Dimitrakopoulou A, Talbot CJ, Bismil Q. Hip pain in young adults and the role of hip arthroscopy. *Orthopaedics and Trauma* 2009; 23: 128–136.

40.   **B**

A low radial clearance and a large diameter femoral head are both crucial factors to achieve fluid film lubrication, which is associated with very low friction and very low wear rates. Lowering the surface roughness also makes fluid film lubrication more likely. Increasing the carbide content of the cobalt chromium alloy increases the hardness of the metal and reduces the wear rate.

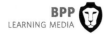

Ref:
1.	Tipper JL, Ingham E, Jin ZM, Fisher J. The science of metal-on-metal articulation. *Current Orthopaedics*, 2005; 19: 280–287.
2.	Roberts P, Grigoris P, Bosch H, Talwaker N. Resurfacing arthroplasty of the hip. *Current Orthopaedics* 2005; 19: 263–279.

## 41.	A

A study on surgical hip dislocation revealed no cases of avascular necrosis in 213 hips.

Ref:

Ganz R, Gill TJ, Gautier E (2001) Surgical dislocation of the adult hip. *J Bone Joint Surg (Br)*; 83: 1119–1124.

## 42.	E

Complication rate in literature has been reported between 14–80% with a median rate of 33%. It has also been found that rheumatoid patients in their fourth decade had no significant difference in incidence of loosening when compared to patients in their sixth decade.

Ref:

Limb D (2007) *The evidence for orthopaedic surgery.* TFM, Malta. p. 153.

## 43.	C

It is the third most common site in the body after distal femur and proximal tibia. They have a poorer prognosis than those around the knee. Alkaline phosphatase is raised in 45–50% of cases. Chemotherapy is first line treatment.

Ref:

Dee R, Hurst L (1997) *Principles of orthopaedic practise.* McGraw Hill, p. 280.

## 44.	D

Scapula thoracic fusion and dynamic muscle transfers (sternal head of pectoralis major, reinforced with autologous fascia lata graft – preferred donors) are also other procedures used for scapula winging. This is usually considered if there is no recovery for more than a year. Post ganglionic reconstruction and repair in brachial plexus injuries should not be delayed as this reduces chances of success.

Ref:

James H (1999) *Orthopaedic Knowledge Update 6.* American Academy of Orthopaedic Surgeons.

## 45.	D

The Arcade of Froche is formed by the proximal edge of the supinator and is a potential site of compression of the radial nerve. The Gantzer's muscle is the accessory head of flexor pollicis longus found under the deep head of pronator teres.

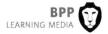

Ref:
Tsai P (2008) Median and radial nerve compression about the elbow. *Journal of Bone and Joint Surgery*; 90: 420–428.

46.   **B**

Long thoracic nerve supplies serratus anterior, subclavius nerve supplies subclavius, musculocutaneous nerve terminates as lateral cutaneous nerve of forearm and thoracodorsal nerve supplies the latissimus dorsi.

Ref:
Snell RS (2003) *Clinical Anatomy*. Lippincott & Wilkins, Williams, Philadelphia, p. 481

47.   **C**

Shoulder arthrodesis should be considered an end-stage salvage procedure. Other indications include failed revision arthroplasty and bone deficiency following resection of proximal humerus tumours. Although controversy exists regarding the ideal position of the limb, it is recommended that 10 degrees to 15 degrees of abduction, 10 degrees to 15 degrees of flexion, and 45 degrees of internal rotation, enables the patient to reach his or her mouth, belt buckles, and contra lateral shoulder and axilla comfortably.

Ref:
Clare DJ Current concepts review shoulder arthrodesis. *J Bone Joint Surg Am* 2001; 83: 593.

48.   **C**

The primary static stabilisers of the elbow are – ulnohumeral articulation, anterior portion of medial collateral ligament and lateral (ulnar) collateral ligament. The secondary stabilisers are the flexor and extensor origin, radial head and anterior capsule. The dynamic stabilisers are the muscles that cross the joint and cause articular compression – triceps, anconeus and brachialis.

Ref:
O'Driscall SW Selected Instructional Course Lecture: the unstable elbow. *J Bone Joint Surg Am* 2000; 82 (5); 724.

49.   **C**

Stage I is disruption of lateral collateral ligament, Stage II is disruption of the anterior and posterior capsule, Stage III is the above and further divided into 3 parts, IIIA with an intact anterior portion of the medial collateral ligament only, IIIB with a complete disruption of the medial collateral ligament complex and IIIC is an unstable elbow even in flexion to 90 degrees in a backslab. The coronoid is most commonly accessible through the posterior approach just lateral to olecranon tip.

Ref:
O'Driscall SW (2000) Selected Instructional Course Lecture: the unstable elbow. *J Bone Joint Surg Am 2000; 82 (5): 724.*

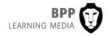

**50.  D**

Scapholunate and lunotriquetral are intrinsic, while the radioscaphocapitate ligament is an extrinsic. The space of Poireur is a weak area in the capsule at the level of the midcarpal joint, between the radioscaphocapitate and long radiolunate ligaments.

Ref:
Gelberman R Instructional course lecture, Carpal instability. *J Bone Joint Surg Am.* 2001; 82(4).

**51.  E**

Plain radiographs taken are usually 6 views: PA, lateral, radial and ulnar deviation, and flexion and extension views. An additional postero-anterior radiograph of the wrist with a clenched and loaded fist is made to rule out scapholunate instability.MRI with gadolinium enhancement is useful for carpal ligament injuries, but consistency with which both the radiocarpal and the interosseous ligaments are demonstrated, however, is not sufficient for this to be a primary method of evaluation. Arthrography is useful for identifying TFCC and intercarpal ligament injuries. Midcarpal, radiocarpal, and distal radioulnar arthrography (triple phase injection) provides definitive data on intercarpal ligaments. However, arthroscopy has now replaced arthrography as the mainstay of diagnosis.

Ref:
Gelberman R Instructional course lecture, Carpal instability. *J Bone Joint Surg Am* 2001; 82 (4).

**52.  D**

Typically seen in volleyball players and other overhead athletes. Cross adduction test puts a strain on the suprascapular nerve. Common sites of entrapment are the scapular notch and the supraglenoid notch.

Ref:
Cummins CA Current concepts review Suprascapular nerve entrapment. *J Bone Joint Surg Am* 2000; 82: 415

**53.  D**

It passes below the superior transverse scapular ligament and the artery and vein pass over it.

Ref:
Cummins CA Current concepts review Suprascapular nerve entrapment. *J Bone Joint Surg Am* 2000; 82: 415.

**54.  B**

Symptoms are exacerbated by abduction and external rotation. The posterior circumflex humeral artery is also compressed as it passes through the quadrilateral space. Thus a subclavian arteriogram showing occlusion of the posterior circumflex humeral artery is considered a positive diagnosis.

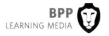

Ref:
Dee R, Hurst L (1997) *Principles of orthopaedic practise*. McGraw Hill. p. 1098.

**55. D**

The functional arc is 100 degrees, but the range of movement (flexion-extension) is 1–146 degrees.

Ref:
Dee R, Hurst L (1997) *Principles of orthopaedic practise*. McGraw Hill. p. –1105.

**56. A**

Attempts should be made to re-implant guillotine or localised crush amputations to thumb, multiple digits, hand or forearm.

Ref:
Dee R, Hurst L (1997) *Principles of orthopaedic practise*. McGraw Hill. p. 1187.

**57. C**

Fracture healing occurs by a process of enchondral ossification with the formation of a cartilaginous precursor. Thus, in the first two weeks collagen type II production is high and type I production is low. As the formed bone is later mineralised, type I collagen production takes over.

Ref:
Buckwalter J, Einhorn T, Simon S (2000) (2nd ed.) *Orthopaedic Basic Science: Biology and Biomechanics of the Musculoskeletal System*. American Academy of Orthopaedic Surgeons.

**58. B**

Enchondral ossification is whereby an intermediate cartilage model is first formed. Examples include

(a)  Embryonic long bone development
(b)  Epiphyseal secondary centres of ossification
(c)  Callus formation in fracture healing
(d)  Heterotopic ossification
(e)  Use of demineralised bone matrix
(f)  Bone formation by chondrosarcomas

Intramembranous ossification ('in membranes') does not have a cartilaginous precursor and is responsible for bone growth seen in the development of flat bones, during bone transport and in perichondrial bone formation.

Ref:
Buckwalter J, Einhorn T, Simon S (2000) (2nd ed.) *Orthopaedic Basic Science: Biology and Biomechanics of the Musculoskeletal System*. American Academy of Orthopaedic Surgeons.

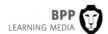
BPP LEARNING MEDIA

**59.** **D**

Isotropic materials are ones where the properties are not influenced by the direction of measurement. When one is considering materials rather than structures, then specimen geometry can be excluded as a factor and one has to essentially consider the directionality of bonding and micro-architecture of the material.

Metals on an atomic scale consist of a sea of electrons isolating positive nuclear cores. Consequently, the atomic bonds are not directional and are very strong. On this scale the material can be thought of as very isotropic. The microscopic structure of metals reveals them to consist of a multitude of grains or crystals which are made evident by the fact that the orientation of the lattice structure within each grain is subtly different to that of its neighbours. However, any directionality of the structure as a whole is eliminated by the fact that there are countless grains whose orientations are in countless different directions. Therefore on a microscopic level, most metals are still considered as isotropic.

Non metal materials are composed of bonds and attractions that are covalent or ionic. Ceramics are principally composed of ionic bonds which are very strong and render a crystalline structure similar to that seen in metals. Consequently, they are also considered to be isotropic. Other non-metal materials may be composed of covalent bonds where certain atoms share electrons. These bonds which can be strong are also highly directional which alters the resistance to different types of force profile. However, when such a material is highly crosslinked, such as the latest generation of polyethylene implants, the properties become independent of direction of measurement.

When bone is considered as a material, the two types have considerably different mechanical properties. Although cortical bone is stronger with a higher modulus of elasticity the directionality of the collagen fibres renders it susceptible to bending and shear type stresses despite being very strong in axial compression. Trabecular bone is composed of interconnecting lamellae in different orientations. Although less dense and less strong than cortical bone, the nature of all the different interconnections gives it comparable resistance to forces in different planes. Thus trabecular bone can be considered as more isotropic than cortical bone.

Ref:

Nordin M, Frankel V (2001) (3rd ed.) *Basic biomechanics of the musculoskeletal system*. Lippincott Williams & Wilkins, Philadelphia.

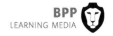

**60.** **E**

It is useful to remember the different groups of antibiotics, their mechanisms of action and examples of each.

| Group | Mechanism | Example |
| --- | --- | --- |
| Cephalosporins | Inhibit cell wall synthesis | Cefuroxime ceftriaxone |
| Carbapenems | Inhibit cell wall synthesis | Imipenem, micropenem |
| Aminoglycosides | Inhibit bacterial protein synthesis Bind to 30s subunit rRNA | Gentamycin, neomycin |
| Macrolides | Inhibit dissociation of peptidyl tRNA from ribosomes during translocation | Erythromycin, clarithromycin |
| Quinolones | Inhibit DNA gyrase | Ciprofloxacin, norfloxacin |
| Glycopeptides | Inhibit cell membrane synthesis | Vancomycin, teicoplanin |
| Tetracyclines | Inhibits bacterial protein synthesis Bind to 30s subunit rRNA | Tetracycline, doxycycline |

Ref:

Ramachandran, M (2007) *Basic Orthhopaedic Sciences: The Stanmore Guide.* Hodder Arnold, London.

**61.** **C**

The biomechanical basis for reverse shoulder arthroplasty in rotator cuff deficient shoulders is that by lowering the centre of rotation and moving it medially, the efficiency of the deltoid lever arm is improved and shear forces on the glenoid are reduced.

Ref:

Buckwalter J, Einhorn T, Simon S (2000) (2nd ed.) *Orthopaedic Basic Science: Biology and Biomechanics of the Musculoskeletal System.* American Academy of Orthopaedic Surgeons.

**62.** **A**

Bisphosphonates are synthetic analogs of inorganic pyrophosphate. However, their most important feature is the presence of a PCP bond which is highly resistant to metabolism by endogenous phosphatases. They are poorly absorbed in the gut especially in the presence of foods rich in calcium and iron. However, once absorbed they are readily taken up by bone where they remain for a long time (half life = 6–11 years). Their chief mode of action is to inhibit the osteoclastic resorption of bone although they also bind to hydroxyapatite crystals and have been shown to inhibit their dissolution invitro.

Ref:

Buckwalter J, Einhorn T, Simon S (2000) (2nd ed.) *Orthopaedic Basic Science: Biology and Biomechanics of the Musculoskeletal System.* American Academy of Orthopaedic Surgeons.

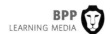

**63.  D**

Magnetic resonance imaging, unlike conventional radiography, is a difficult image modality to explain. There are three essential concepts:

1.  Strong magnetic fields
2.  Excitatory radiofrequency pulses
3.  Relaxation causing emission of radiofrequency signals

The normal magnetic field of the body is equivalent to zero. The water in our bodies is composed of hydrogen nuclei which are in effect protons. These are all spinning on their central axes. There is no net magnetic field as all of these axes are randomly orientated. In addition each of these protons are wobbling as well as rotating on their axes. This wobble is known as precession and like the axes the wobbles are out of sync with each other. The application of a strong magnetic field in the scanner causes all of the long axes of the protons to be aligned with the long axis of the magnet. The precessions are still out of step.

The body is then struck by excitatory radiofrequency pulses. The longitudinal axes of the protons are thrown off course and are now at an angle to the long axis of the magnet. However, the pulse also causes the precessions to pull into step with each other.

As the pulse stops, the protons are drawn back to their original behaviour while under the influence of the magnetic field and this reversion releases a radiofrequency signal based on two aspects:

(a)  Protons realign themselves with the long axis of the magnet. This is known as the longitudinal magnetisation vector. T1 is the time for the longitudinal magnetisation vector to increase up to 63% of its maximal value.
(b)  Protons wobbling ie precessions fall out of step with each other. This is expressed as the transverse magnetisation factor. T2 is the time taken for the transverse magnetisation factor to fall to 37% of its maximum value.

Therefore the appearance on MRI is dictated by three aspects

(a)  Longitudinal relaxation properties
(b)  Transverse relaxation properties
(c)  Proton density

The difference in T1 and T2 weighted sequences is based on altering 2 aspects:

(a)  TR – repetition time between radiofrequency pulses (time to repetition)
(b)  TE – time between application of pulses and recording signal (time to echo)

Ref:
Ramachandran, M (2007) *Basic Orthhopaedic Sciences: The Stanmore Guide*. Hodder Arnold, London.

**64.  D**

Bone densitometry using dual energy X-ray relies on X-rays with 2 different energies which have different attenuation characteristics in bone and soft tissues. Consequently, bone density can be determined by a process analogous to digital subtraction radiography.

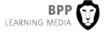

The commonest sites to be assessed are the proximal femur and the lumbar spine although more recent advances have allowed measurements from the forearm and the os calcis.

Ref:
Buckwalter J, Einhorn T, Simon S (2000) (2nd ed.) *Orthopaedic Basic Science: Biology and Biomechanics of the Musculoskeletal System*. American Academy of Orthopaedic Surgeons.

**65. B**

Tuberculosis is most commonly caused by M. tuberculosis although it can also be caused by M Africanum and M Bovis. All of these micro-organisms are mycobacteria which are aerobic acid fast bacilli (rods). They are acid fast because they resist decolourisation with acids after staining with Ziehl Nielsen or carbol-fuschin. They are also aerobic bacteria and growth is related to oxygen tension. This makes the pulmonary bed a very attractive site for growth and this is the most common site. In the skeletal system the most common site of disease is the thoracic spine with abscess formation causing bony and soft tissue destruction. When suitable specimens are obtained culture is usually done in Lowenstein-Jensen medium for at least 6 weeks as it can take some time before visible colonies form. Gross histology of involved tissues shows classical caseating granulomas with central regions of necrosis.

Ref:
Buckwalter J, Einhorn T, Simon S (2000) (2nd ed.) *Orthopaedic Basic Science: Biology and Biomechanics of the Musculoskeletal System*. American Academy of Orthopaedic Surgeons.

**66. C**

A triple phase bone scan involves intravenous administration of a radioactive isotope, most commonly a 99m Technetium – labelled phosphonate complex. Images are taken during three phases to aid diagnosis.

(a) Dynamic flow phase – 1–2 minutes. Images are taken every 2–5 seconds. At this time the radioisotope is found in the blood vessels.
(b) Blood pool phase – 2–5 minutes. This is usually a static scan taken after the flow phase and within 5 minutes of administration. Much of the radioisotope is in the extravascular space.
(c) Static phase – these are usually taken 2–4 hours after injection by which time the radioisotope is cleared from the soft tissues and taken up by the bone. Occasionally a delayed image has to be taken after 24 hours after urinary excretion has cleared accumulated radioisotope from the bladder where it may be obscuring uptake in the pelvis.

Ref:
Buckwalter J, Einhorn T, Simon S (2000) (2nd ed.) *Orthopaedic Basic Science: Biology and Biomechanics of the Musculoskeletal System*. American Academy of Orthopaedic Surgeons.

**67. E**

Hereditary motor sensory neuropathy presenting in early childhood may progress very rapidly resulting in severe foot deformity. The result of intrinsic and extrinsic muscle imbalance requires balancing of the foot musculature in particular during during the growth of the foot. Some of the bony correction can be deferred until the foot is closer to

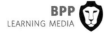

skeletal maturity. Triple fusions are contraindicated in children under the age of 8 and do poorly, since foot size mismatch over 25% is poorly tolerated.

Ref:
Beals TC, Nickisch F. Charcot-Marie-Tooth Disease and the Cavovarus Foot. *Foot Ankle Clin N Am* 2008; 13: 259–274.

**68.  D**

Correction may be achieved with hemivertebral resection. Future progression is of concern and prevention of secondary curves may be avoided.

Convex hemiepiphyseodesis is best suited for patients young who present with a fully segmented hemivertebrae. Hemiepiphyseodesis and posterior fusion are not indicated.

Ref:
Bradford DS, Boachie-Adjei O. One-stage anterior and posterior hemivertibral resection and arthrodesis for congenital scoliosis. *J Bone Joint Surg [Am]* 1990; 72: 536–540.

**69.  C**

Ref:
The Ponseti IV *et al*. The Ponseti technique for correction of congenital clubfoot. *J Bone Joint Surg [Am]* 2002; 84: 1889–1890.

**70.  B**

Acute hematogenous osteomyelitis signs and symptoms vary but include fever, bone pain, and impaired use of the involved extremity. The child may refuse to use the arm. Examination often reveals bone tenderness. In more advanced cases, erythema, warmth, and swelling may be present. If presentation is early, before a subperiosteal collection has formed, antibiotics alone may be adequate to treat the infection.

This child has a more advanced infection. When an abscess is present, surgical drainage is generally indicated to remove devitalised tissue and to enhance the efficacy of the antibiotics. Bone scans cause delay and are not necessary.

Ref:
1.  Scott RJ, Christofersen MR, Robertson WW Jr *et al*. Acute osteomyelitis in children: A review of 116 cases. *J Pediatr Orthop* 1990; 10: 649–652.
2.  Vaughan PA, Newman NM, Rosman MA. Acute hematogenous osteomyelitis. *J Pediatr Orthop* 1987; 7: 652–655.

**71.  E**

Shoe wear modification is the most appropriate management based on the patient's age, activity level and minor symptoms. She also has a mild hallux valgus.

Normal radiographic measurements are IM angle of < 9 degrees, a HVA < 15 degrees, and a distal DMAA < 9 degrees.

Surgical procedures should be reserved for older patients with more severe or progressive deformities. Recurrence in this age group is approximately 30%.

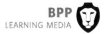

Ref:
1. Myerson MS. Surgery of the Foot and Ankle.
2. Mann RA, Rudicel S, Graves SC. Repair of hallux valgus with a distal soft-tissue procedure and proximal metatarsal osteotomy. A long-term follow-up. *J Bone Joint Surg [Am]* 1992; 74: 124–129.

**72. B**

Granulation tissue, has been noted between the columns in the zone of hypertrophy, leading to the theory of microtrauma as an aetiology in non renal SCFE. SCFE in patients with renal disease slippage tends to occur through the metaphyseal spongiosa.

Ref:

Miller MD (2008) *Review of Orthopaedics*. Saunders Elsevier, Philadelphia.

**73. B**

Neurological deficit does not constitute as one of the diagnostic criteria although it may be associated with some of the spinal deformities in neurofibromatosis (NF-1).

The diagnostic criteria for NF-1 were established by The Consensus Development Conference on Neurofibromatosis at the National Institutes of Health in 1987.

1. Six or more café au lait spots, at least 15mm in diameter in adults and 5mm in children.
2. Two or more neurofibromas of any type or one plexiform neurofibroma.
3. Freckling in the axillae or inguinal regions (Crowe sign).
4. Two or more iris hamartomas (Lisch nodules).
5. A distinctive osseous lesion, such as sphenoid dysplasia or thinning of long bone cortex, with or without pseudarthrosis.
6. A first-degree relative with NF-1 by the above criteria.

Ref:

Riccardi VM. (1992) (2nd ed.) *Neurofibromatosis; phenotype, natural history and pathogenesis.* The Johns Hopkins University Press.

**74. E**

It is the 'push me, pull you' relationship of weak dorsiflexion power of the tibialis anterior muscle and the strongly plantar-flexing peroneus longus acting on the medial midfoot that is felt to be the primary driver of the cavus deformity once the intrinsic musculature is dysfunctional. Hence, a forefoot driven hindfoot varus which develops to counter the forefoot plantar flexed first ray. This is pronounced as the intrinsics further weaken and the plantar fascia further contracts

Ref:

Aminian A, Sangeorzan B. The Anatomy of Cavus Foot Deformity. *Foot Ankle Clin N Am 2008*; 13: 191–198.

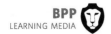

75. **E**
    Ref:
    Miller MD (2008) *Review of Orthopaedics*. Saunders Elsevier, Philadelphia.

76. **B**
    Cervical instability is not a feature of Klippel-Feil syndrome.

    Ref:
    Miller MD (2008) *Review of Orthopaedics*. Saunders Elsevier, Philadelphia.

77. **D**
    The zone of provisional calcification is affected in rickets. There is a deficiency of calcium and/or parathyroid hormone leading to abnormal calcification of the matrix.

    Ref:
    Miller MD (2008) *Review of Orthopaedics*. Saunders Elsevier, Philadelphia.

78. **E**
    Bacteria settle in the slow moving, poorly oxygenated blood in the terminal branches of the metaphyseal arteries area of the primary spongiosa.

    Ref:
    Miller MD (2008) *Review of Orthopaedics*. Saunders Elsevier, Philadelphia.

79. **D**
    Duchenne Muscular Dystrophy (DMD) is the most common and most severe muscular dystrophy of childhood. It is an X-linked recessive disorder and is progressive resulting in respiratory or cardiac failure and death in the early twenties. At present there is no cure. The diagnosis is made by the absence of the protein dystrophin on immunohistochemical analysis by immunoperoxidase staining of a muscle biopsy. Family counselling and prenatal diagnosis of DMD is advised.

    Ref:
    Jay V, Vajsar J. The Dystrophy of Duchenne. *Lancet* 2001; 357: 550–552.

80. **A**
    The Milch classification for lateral condylar fractures of the distal humerus I children:

    Type I: Fracture through the ossification center of the capitellum, lateral to the capitello-trochlear groove, Salter-Harris type 4 injury. The elbow is usually stable and the relationship between the forearm and the humerus remains intact.

    Type 2: The most common type of injury. Fractures through the capitello-trochlear groove, Salter-Harris type 2 injury. Unstable. Peak incidence is at age 6 years.

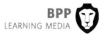

Treatment : Undisplaced: controversial. Some authors advocate operative fixation, others suggest cast immobilisation and weekly radiographs with reduction and fixation if there is subsequent loss of position. Displacement – manipulation under anaesthesia (flexion and pronation) and percutaneous wires or open reduction and internal fixation through a lateral approach as appropriate.

Ref:
Brinker M (2001) *Review of Orthopaedic Trauma*. Saunders, Philadelphia.

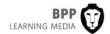

BPP
LEARNING MEDIA

# MCQ Paper 2

## Question Bank

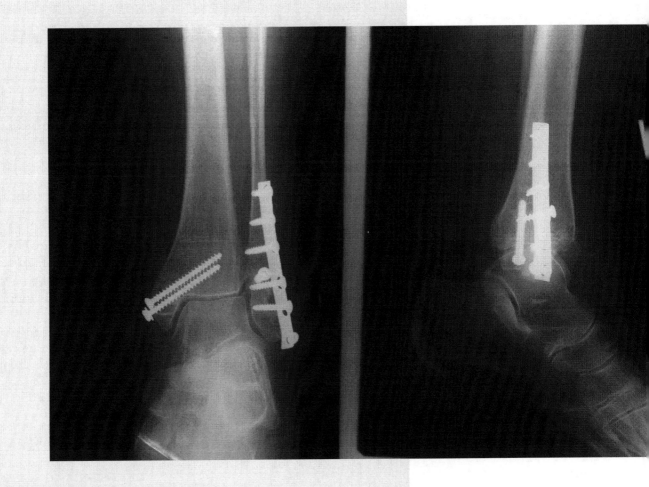

1.  The obturator oblique view of the acetabulum provides information on which of the following?
    A.  Anterior column and anterior wall
    B.  Posterior column and posterior wall
    C.  Anterior wall and posterior column
    D.  Posterior wall and anterior column
    E.  Anterior wall and posterior wall

2.  The following statement accurately describes a Type III fracture of the femoral head based on the Pipkin classification:
    A.  Femoral head fracture cephalad to the fovea
    B.  Femoral head fracture caudad to the fovea
    C.  Femoral head fracture caudad to the fovea and minor acetabular rim fracture
    D.  Femoral head fracture cephalad to the fovea and minor acetabular rim fracture
    E.  Femoral head fracture with femoral neck fracture

3.  The following statements are **true** for the use of anterior approach in treatment of femoral head fracture in a posterior dislocation of the hip, except:
    A.  It allows direct visualisation of the femoral head fragment
    B.  Re-dislocation and external rotation of the hip allows for cleaning of the fracture bed
    C.  There is no increase in the incidence of avascular necrosis of the femoral head
    D.  There is an increase in the rate of heterotrophic ossification
    E.  There is concern of damaging the vascular supply to the femoral head

4.  All of the following statements are **true** with respect to a greater tuberosity fracture following an anterior dislocation of the humerus, except:
    A.  It is associated with 10–15% of anterior dislocation of humerus
    B.  Malunion results in limited motion and / or pain.
    C.  The anterior rotator cuff bony insertion is avulsed
    D.  Closed reduction usually reduces the greater tuberosity to an acceptable position following dislocation
    E.  <5cm of displacement of the greater tuberosity can acceptably be treated conservatively

5.  The following is **true** regarding four part proximal humeral fractures:
    A.  The articular segment is isolated from the greater tuberosity and the humeral shaft
    B.  The articular segment typically dislocates posteriorly while the shaft lies laterally
    C.  Most cases requires open reduction and internal fixation as the treatment of choice
    D.  Valgus impacted four part fracture have good results with both percutaneous pinning technique and open reduction
    E.  Open reduction internal fixation have good outcome due to low incidence of osteonecrosis and post-traumatic arthritis

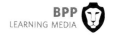

6.  The following statements are **true** regarding Type II (diaphyseal) peri-prosthethic fractures around the elbow, except:
    A.  Can occur intra-operatively or are associated with trauma
    B.  Most commonly associated with well fixed implants
    C.  The fracture requires stabilisation despite the type of implant (linked or unlinked)
    D.  Cerclage wires and strut grafts are the most reliable methods in the management of these fractures
    E.  Revision surgery with longer prosthesis is considered for loose implants

7.  Wright & Cofield Type A periprosthethic fracture around the proximal humerus prosthesis is pertinently described by which of the following statements:
    A.  Fracture around the proximal prosthesis
    B.  Fracture around the tip of the prosthesis and extending proximally
    C.  Fracture distal to the tip of the prosthesis
    D.  Fracture around the tip of the prosthesis and extending distally
    E.  Fracture at the tip of the prosthesis without extension

8.  The following periprosthethic humeral fractures are amenable to non-operative treatment:
    A.  Displaced fracture around a loose prosthesis
    B.  Undisplaced fracture through an osteolytic area
    C.  Fracture distal to the tip of the prosthesis
    D.  Fracture through bone and cement limiting the area of bone contact
    E.  Transverse displaced fracture at the tip of prosthesis

9.  Based on Vancouver classification for post-operative periprosthethic fractures, a comminuted fracture involving the tip of the femoral stem is classified as:
    A.  Type A fracture
    B.  Type B1 fracture
    C.  Type B2 fracture
    D.  Type B3 fracture
    E.  Type C fracture

10. The following technical details should be observed with in use of strut graft in treatment of Type B1 periprosthetic fracture of femoral stem:
    A.  Up to four cables/wires should be used for stable fixation
    B.  Preferred placement of the strut graft is antero-medial on femoral shaft
    C.  Soft tissue dissection and elevation of muscular attachment from the posterior femur allows greater access to the fracture
    D.  Morsellised bone graft applied at graft-host junction allow healing
    E.  All of the above

11. An intra-operative periprosthetic fracture adjacent to the stem of a well fixed tibial tray in total knee replacement is classified as:
    A.  Type 1 A fracture
    B.  Type 2 C fracture
    C.  Type 3 B fracture
    D.  Type 3 C fracture
    E.  Type 4 A Fracture

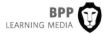

12. A Vancouver Type B2 periprosthetic fracture noted intra-operatively is best treated with:
    A. Bone graft
    B. Cerclage wire
    C. Longer stem implant bypassing the fracture
    D. Longer stem implant & Cerclage wire
    E. Bone graft & cortical strut graft

13. The most suitable treatment option for a Type C Vancouver postoperative periprosthetic fracture is:
    A. Symptomatic treatment unless involvement of substantial medial cortex
    B. Cerclage wires, cortical strut grafts and plates
    C. Revision to long stem
    D. Revision and augmentation with allograft
    E. Primary fracture fixation

14. The highest rate of dural tear is seen after which one of the following procedures?
    A. Lumbar discectomy
    B. Lumbar decompression
    C. Revision lumbar discectomy
    D. Lumbar decompression and instrumented fusion
    E. Anterior cervical discectomy and fusion

15. The acute management of a patient with a cervical spinal cord injury includes all of the following except:
    A. Maintenance of perfusion systolic pressure >90mmHg
    B. Administering 100% $O_2$
    C. Immobilisation of spine
    D. MRI scan
    E. Flexion/extension radiographs

16. Atlantoaxial instability is associated with which one of the following conditions?
    A. Arthrogryphosis
    B. Achondroplasia
    C. Morquio syndrome
    D. Turner syndrome
    E. Ostepetrosis

17. A 73-year-old man presents with symptoms of left leg pain made worse by walking and eased by resting. On examination he is found to have an ataxic gait and a positive Hoffmann's reflex. MRI scan of the lumbar spine shows central and left L4/5 lateral recess stenosis. The most appropriate next step in management is:
    A. Left L4/5 root canal steroid injection
    B. Epidural steroid injection
    C. Cervical spine MRI scan
    D. L4/5 undercutting facetectomy
    E. L4/5 decompression and fusion

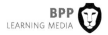

18. A 38-year-old lady presents with severe mid axial neck pain of 2 weeks' duration. The pain radiates down to the left shoulder. She has associated neck spasm and headaches and has been on non-narcotic analgesics with little improvement in her symptoms. There are no red flags in the history. On examination cervical spine movements are painful especially extension and reduced to half normal, but there is no neurological deficit. The most appropriate next step in management is:
    A. Continue oral analgesics and refer for physiotherapy
    B. MRI scan
    C. Flexion/extension radiographs
    D. Epidural steroid injection
    E. Plain radiographs of cervical spine

19. What percentage of slipped upper femoral epiphyses are bilateral and what percentage present with simultaneous involvement?
    A. 10% bilateral        0% simultaneous presentation
    B. 25% bilateral        50% simultaneous presentation
    C. 25% bilateral        100% simultaneous presentation
    D. 50% bilateral        50% simultaneous presentation
    E. 50% bilateral        100% simultaneous presentation

20. Which of the following conditions is not associated with slipped upper femoral epiphysis?
    A. Renal osteodystrophy
    B. Juvenile rheumatoid arthritis
    C. Hypogonadism
    D. Obesity
    E. Hypopituitarism

21. Which of the following statements regarding botulinum toxin and its use in cerebral palsy is **false**?
    A. The toxin is produced by anaerobic bacterium
    B. The mechanism of action is blockade of the release of acetylcholine at the neuromuscular junction
    C. The onset of action takes 12 hours with the effect typically lasting two to three months
    D. Treatment by injection is best directed at dynamic deformities in the absence of fixed contractures
    E. The weakness in the muscle resolves as the neuromuscular junction sprouts new nerve endings

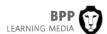

22. Which of the following statements regarding hip subluxation or dislocation in cerebral palsy is **true**?
    A. The risk of dislocation is higher in hemiplegia compared with total body involvement
    B. The risk of dislocation is lower in ambulatory patients compared with non-ambulatory patients
    C. Quadriplegic patients do not require follow up after 6 years of age if radiographs at this time show both hips to be reduced
    D. Hip dislocation does not arise from laxity
    E. A migration index of greater than 60% is associated with eventual dislocation

23. Which of the following statements is **false** regarding Type I Scheurmann's disease?
    A. The condition is more common in males and usually presents in adolescence
    B. There may be associated pectus carinatum
    C. The deformity may be flexible or rigid
    D. There is associated hamstring tightness
    E. Neurological involvement is rare

24. The following are all associated with less successful outcomes after knee arthrodesis, except:
    A. Tumour resection
    B. Previous deep implant infection
    C. Massive bone loss
    D. A larger number of procedures prior to arthrodesis
    E. The use of constrained knee implants

25. Degenerate valgus deformity of the knee is best treated with:
    A. Varus high tibial osteotomy
    B. Distal femoral varus osteotomy
    C. Coventry high tibial osteotomy
    D. Valgus high tibial osteotomy
    E. Proximal femoral varus osteotomy

26. Valgus knee deformities are positively associated with all of the following, except:
    A. Trauma
    B. Rheumatoid arthritis
    C. Renal osteodystrophy
    D. Infantile poliomyelitis
    E. Syphilis

27. Regarding rupture of the quadriceps tendon:
    A. It is most common in the 30–40 years age group:
    B. Partial tears can be treated non operatively
    C. Requires ultrasound to confirm diagnosis
    D. Has equal incidence in males and females
    E. Is confirmed by the absence of a straight leg raise in the supine patient

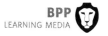

28. The following are all **true** regarding a discoid meniscus, except:
    A. They occur in up to 5% of the population
    B. Usually involve the lateral meniscus
    C. Are rarely bilateral
    D. Normally present with symptoms of 'popping'
    E. Can be treated nonoperatively in the absence of pain or swelling

29. With regards to osteoarthritic related changes in articular cartilage, the following statement is **false**:
    A. Increased water content
    B. Reduced proteoglycan content
    C. Increased modulus of elasticity
    D. Increased chondroitin 4 sulphate concentration
    E. Increased proteoglycan synthesis

30. Which of the statements is **true** regarding the mechanical characteristics of IM nails?
    A. Tortional rigidity depends only on the shear modulus
    B. Bending rigidity is related to the third power of the nail's radius
    C. Increasing the nail diameter by 10% increases bending rigidity by 50%
    D. Tortional rigidity depends only on polar moment of inertia
    E. The greatest mechanical advantage of closed section IM nails over slotted nails is decreased tortional stiffness

31. Arthrodesis of the ankle should be performed in:
    A. 5–10 degrees of internal rotation, neutral dorsiflexion, 5 degrees of hindfoot valgus
    B. Neutral dorsiflexion, 5 degrees of hindfoot valgus, 5–10 degrees of external rotation
    C. 5–10 degrees of dorsiflexion, 5–10 degrees internal rotation and 5 degrees of hindfoot varus
    D. Neutral dorsiflexion, 5 degrees of external rotation and 5 degrees of hindfoot varus
    E. 5–10 degrees of external rotation, 5 degrees of hindfoot varus and 5–10 degrees of plantar flexion

32. Regarding screws:
    A. Lead is distance between threads
    B. Pitch is the distance advanced in one revolution
    C. To maximise pull out strength, the screw should have a small outer diameter and large root diameter
    D. To maximise pull out strength, the screw should have a large outer diameter and a small root diameter
    E. Pull out strength of a screw is not related to the pitch

33. Regarding hip arthrodesis, which of the following statements is **false**?
    A. Position of hip arthrodesis should be in 25 degrees of flexion and 15–20 degrees of abduction.
    B. Hip arthrodesis increases oxygen consumption
    C. Hip arthrodesis increases transpelvic rotation of the contralateral hip
    D. Hip arthrodesis decreases gait efficiency
    E. Position of hip arhrodesis should be in 30 degrees of flexion, no abduction and no rotation.

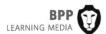

34. Which of the following statements regarding ACL reconstruction is **true**?
    A. Right knee femoral tunnel placement should be in the 1 o'clock position
    B. Bone patella bone grafts results are inferior to Hamstring tendon grafts
    C. Ultimate tensile strength of the untorn anterior cruciate ligament is greater than 1800 Newtons
    D. Tibial tunnel placement should be in the anterior half of the Blumensaat's line
    E. ACL reconstruction reduces the risk of degenerative changes in the knee

35. A requirement for high tibial osteotomy for varus knee osteoarthritis is:
    A. lateral compartment involvement
    B. Preoperative range of motion greater than 90 degrees
    C. Inflammatory arthritis
    D. instability of the knee
    E. Medial tibial subluxation

36. A 25-year-old patient undergoing arthroscopy is found to have a buck-handle tear of the peripheral third of the anterior horn and body of the lateral meniscus. Management should consist of:
    A. Meniscal trephination
    B. Meniscal repair
    C. Partial meniscectomy
    D. Total meniscectomy
    E. Resecting the anterior horn and repairing the body

37. Polymer chain cross-links may be increased in ultra-high molecular weight polyethylene bearing surfaces by:
    A. Heat annealing
    B. Smelting
    C. High-pressure molding
    D. Gamma irradiation in vacuum
    E. Ethylene oxidisation

38. One of the commonest pathogens in post surgical site infection following total knee replacement is:
    A. E Coli
    B. Coagulase negative staphylococci
    C. Enterococcus
    D. Streptococcus
    E. Klebsiella

39. The principal collagen in knee menisci is:
    A. Type I
    B. Type II
    C. Type III
    D. Type IV
    E. Type V

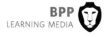

40. Which of the following factors can help reduce the rate of dislocation following the posterior approach?
    A. Using a long femoral neck
    B. Performing a formal posterior soft tissue repair during closure
    C. Inserting the acetabular component in 0–10 degrees anteversion
    D. Medialising the acetabular component
    E. Using a smaller femoral head

41. Which of the following factors is important for successful osseointegration of a hydroxyapatite coated porous stem?
    A. No gap between prosthesis and bone
    B. Micromotion of >500$\mu$m of implant
    C. Pore size 100–400$\mu$m
    D. Proximal hydroxyapatite coating only
    E. Presence of a femoral collar

42. Which of the following occur when using large metal on metal bearing surfaces for total hip arthroplasty compared to standard metal on polyethylene?
    A. Smaller number of wear particles
    B. Larger size of wear particles
    C. Increased volumetric wear
    D. Lower number of cobalt ions in urine
    E. Fluid film lubrication

43. Reducing the rate of dislocation due to impingement of the components in total hip arthroplasty can be achieved by which of the following?
    A. Using an elevated rim liner
    B. Using lateral approach
    C. Increasing head-neck ratio
    D. Increasing femoral offset
    E. Using smaller femoral head

44. In patients undergoing total hip arthroplasty with a high hip dislocation placing the hip in a high hip centre compared to a normal hip centre results in which of the following?
    A. Increased aseptic loosening
    B. Increased risk of sciatic nerve palsy
    C. Reduced risk of dislocation
    D. Use of larger acetabular component
    E. Lower risk of impingement

45. In hand re-plantation surgery, which statement is **false**?
    A. Surgery is contraindicated if cold ischaemia time is greater than 24 hours
    B. Surgery is contraindicated if warm ischaemia time is greater than 12 hours
    C. Survival results are around 80% in adults and 70% in children
    D. Caffeine-free diet post-operatively
    E. Continuous temperature monitoring of replants post op is not common

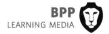

46. In differentiating pronator syndrome from carpal tunnel syndrome, which statement is **false**?
    A. The two conditions are commonly confused
    B. Nocturnal symptoms are more commonly seen in pronator syndrome than carpal tunnel syndrome
    C. Electromyography studies are not usually helpful in pronator syndrome
    D. Thenar atrophy is more commonly seen in carpal tunnel syndrome
    E. Muscle fatigue is more commonly seen in pronator syndrome
    F. Medial hypohidrosis is more commonly seen in carpal tunnel syndrome

47. The initial management of de Quervain's disease is:
    A. Aggressive physiotherapy
    B. Surgical decompression of the first dorsal compartment
    C. Activity modification, steroid injection and splinting
    D. Release of extensor pollicis longus
    E. Steroid injection of second dorsal compartment followed by splinting

48. Horner's syndrome is characterised by all these except:
    A. Meiosis
    B. Enophthalmos
    C. Diplopia
    D. Ptosis
    E. Exophthalmos

49. The principal nerve which supplies the wrist joint is:
    A. Palmar cutaneous branch of median nerve
    B. Posterior interosseous nerve
    C. Lateral antebrachial nerve
    D. Anterior interosseous nerve
    E. Recurrent motor branch of median nerve

50. The anterior interosseous nerve, a branch of the median nerve, originates at:
    A. 5cm distal to medial epicondyle
    B. 5cm proximal to medial epicondyle
    C. 10cm distal to medial epicondyle
    D. At level of medial epicondyle
    E. Has an extremely variable origin

51. Operative indications for Dupuytren's include:
    A. Painful cord
    B. Dupuytrens diathesis
    C. Proximal interphalangeal joint contracture of >30 degrees
    D. Bilateral disease
    E. Metacarpophalangeal joint contracture of 15 degrees

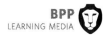

52. Which of the pulleys are most important in preventing tendon bowstringing?
    A. A1 and A3
    B. A2 and A3
    C. A2 and A4
    D. A3 and A4
    E. A2 and A5


53. Which of the following tests describe an Intrinsic-Plus deformity?
    A. PIPJ cannot be flexed with the MCPJ held in extension
    B. PIPJ cannot be flexed with the MCPJ held in flexion
    C. MCPJ flexion causes extension of the PIP
    D. MCPJ extension causes flexion of the PIPJ
    E. None of the above


54. All of the following statements are **true** for the interossei of the hand except:
    A. It includes 4 dorsal interossei muscles that abduct the index, middle and ring finger
    B. It includes 3 dorsal interossei muscles that adduct index, middle and ring finger
    C. All interossei allow effective flexion of MCPJ
    D. All interossei are innervated by the deep branch of ulnar nerve
    E. All interossei pass volar to the axis of MCPJ


55. All of the following statements are **true** about the triangular fibro cartilage in the wrist except:
    A. This forms the load bearing area of the triangular fibro cartilage cmplex allowing transmission of compressive forces between carpus and ulna
    B. The blood supply to TFC is from the volar and the dorsal branches of the anterior interosseous artery
    C. The thickness of TFC varies from 2mm to 5mm and this is directly proportional to the ulnar variance
    D. It attaches to the distal radius at the sigmoid notch and runs to the fovea at the base of the ulnar styloid
    E. Volar and dorsal radioulnar ligaments are associated with tri-fibrocartilage and stabilise the distal radioulnar joint


56. The following statements are **true** with respect to the mobility at the carpus bones except:
    A. 50% of movement occur within the proximal row
    B. Distal row is fixed
    C. Scaphoid acts as a link between the two rows
    D. The midcarpal joint is spanned by extrinsic ligaments
    E. Extensive excursion occurs due to variable geometry of proximal row

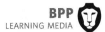

57. In Kienbock's disease, the treatment for the stage of collapse is:
    A. Splinting and rest
    B. Joint levelling procedure
    C. Scaphotrapezial – trapezoid fusion
    D. Proximal row carpectomy
    E. Wrist fusion

58. At the finger tips, the normal value of two point discrimination is:
    A. 5–6mm
    B. 2–3mm
    C. 9–10mm
    D. 3–4mm
    E. 7–8mm

59. Which of the following statements is **false** in Wartenberg's syndrome?
    A. It is a compressive neuropathy
    B. The clinical test includes forceful forearm pronation
    C. There may be a positive Tinel's sign
    D. Surgical decompression is warranted early for good outcome
    E. Involves the sensory branch of the radial nerve only

60. Which of the following statements regarding tendons is **false**?
    A. Paratenon covered tendons heal better than other tendons
    B. Type III collagen constitutes less than 10%
    C. Fibrocartilage is found within the enthesis
    D. The stress strain curve for tendon has a characteristic concave toe region
    E. An increasing strain rate leads to a decrease in the modulus of elasticity

61. In which layer of healthy articular cartilage is type X collagen most commonly found?
    A. Superficial zone
    B. Middle zone
    C. Deep zone
    D. Calcified zone
    E. Subchondral bone

62. Which of the following is not a proteoglycan?
    A. Aggrecan
    B. Decorin
    C. Superficial zone protein
    D. Keratan sulphate
    E. Fibromodulin

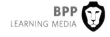

63. Which of the following statements regarding aggrecan structure is **false**?
    A. Aggrecans are a diverse population of proteoglycans
    B. The protein core attaches to a hyaluronate molecule via a specific binding domain
    C. The link protein stabilises the attachment of individual glycosaminoglycan chains to the protein core
    D. The ratio of chondroitin sulphate to keratin sulphate decreases with age
    E. The ratio of chondroitin sulphate 4 to chondroitin sulphate 6 decreases with age

64. Which of the following is not a biomechanical property of articular cartilage?
    A. Stress relaxation
    B. Anisotropicity
    C. Decreased stiffness due to a compressive load
    D. Elastohydrodynamic lubrication
    E. Boundary lubrication

65. Which of the following types of lubrication describes the theorised phenomenon of articular cartilage loading causing the formation of a concentrated gel of lubricating molecules between the two articular surfaces?
    A. Hydrodynamic
    B. Boundary
    C. Squeeze film
    D. Weeping
    E. Boosted

66. In skeletal muscle, how many subunits are there in the troponin protein?
    A. 2
    B. 3
    C. 4
    D. 5
    E. 8

67. Which of the following is not a characteristic of Type I muscle fibres?
    A. Slow speed of contraction
    B. High anaerobic capacity
    C. Small motor unit size
    D. Fatigue resistant
    E. Slow speed of contraction

68. In circular frame external fixators, which of the below measures does not improve stiffness of the bone-fixator construct?
    A. Larger wire diameter
    B. Use of olive wires
    C. Increased distance between adjacent rings
    D. Placing wires at 90 degrees to each other
    E. Adopting eccentricity of the bone within the frame

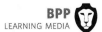

69.  Regarding hip joint sagittal kinetics and kinematics, which of the below statements best describes the events in the gait cycle from heel strike to foot flat?
A.  The hip is flexed 25–30 degrees; the ground reaction force is anterior to the hip joint
B.  The hip is flexed 25–30 degrees; the ground reaction force is posterior to the hip joint
C.  The hip passes from flexion to 15 degrees extension, the ground reaction force is anterior to the joint
D.  The hip passes from flexion to 15 degrees extension; the ground reaction force is posterior to the joint
E.  The hip passes from flexion to 15 degrees extension, the ground reaction force passes from anterior to posterior to the hip joint

70.  The following approach is through a true internervous plane:
A.  Anterolateral: Watson-Jones
B.  Lateral: Hardinge
C.  Posterior: Moore/Southern
D.  Anterior: Smith-Petersen
E.  Medial: Ludloff

71.  Which of the following statements is **true** regarding osteogenesis imperfecta (OI)?
A.  It is a disorder of collagen Type II
B.  The most common type of osteogenesis imperfecta is Type 3
C.  Bisphosphonates are administered to increase bone mass and reduce the incidence of fracture
D.  The gene responsible is COL1A3
E.  Radiographs demonstrate thickened cortices with generalised osteopenia

72.  Which feature indicates the likelihood of curve progression in adolescent idiopathic scoliosis?
A.  Risser sign 1
B.  A lumbar curve
C.  Male gender
D.  Risser sign 5
E.  Concomitant Marfan's syndrome

73.  Regarding supracondylar fractures of the humerus in children, the following statement is **true**:
A.  Peak incidence occurs in those over 11 years of age
B.  Posterior intraosseous nerve (PIN) is commonly injured
C.  Interphalangeal joint of the thumb and the distal interphalangeal joint of the little finger are weak following nerve injury
D.  The Gartland Classification is based on the degree of fracture displacement
E.  Injury is suspected radiographically if the posterior humeral line does not bisect the capitellum

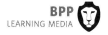

74. A triangular ossification defect in the inferomedial femoral neck is seen commonly in:
    A. Congenital coxa vara
    B. Slipped upper femoral epiphysis
    C. Osteomyelitis of the hip
    D. Transient synovitis
    E. Legg-Calve–Perthes' disease

75. Clinical features of achondroplasia include the following except:
    A. Inability to approximate extended middle and ring fingers
    B. Bilateral leg pain
    C. Rhizomelic dwarfism
    D. Genu varum
    E. Short trunk

76. A 2-year-old child with in-toeing gait and internal rotation of feet with patella facing forwards is most likely due to:
    A. Tibial torsion
    B. Down syndrome
    C. Coxa plana
    D. Coxa vara
    E. Femoral anteversion

77. Which of the following statements is **false**?
    A. Developmental dysplasia of the hip (DDH) is commonly seen in females
    B. Slipped upper femoral epiphysis (SCFE) is seen commonly in Caucasian children
    C. Forefoot adductus is a component of clubfoot
    D. Radiographs are helpful in children over 3 months old with developmental dysplasia of the hip
    E. Kohler's disease involves the navicular bone

78. Improved prognosis in obstetric brachial plexus injury includes the return of biceps function within:
    A. 9 months
    B. 12 months
    C. 3 months
    D. 18 months
    E. 24 months

79. The alignment of a 2-year-old child's knee would normally show:
    A. Varus of 20 degrees
    B. Varus of 10 degrees
    C. Neutral alignment
    D. Valgus of 5 degrees
    E. Valgus of more than 20 degrees

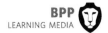

BPP
LEARNING MEDIA

# MCQ Paper 2

## Answers

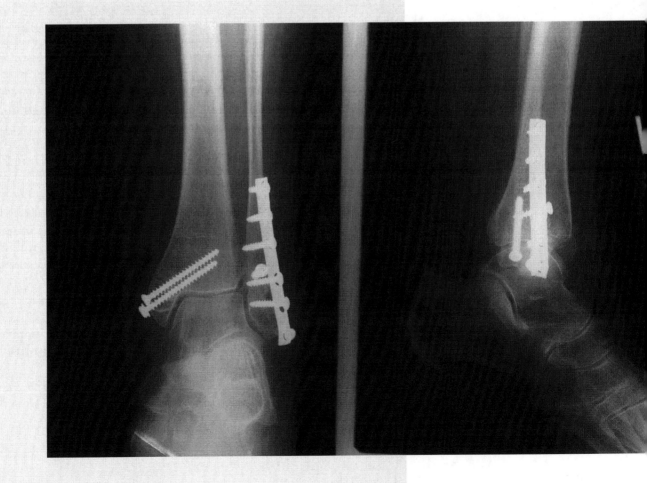

1. **D**

   The obturator oblique view is obtained with pelvis rotated 45 degrees with the injured side up. The anterior column and posterior wall is well visualised with this view along with the obturator foramen and ischial ramus.

   Ref:
   Reilly MC. Fractures of the Acetabulum. In Rockwood & Wilkins. *Fracture in Adults* (6th ed) (2006) Lippincott Williams & Wilkins, Philadelphia.

2. **E**

   The femoral head fractures have been classified by Pipkin into four types. This classification is commonly used and is important in decision making in the management of femoral head fractures.

   Type 1 – Posterior dislocation of head with femoral head fracture caudad to the fovea
   Type 2 – Posterior dislocation of head with femoral head fracture cephalad to the fovea
   Type 3 – Femoral head fracture with associated femoral neck fracture
   Type 4 – Any of the above type with associated acetabular fracture.

   Ref:
   1. Pipkin G. Treatment of grade IV fracture dislocation of the hip. *JBJS Am*. 1957; 39: 1027–1042.
   2. Reilly MC. Fractures of the Acetabulum. In Rockwood & Wilkins. *Fracture in Adults* (6th ed) (2006) Lippincott Williams & Wilkins, Philadelphia.

3. **B**

   The approach for a posterior fracture dislocation of the hip is an issue that is highly debated. As the fracture of the femoral head is caused by impinging on the posterior wall of the acetabulum in an internally rotated position, the fracture fragment is anteromedial. Hence, use of posterior approach through an already damaged capsule does not provide with enough access to the fracture fragment. The posterior approach also demands for re-dislocation of the head for fixation of anteromedial fragment.

   An anterior approach allows for direct visualisation and fixation of anteromedial fragment without re-dislocation of the hip. The fracture bed can be cleaned by mere external rotation of the hip and this also allows for anatomical reduction of the fracture. There has been no increased incidence of avascular necrosis with the anterior approach in comparison to the posterior. There is however higher incidence of heterotrophic ossification with anterior approach compared to the posterior. Also there is concern raised towards disruption of the anterior blood supply due to approach as the main posterior blood supply has been disrupted due to the dislocation.

   Ref:
   1. Swiontkowski MF, Thorpe M, Seller JG *et al*. Operative management of displaced femoral head fractures, case match comparison of anterior versus posterior approaches for Pipkin I & II fractures. *J Orthop Trauma* 1992; 6: 437–442.
   2. Reilly MC. Fractures of the Acetabulum. In Rockwood & Wilkins. *Fracture in Adults* (6th ed) (2006) Lippincott Williams & Wilkins, Philadelphia.

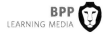

4.  **C**

    Isolated greater tuberosity fracture of the humerus is not uncommon. 7–15% of these fractures are associated with anterior dislocation of the shoulder. With anterior dislocation, the posterior rotator cuff bony attachment is avulsed in this type of fracture. Malunion of untreated grater tuberosity fracture results in limited motion and / or pain. Closed reduction adequately reduces the fracture of the greater tuberosity as the remaining attachment of the rotator cuff tethers the fragment back to its bed, however extra care must be taken to identify a minimally displaced anatomical or surgical neck fracture as this gets displaced following closed reduction invariably then requiring open reduction. Less than 5mm of displacement is generally used as a criterion for conservative management.

    Ref:
    1.  Green A, Izzi JJ. Isolated fractures of greater tuberosity of the proximal humerus. *J Shoulder Elbow Surg* 2003; 12(6): 641–649.
    2.  Warnar JJP, Costouros JG, Gerber C. Fractures of the proximal humerus. In Rockwood & Wilkins. *Fracture in Adults* (6th ed) (2006) Lippincott Williams & Wilkins, Philadelphia.

5.  **D**

    By definition, a 4-part fracture has the articular segment isolated from both the tuberosities and the humeral shaft. A typical pattern is when the articular fragment dislocates anteriorly in the axillary pouch and the shaft lies laterally. Open reduction internal fixation leads to poor outcome as a result of loss of fixation, osteonecrosis, post traumatic arthritis and stiffness. However, the valgus impacted 4 part fracture have good outcomes both with percutaneous pinning and open reduction due to preservation of medial soft tissue hinge, leading to preserved blood supply to the articular segment.

    Ref:
    1.  Gerber C, Hersche O, Berberat C. The clinical relevance of post traumatic avascular necrosis of the humeral head. *J Shoulder Elbow Surgery* 1998; 7: 586–590.
    2.  Gerber C, Werner CM, Vienne P. Internal fixation of complex fractures of proximal humerus. *JBJS Br* 2004; 86(6): 848–855.
    3.  Warnar JJP, Costouros JG, Gerber C. Fractures of the proximal humerus. In Rockwood & Wilkins. *Fracture in Adults* (6th ed) (2006) Lippincott Williams & Wilkins, Philadelphia.

6.  **B**

    The diaphyseal peri-prosthetic fracture of the humeral shaft commonly occurs following trauma, but can occur intra-operatively in a revision procedure. Most commonly the post-operative fractures occur around a loose implant, this is determined as subtype B fractures. A diaphyseal fracture irrespective to the type of implant used requires stabilisation and with a loose implant requires implant revision with a longer implant. In presence of good quality bone, Cerclage wire and cortical strut graft is the most reliable means of achieving stabilisation.

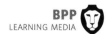

Ref:
1.  Kamineni S, Morrey BF. Proximal ulnar reconstruction with strut allograft in revision total elbow arthroplasty. *JBJS* 2004; 86(6): 1223–1229.
2.  Sanchez-Sotelo J, O'Driscoll SW, Morrey BF. Peri-prosthetic humeral fracture after total elbow arthroplasty: treatment with implant revision and strut allograft augmentation. *JBJS* 2002; 84(9): 1642–1650.

7.  **B**

Wright & Cofield described a system for classification of peri-prosthetic fractures around the proximal humerus. The fractures are classified in relation to their location to the distal tip of the humeral implant.

Type A – Fracture at the prosthesis tip and extending proximally.
Type B – Fracture at the prosthesis tip without extension, or minimal extension proximally and variable extension distally
Type C – Fracture distal to the tip of the prosthesis.

Ref:
Wright T, Cofield RH. Humeral fractures after shoulder arthroplasty. *JBJS* 1995; 77: 1340–1346.

8.  **C**

The specific indication for operative treatment of peri-prosthetic humeral fracture include: substantially displaced or unstable fracture pattern, fracture through the bone cement reducing the area of bone contact, displaced fracture at the tip of prosthesis, displaced fracture surrounding a loose prosthesis and crack through an area of osteolytic bone. The fracture located distal to the tip of the prosthesis should be treated as closed humeral fracture and responds well to non-operative treatment.

Ref:
1.  Cofield RH *et al*. Periprosthetic Fractures. In Rockwood & Wilkins. *Fracture in Adults* (6th ed) (2006) Lippincott Williams & Wilkins, Philadelphia.
2.  Campbell J, Moore R, Iannoti J *et al*. Peri-prosthetic humeral fractures: mechanism of fractures and treatment options. *J Shoulder Elbow Surg* 1998; 7: 406–413.

9.  **D**

Vancouver classification developed by Duncan and Masri is universally used for assessing and reporting of peri-prosthetic femur fractures and includes fracture configuration, implant stability and bone quality. It is recommended for guiding treatment and outlining prognosis. The classification was initially developed for postoperative peri-prosthetic femur fracture but has been recently expanded to include intra-operative peri-prosthetic femur fractures.

The classification consists of following types:

Type A – Fracture confined to trochanteric region, subdivided into type $A_L$ and $A_G$ based on the associated of the lesser or Greater trochanter respectively.
Type B1 – Fracture around the stem, good bone stock, solidly fixed implant
Type B2 – Fracture around the stem, good bone stock, and loose implant

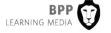

Type B3 – Fracture around the stem, severe bone stock deficiency, and loose implant. This also includes (poor bone stock due to comminution, osteopenia and osteolysis)
Type C – Fracture distal to the stem (enough distal for the treatment to be considered independent of hip replacement)

Ref:

Masri BA, Meek RM, Duncan CP. Peri-prosthetic fracture evaluation and treatment. *Clin Orthop* 2004; (420): 80–95.

**10. D**

The four important technical points for treatment of Type B1 periprosthetic femur fractures with cortical on lay strut graft, as suggested are:

1. As many cable/wires as necessary should be used to establish stable fixation.
2. The struts must be contoured to allow maximum graft/host contact.
3. Preservation of the blood supply of the femur is critical and the linea aspera should not be stripped of its soft tissue attachment.
4. Autograft or morsellised allograft applied at the strut/host junction enhances healing.

Ref:

Haddad FS, Duncan CP, Berry DJ *et al.* Peri-prosthetic femoral fractures around well fixed implants: use of cortical on lay graft with or without a plate. *JBJS Am.* 2002; 84(6): 945–950.

**11. B**

The periprosthetic tibial fracture around total knee replacement are classified according to Felix *et al.* and are described as follows

Type I – fracture around tibial plateau
Type II – Fracture around the stem
Type III – Fracture distal to the prosthesis
Type IV – Fractures involving tibial tubercle.

Each type then has a further subtype: subtype A – well fixed implant. Subtype B- loose implant and Subtype C – intra-operative fracture.

Ref:
Felix NA, Stuart MJ, Hassen AD. Peri-prosthetic fractures of the tibia associated with total knee arthroplasty. *Clin Orthop* 1997; 345: 113–124.

**12. D**

The management of an intra-operatively sustained Vancouver type B2 periprosthetic femur fracture is with Cerclage wire and longer stem implant bypassing the fracture or use of cortical strut graft with or without plates and screws.

Ref:
Masri BA, Meek RM, Duncan CP. Peri-prosthetic fracture evaluation and treatment. *Clin Orthop* 2004; (420): 80–95.

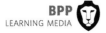

13. **E**

The most suitable management for a Vancouver type C post-operative periprosthetic femur fracture is primary fracture fixation. The implant should be ignored and if revision is required it should be considered after the fracture has united. Symptomatic treatment is opted for type A fractures. Type B1 fractures require Cerclage wire, cortical struts with or without plates. Type B2 fractures require revision to long stem and type B3 require revision and augmentation with allograft or tumour prosthesis.

Ref:

Masri BA, Meek RM, Duncan CP. Peri-prosthetic fracture evaluation and treatment. *Clin Orthop* 2004; (420): 80–95.

14. **C**

Revision spinal surgery carries the highest risk of dural tear due to the increased scarring seen intra-operatively in such cases, with a reported incidence of 13.2%. Primary lumbar discectomy has been associated with a 3.5% risk of dural tear and an 8.5% risk in those undergoing a lumbar decompression. Anterior cervical spine surgery has been associated with a reported incidence of 1%.

Ref:
1. Tafazal SI, Sell P. Incidental durotomy in lumbar spine surgery: incidence and management. *Eur Spine J*. 2005; 14: 287–90.
2. Hannallah D, Lee J, Khan M. Cerebrospinal fluid leak following cervical spine surgery. *J Bone Joint Surg (Am)*, May 2008; 90: 1101–1105.

15. **E**

The management of a patient presenting with an acute spinal cord injury is directed at protecting the spine to prevent further injury, prevention of secondary hypoxia and ischaemia at the site of injury by controlling haemodynamic status and oxygenation and obtaining appropriate imaging to visualise the spinal cord and surrounding structures. Flexion/extension radiographs are useful in determining dynamic instability in patients with a cervical spine injury with normal initial plain radiographs and persistent pain or tenderness of the cervical spine. It has been suggested that they are of limited use in the acute setting where MRI scanning can detect ligamentous instability.

Ref:
1. Delamarter RB, Coyle J. Acute Management of spinal cord injury. *J Am Acad Orthop Surg*, 1999; 7: 166–175.
2. Pollack CV, Hendey GW, Martin DR *et al.* (2001): Use of flexion-extension radiographs of the cervical spine in blunt trauma. *Ann Emerg Med*, 2001; 38: 8–11.

16. **C**

Patients with Morquios syndrome have been shown to have a 100% risk of upper cervical spine anomalies and a very high risk of instability and therefore routine screening of these children is advised.

Ref:

Frymoyer JW, Wiesel SW, An HS *et al.* (eds.) (2004) Congenital anomalies of the cervical spine. *In The Adult and Paediatric Spine*. Lippincott Willians & Wilkins, Philadelphia.

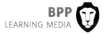

17. **C**

The patient most likely has a double-crush phenomenon with cervical spinal stenosis as well as lumbar spinal stenosis. He has signs of cervical spine compression and needs an MRI scan of the cervical spine to further investigate this prior to instituting any treatment.

Ref:
Frymoyer JW, Wiesel SW, An HS *et al.* (eds.) (2004) Congenital anomalies of the cervical spine. *In The Adult and Paediatric Spine*. Lippincott Willians & Wilkins, Philadelphia.

18. **A**

The initial management of axial cervical spine pain is always conservative and includes NSAIDs, early mobilisation and physiotherapy including stretching and strengthening exercises to help reduce muscle spasm. There is no evidence that a soft cervical collar speeds recovery and may lead to considerably cervical muscle atrophy if used for more than a few days. Epidural steroids have not shown any benefit in this group of patients. In a patient complaining mainly of pain and no neurological deficit and no red flags it is reasonable to try conservative treatment for a period of 6 weeks and if there is no improvement to consider further imaging, such as plain radiographs, flexion/extension views and MRI scan.

Ref:
Frymoyer JW, Wiesel SW, An HS, *et al.* (eds.) (2004) Axial mechanical neck pain and cervical degenerative disease. In *The Adult and Paediatric Spine*. Lippincott Williams & Wilkins, Philadelphia.

19. **B**

Twenty-five percent of slips are bilateral with 50% presenting with simultaneous involvement. The remaining 50% present within 18 months of each other. There is considerable debate over whether prophylactic pinning should be undertaken of the unaffected side in cases of unilateral presentation. The consensus opinion is that this should be offered if there is a high risk of an opposite slip occurring due to the presence of risk factors eg obesity, endocrinopathies, metabolic disorders or the slip has occurred at an early age (less than 10 years). A relative indication is if there are perceived difficulties with attendance at follow up or likelihood of late presentation despite symptoms.

Ref:
Staheli LT (2007) (4th ed) *Fundamentals of Pediatric Orthopaedics*. Lippincott Williams & Wilkins, Philadelphia.

20. **B**

Important predisposing factors in developing a slipped upper femoral epiphysis are:

- Obesity
- Endocrinopathy
  - Hypopituitarism
  - Hypothyroidism
  - Hypogonadism
- Metabolic causes
  - Renal oteodystropy
  - Rickets

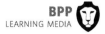

- Trauma
- Radiotherapy / Chemotherapy

Ref:

Staheli LT (2007) (4th ed) *Fundamentals of Pediatric Orthopaedics*. Lippincott Williams & Wilkins, Philadelphia.

**21.    C**

Two preparations of botulinum toxin are commonly used in the treatment of cerebral palsy associated deformities – Dysport and Botox. The drug is delivered by injection into the substance of the muscle and usually takes 2–3 days to take effect which wears off after approximately 3 months although with repeated treatment the effect may last a shorter time. There is an upper limit to how much can be administered and therefore it is rarely injected into more than two muscle groups at one time. Patients and parents need to be advised that a 'spill over' effect may occur with excessive weakness and that it is difficult to predict an individual patient's response to treatment. Treatment is best directed at dynamic deformities in the absence of fixed contractures.

Ref:

Herring JA (2008) (4th ed) *Tachdjian's Paediatric Orthopaedics*. Saunders, Philadelphia.

**22.    C**

Hip subluxation and dislocation in cerebral palsy does not arise as a result of laxity but rather it occurs due the deforming forces of spastic muscles. Consequently, hip subluxation is more common in non-ambulators and patients with greater involvement. Bony deformity eventually results from the action of the spastic muscles and these patients require close surveillance to adulthood to ensure the hips are not subluxing. Late diagnosis can increase the scale and difficulty of corrective surgery and may lead to problems with patient comfort and sitting balance. Reimer's migration index quantifies the percentage of the transverse diameter of the femoral head protruding past Perkins line i.e. the lateral border of the acetabulum. Follow up studies have shown that all hips with a migration index of greater than 60% eventually dislocate.

Ref:

Herring JA (2008) (4th ed) *Tachdjian's Paediatric Orthopaedics*. Saunders, Philadelphia.

**23.    C**

Type I Scheurmann's disease commonly presents 2 years before skeletal maturity and tends to occur in males. It can be differentiated from benign postural round back by the fact that it is a rigid deformity and on forward bending there is a definite apex to an angular kyphosis as opposed to a smooth kyphosis. The kyphosis leads to varying degrees of anterior chest wall defect as these structures come under compression. Although the hamstrings are frequently tight, neurological involvement of the lower limbs is rare. Conservative management is the mainstay of treatment with most patients experiencing an improvement in saggittal profile with extension bracing followed by spinal extension exercises. Occasionally surgical correction is necessary in severe deformities which present after skeletal maturity and are refractory to conservative management.

Ref:

Benson MKD (2nd ed)(2002) *Children's Orthopaedics and Fractures*. Harcourt Publishers, London.

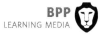

**24.    A**

Successful outcomes following knee arthrodesis are reduced in the presence of massive bone loss and significant previous infection, and are inversely proportional to the number of previous surgical procedures. The use of constrained knee implants are associated with increased bone loss and lower rates of fusion. Knee arthrodesis following tumour resection is associated with excellent results, with fusion rates between 80–100%.

Ref:

Conway JD, Mont MA, Bezwada HP. Arthrodesis of the knee. *J Bone Joint Surg Am*, 2004; 86-A 4: 835–48.

**25.    B**

Lateral tibiofemoral compartment osteoarthritis with an associated valgus deformity is best treated with a distal femoral varus osteotomy. High tibial osteotomy is unsuitable in such cases as it would tend to cause an oblique joint line. The Coventry HTO is a closing wedge osteotomy, above the level of the tibial tubercle.

Ref:

Wang JW, Hsu CC. Distal Femoral Varus Osteotomy for Osteoarthritis of the Knee. *J Bone Joint Surg Am*, 2006; 88 1: 100–108.

**26.    E**

Genu valgum is more common in patients with a history of trauma, rheumatoid arthritis, renal osteodystrophy, rickets, and infantile poliomyelitis.

Ref:

Wang JW, Hsu CC. Distal Femoral Varus Osteotomy for Osteoarthritis of the Knee. *J Bone Joint Surg Am*, 2006; 88 1: 100–108.

**27.    B**

Rupture of the quadriceps tendon is a clinical diagnosis. It is more common after 40 years of age and in the male population, and is associated with steroid use, diabetes, gout and renal failure. Patients normally present with pain and an inability to walk. Examination findings include a palpable gap in the extensor apparatus, and often an inability to straight leg raise when the hip is flexed. When lying supine, straight leg raise can be assisted by an intact lateral retinaculum (in partial tears) and the iliotibial band. Partial tears can be treated non operatively.

Ref:

Ilan DI, Tejwani N, Keschner M, Leibman M. Quadriceps tendon rupture. *J Am Acad Orthop Surg*, 2003; 11 3: 192–200.

**28.    C**

The discoid meniscus is a thickened and wafer shaped variant of the normal meniscus, which varies in shape from a complete disc to a ring shaped meniscus. It occurs in up to 5% of population, but only a small percentage of these are symptomatic. It usually involves the lateral meniscus and is bilateral in 20% of patients. Clinically patients may complain of pain, swelling, and snapping. They can be classified as complete and incomplete, and

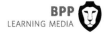

this refers to the shape of the discoid meniscus (incomplete having a more semilunar shape). Patients complaining of popping and no further symptoms can be treated non operatively, as long as they do not develop pain or swelling of the knee.

Ref:
Miller MD (ed.) (2008) *Review of Orthopaedics*. Saunders Elsevier, Philadelphia.


29. **C**

Osteoarthritic cartilage is characterised by: increased water content, loss of proteoglycans, increase in relative concentration of collagen, increase in proteoglycan synthesis and degradation, increase in chondroitin 4 sulphate concentration, reduction in keratin sulphate concentration and reduction in modulus of elasticity.

Ref:
Mankin, HJ. Current concepts review: The response of articular cartilage to mechanical injury. *J Bone Joint Surg Am*. 1982; 64: 460–466.


30. **C**

Tortional rigidity of an IM nail depends on both material properties (shear modulus) and structural properties (polar moment of inertia). Bending rigidity of a nail is related to the 4th power of the nails radius and depends on both the material properties and structural properties (area moment of inertia). IM nails are load sharing devices.

Ref:
Miller MD (ed.) (2008) *Review of Orthopaedics*. Saunders Elsevier, Philadelphia.


31. **B**

Arthrodesis of the ankle should be performed in neutral dorsiflexion, 5–10 degrees of external rotation, 5 degrees of hindfoot valgus. Arthrodesis of the knee should be performed in 0–7 degrees of valgus, 10–15 degrees of flexion.

Ref:
Buckwalter JA, Einhorn TA, Simon SR (eds.) (2000) (2nd ed.) *Orthopaedic Basic science: Biology and Biomechanics of the musculoskeletal system*, American Academy of Orthpaedic Surgeons.


32. **D**

Pitch is the distance between the threads. Lead is distance advanced in one revolution. Root diameter (inner diameter) is proportional to tensile strength. To maximise pullout strength, a screw should have a large outer diameter, a small root diameter and a fine pitch.

Ref:
Friedman RJ, Black J, Galante JO *et al.* Current concepts in orthopaedics biomaterials and implant fixation. *J Bone Joint Surg Am* 1993; 75: 1086–1109.

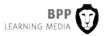

**33.    A**

The position of hip arthrodesis should be 25–30 degrees of flexion, 0 degrees of abduction and rotation (external rotation is better than internal rotation). If the hip is fused in an abducted position, the patient will lurch over the affected lower extremity with an excessive trunk shift, which will later result in lower back pain. Hip arthrodesis decreases gait efficiency to approximately 50% of normal.

Ref:

Buckwalter JA, Einhorn TA, Simon SR (eds.) (2000) (2nd ed.) *Orthopaedic Basic science: Biology and Biomechanics of the musculoskeletal system.* American Academy of Orthpaedic Surgeons.

**34.    C**

Ref:

1.    Muadi QI *et al.* Prognosis of conservatively managed anterior cruciate ligament injury: a systematic review. *Sports Med* 2007; 37(8): 703–16.

2.    Cyril TB *et al.* The Science of Reconstruction of the Anterior Cruciate Ligament. *Bone Joint Surg [Am]* 1997; 79: 1556–76.

**35.    B**

Indications for high tibial osteotomy:

*   Medial compartment arthritis
*   10–15 degrees of varus alignment on weight-bearing X-rays
*   Physiologically young
*   A preoperative range of motion of at least 90 degrees.

Ref:

Grelsamer RP. Unicompartmental Osteoarthrosis of the Knee. *J Bone Joint Surg [Am]* 1995; 77: 278–292.

**36.    B**

The meniscus is divided into 3 parts by its blood supply. The peripheral third is the red-red zone and is well vascularised. The middle zone is the red-white zone with a limited healing potential. The central third is the white-white zone which has no blood flow and no ability to heal. Tears in the peripheral third will heal and should be repaired. The Fairbanks article describes the classic arthritic changes after total meniscectomy: development of an antero-postero ridge, flattening of the femoral condyle, and narrowing of the joint space.

Ref:

1.    Fairbanks TJ. Knee joint changes after meniscectomy. *J Bone Joint Surg Br* 1948; 30: 664–670.

2.    Cannon WD Jr, Morgan CD. Meniscal repair Part II: Arthroscopic Repair Techniques. *J. Bone Joint Surg [Am]* 1994; 43: 77–96.

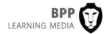

37. **D**

Alloys and ultrahigh molecular weight polyethylene form the components for hip and knee arthroplasty. Polymethylmethacrylate (PMMA) or bone cement is also often used. It is the polyethylene that eventually undergoes wear to produce wear debris, osteolysis, loosening of the prosthetic device and revision surgery.

Gamma radiation is used on polyethylene components to sterilise them before implantation. Recent research has discovered that the radiation process produces free radicals. This has 2 effects: 1) it cross-links polyethylene 2) it oxidises polyethylene. The cross-linking of polyethylene has favorable advantages including prolonging durability and producing less wear debris. This could increase the life of total joints. Specially designed cross-linked polyethylene components are currently being investigated. However, gamma radiation of polyethylene in the presence of oxygen produces oxidised products. The areas of oxidation have been found to be sources of wear debris.

Recent attempts have been made to use gamma radiation in a vacuum to retain the positive cross-linking effects and forgo the negative oxidation effects. Other processes to sterilise polyethylene have also been developed including ethylene oxide gas and gas plasma. Certain thermal processing of parts after gamma radiation can result in the combination of free radicals and a reduction in their number. High pressure forms of polyethylene have also been developed to produce a product with a higher degree of crystallinity and mechanical properties. However, recent clinical results indicate that the linear wear rate, incidence of osteolysis, and revision rates are greater than for conventional polyethylene for unclear reasons.

Ref:

Barrack MD *et al.* (2006) *Orthopaedic Knowledge update: Hip and Knee Reconstruction 3*. American Academy of Orthopaedic Surgeons.

38. **B**

Ref:

Blom AW *et al.* Infection after total knee arthroplasty. *J Bone Joint Surg [Br]* 2004; 86: 688–691.

39. **A**

Ref:

Miller MD (ed.) (2008) *Review of Orthopaedics*. Saunders Elsevier, Philadelphia.

40. **B**

This has been shown to reduce the rate of dislocation to <1% following a posterior approach. Along with this using a large femoral head can also help to reduce the rate of dislocation following either the posterior or lateral approach.

Ref:
1. Pellicci PM, Bostrom M, Poss R. Posterior approach to total hip replacement using enhanced posterior soft tissue repair. *Clin Orthop*, 1998; 355: 224–228.
2. Berry DJ, Von Noch M, Schleck CD, Harmsen WS. Effect of femoral head diameter and operative approach on risk of dislocation after primary total hip arthroplasty. *J Bone Joint Surg (Am)*, 2005; 87: 2456–2463.

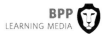

**41. C**

This pore size has been shown to be optimal for bone ingrowth. Bone growth across a gap of 1mm has been shown for HA coated implants. Micromotion should be kept <150μm (preferably 50–100μm).

Ref:

1.  Dumbleton J, Manley MT. Hydroxyapatite- coated prostheses in total hip and knee arthroplasty. *J Bone Joint Surg (Am)*, Nov 2004; 86: 2526–2540.
2.  Miller MD (ed.) (2008) *Review of Orthopaedics*. Saunders Elsevier, Philadelphia.

**42. E**

With large metal on metal bearing surfaces true fluid film lubrication can occur. There is generation of a large number of very small sized particles (<50nm compared to >0.1μm particles for metal on polyethylene) and lower volumetric wear rates most likely due to the fluid film lubrication that occurs and the very small size of wear particles generated. In patients with metal on metal bearings cobalt and chromium ions are detected in serum and urine.

Ref:

1.  Roberts P, Grigoris P, Bosch H, Talwaker N. Resurfacing arthroplasty of the hip. *Current Orthopaedics* 2005; 19: 263–79
2.  McWilliams TG, Parker JR. Alternative bearing surfaces for hip arthroplasty. *Orthopaedics and Trauma* 2009; 23: 2–7.
3.  Keegan GM, Learmonth ID, Case CP. Orthopaedic metals and their potential toxicity in the arthroplasty patient. *J Bone Joint Surg (Br)*, 2007; 89: 567–573.

**43. C**

Impingement of components in total hip arthroplasty occurs when two non-articulating components come into contact during joint range of motion eg femoral neck and rim of acetabular component. This can be reduced by maximising the head-neck ratio of the components, which can also increase range of motion. Elevated rim liners usually have an elevated posterior rim improving femoral head contact during flexion, but these can increase impingement in extension.

Ref:

Soong M, Rubash HE, Macaulay W. Dislocation after total hip arthroplasty. *J Am Acad Orthop Surg*, 2007; 12: 314–321.

**44. A**

Higher forces are generated with superior and lateral placement of the hip centre and studies have shown an increased risk of loosening of both the acetabular and femoral components when the hip is placed in a high hip centre. The acetabular components used in a high hip centre are also very small and so thinner polyethylene is also used. Less lengthening of the leg can be achieved and hip biomechanics are altered.

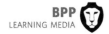

Ref:
1.   Haddad FS, Masri BA, Garbuz DS, Duncan CP. Primary total replacement of the dysplastic hip. *J Bone Joint Surg (Am)* 1999; 81: 1462–1482.
2.   Sanchez-Sotelo J, Berry DJ, Trousdale RT, Cabanela ME. Surgical Treatment of developmental dysplasia of the hip in adults: II. Arthroplasty Options. *J Am Acad Orthop Surg,* 2002; 10: 334–344.

**45.   E**

Temperature monitoring is the most popular type for replants. Caffeine is avoided to prevent vasospasm. Routinely if there is a large amount of muscle in the part to be replanted, the ischaemia time is reduced.

Ref:

Dee R, Hurst LC (1997) (International ed.) *Principles of orthopaedic practise.* McGraw Hill.

**46.   B**

These two conditions are commonly confused. Pronator syndrome is seen in individuals exposed to highly repetitive activities. Diagnosis of pronator syndrome is usually delayed due to the vague poorly related history. Compression is usually due to lacertus fibrosus.

Ref:

Morrey BF (2000) *The elbow and its disorders.* Saunders, Philadelphia.

**47.   C**

The extensor pollicis longus can be a source of pain as it wraps over the wrist extensors giving the classic symptoms of intersection syndrome between the second and third dorsal compartments. This could be confused with de Quervain's disease.

Ref:

Dee R, Hurst LC (1997) (International ed.) *Principles of orthopaedic practise.* McGraw Hill.

**48.   E**

It is characterised by enophthalmos not exophthalmos. Other symptoms include ptosis

Ref:

Dee R, Hurst LC (1997) (International ed.) *Principles of orthopaedic practise.* McGraw Hill.

**49.   B**

The PIN neurectomy is performed during wrist fusion to prevent post operative pain.

Ref:

Snell RS (2003) *Clinical Anatomy.* Lippincott Williams & Wilkins, Philadelphia.

**50.   A**

It normally originates 5cm distal to epicondyle. Compression can give rise to anterior interosseous syndrome, which causes mainly motor symptoms.

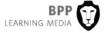

Ref:
Tsai P. Median and Radian nerve compression about the elbow. *Journal of Bone and Joint Surgery*, 2008; 90: 420–428.

**51.  C**

The tabletop test when positive is an indication for surgery. Functional problems are also an indication.

Ref:
Shaw RB. Dupuytren's disease: History, diagnosis and treatment. *Plastic and Reconstructive Surgery* 2007; 120(3).

**52.  C**

The A2 and A4 pulleys are located at the proximal and middle phalanges.

Ref:
Strickland JW. Flexor Tendon Injuries: I. Foundations of Treatment. *J Am Acad Orthop Surg*, 1995; 3(1): 44–54.

**53.  A**

The late effect of traumatic injuries can be described into:

Intrinsic – Plus deformity: Occurs due to foreshortening of the intrinsic muscles. There is intrinsic muscle tightness and hence the PIPJ cannot be flexed with the MCPJ held in extension.

Intrinsic- minus deformity: It is seen following an injury to the ulnar nerve that causes a claw hand deformity. This includes hyperextension of the MCPJ and flexion at the PIPJ.

Extrinsic tightness – This is caused by scarring of the extensor digitorum communis. Hence with PIPJ can be passively flexed with the MCPJ extension; however the PIPJ cannot flex passively with MCPJ in flexion.

Lumbrical-plus deformity: this leads from lumbrical tightness. This leads to paradoxical extension of PIPJ when MCPJ is actively flexed.

Ref:
Schneider LH. Extensor tendon injuries. *Hand Clin* 1995; 11(3).

**54.  B**

The interosseous muscles of the hand includes 4 dorsal interossei, these muscles abduct the the index, middle and ring finger. The little finger is abducted by the abductor digiti minimi. The 3 volar interossei adducts the index, ring and little finger; it does not adduct the middle finger. All the interossei pass volar to the MCP allowing effective flexion of the MCPJ. All the interossei are innervated by deep branch of ulnar nerve.

Ref:
Schneider LH. Extensor tendon injuries. *Hand Clin* 1995, 11(3).

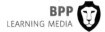

55.   **C**
The most important ligamentous stabiliser for the DRUJ is the TFCC. This TFCC is composed of the following structures – TFC, ulnocarpal ligaments, volar and dorsal radio-ulnar ligaments, meniscal homologue, sheath of ECU tendon and ulnar collateral ligament. The TFC is the heart of the complex and forms the load-bearing component which transmits the compressive forces between the carpus and ulna. The thickness varies between 2mm to 5mm and is inversely proportional to the ulnar variance. The ulnar negative wrists have a thick TFC and the ulnar positive wrists have a thinner TFC. The blood supply is from the volar and dorsal branch of the anterior interosseous artery, which supplies the 20% of the periphery and the central area is avascular. It attaches to the distal radius at the sigmoid notch and runs to the fovea at the base of the ulnar styloid.

Ref:
Melone CP Jr, Nathan R. Traumatic disruptions of triangular fibrocartilage complex, pathoanatomy. *Clin Orthop Rel Res* 1992; 275: 65–73.


56.   **A**
The midcarpal joint is spanned by the extrinsic ligaments and accounts for 50–60% of movement at the wrist joint. There is some movement within the proximal row and fixed distal row. Scaphoid acts as the link and provides stability and integrating motion between the two rows.

The proximal row is described to have a 'variable geometry' of the carpal bones allow it a stable extensive excursion.

Ref:
Linscheid RL. Kinematics consideration of the wrist. *Clin Orthop* 1986; 202: 27–39.


57.   **C**
Osteonecrosis of lunate or Kienbock's disease follows a predictable pattern of degeneration described in 4 stages. The treatment of the disease is based on the stage of the disease at the time of diagnosis. Stage 1 is described by sclerosis seen radiologically and treated with splinting and rest. Stage 2 is described by fragmentation seen radiologically and treated by joint levelling procedures like radial shortening or ulnar lengthening. Stage 3 is described by the radiological appearance of collapse and despite there being controversy on the treatment this stage, scophotrapezial – trapezoid fusion or lunate excision arthroplasty or combined procedures are chosen. Stage 4 is described by radio carpal and intercarpal degenerative joint disease and the treatment at this stage is limited to salvage procedures like proximal row carpectomy or complete wrist fusion.

Ref:
Bruce JF. Hand. In Miller MD (ed.) *Review of Orthopaedics*. Saunders Elsevier, Philadelphia.


58.   **A**
The normal value for static two point discrimination is 6mm and for moving two point discrimination is 5mm. Static two point discrimination and Semmes Weinstein monofilament tests evaluate the slowly adapting fibres (merkle cell receptor) and moving two point discrimination tests evaluate the quickly adapting fibres (meissner corpuscle).

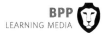

Ref:
Szabo RM. Nerve compression syndromes. In *Hand surgery update* (1996) American Society for Surgery of the Hand. pp. 221–231.

**59.  D**

Wartenberg's syndrome (cheiralgia paresthetica) is a compressive neuropathy of the sensory branch of the radial nerve. It is compressed between the brachioradialis and ECRL. Surgical decompression is warranted if a 6 month trial of non-operative treatment fails; this involves rest, NSAIDs, avoiding aggravating activities and wrist splints.

Ref:
Szabo RM. Nerve compression syndromes. In *Hand surgery update* (1996) American Society for Surgery of the Hand. pp. 221–231.

**60.  E**

The paratenon is a sheath found in certain larger tendons composed of loose areolar tissue which reduces friction and contains abundant fibroblasts and vessels. Tendons lined by a synovial sheath alone may have a blood supply from vincula but derive most of their nourishment from synovial fluid imbibition as a result of motion. For this reason, paratenon covered tendons tend to heal better than those without.

The collagen content of tendons is very high (up to 75–99% of the dry weight) and the vast majority of this is type I collagen. Types III and types IV are also found to a far lesser extent. The site of insertion of tendons into bone is composed of four zones where there is a gradual transition in tissue type from tendon to bone to minimise any stress riser effect and to minimise friction in this region. Zone 1 consists of parallel collagen fibres (Sharpey's fibres) which usually insert at 45 degrees to the bone surface to minimise stress concentration. In zone II we also find unmineralised fibrocartilage which becomes calcified in zone III. Zone IV is bone with trabeculae orientated according to tension and compression that the tendon may impart to different regions of the bone.

The stress strain curve of tendons shows a characteristic concave region at the beginning before adopting the familiar steep ascent of the linear elastic region. This early 'toe' region is ascribed to both tension on the collagen fibres pulling them taut ie taking up the slack in the system and ground substance shear because of interfibrillar sliding. Little dips occur later on in the curve due to partial fibre failure until a point is reached where the whole structure fails which defines the ultimate tensile strength of the tendon.

Ref:
Nordin M, Frankel V (2001) (3rd ed.) *Basic biomechanics of the musculoskeletal system*. Lippincott Williams & Wilkins, Philadelphia.

**61.  D**

Type X collagen is mainly present in the calcified cartilage layer and is associated with cartilage calcification. It is produced by hypertrophied chondrocytes during enchondral ossification and is therefore found in:

(a)  Degenerate calcified cartilage
(b)  Growth plate

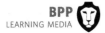

(c)   Fracture callus

(d)   Calcifying cartilaginous tumours

Ref:

Buckwalter J, Einhorn, T, Simon S (2000) (2<sup>nd</sup> ed.) *Orthopaedic Basic Science: Biology and Biomechanics of the Musculoskeletal System*. American Academy of Orthopaedic Surgeons.

**62.   D**

Proteoglycans are large protein-polysaccharide molecules. Essentially they consist of a protein core attached to chains of glycosaminoglycans. Examples of proteoglycans include aggrecan (the predominant type found in articular cartilage), decorin, superficial zone protein, biglycan and fibromodulin.

Glycosaminoglycans are polysaccharide molecules which attach to the protein core. Examples of glycosaminoglycans include chondroitin sulphate, keratin sulphate and dermatin sulphate. These polysaccharide molecules have a highly negative charge which pulls in water molecules. This accounts for the high level of hydration of articular cartilage. However, the proteoglycan molecules which make up much of the ground substance are not able to pull in water indefinitely due to the restraining effect of the collagen network which limits articular cartilage hydration to 40%.

Ref:

Nordin M, Frankel V (2001) (3<sup>rd</sup> ed.) *Basic biomechanics of the musculoskeletal system*. Lippincott Williams & Wilkins, Philadelphia.

**63.   C**

Aggrecans are proteoglycans and are a diverse population whose individual identity is determined by the number, type and sulphation pattern of the attached glycosaminoglycans. Typically they consist of a protein core with attached glycosaminoglycans radiating out. These aggrecan are attached to a long hyaluronate molecule to form a superstructure. The aggrecan molecules are anchored to the hyaluronate molecule by virtue of a specific binding domain which is stabilised by a link protein and both of these are vital to function. The ratio of individual glycosaminoglycan populations in aggrecans changes with ageing. The ratio of chondroitin sulphate to keratin sulphate decreases and sulphation patterns change for individual glycsaminoglycans. The proportion of chondroitin sulphate 6 to chondroitin sulphate 4 increases with age and also in osteoarthritis.

Ref:

Nordin M, Frankel V (2001) (3<sup>rd</sup> ed.) *Basic biomechanics of the musculoskeletal system*. Lippincott Williams & Wilkins, Philadelphia.

**64.   C**

Articular cartilage is a highly anisotropic material principally due to the collagen fibre arrangement which superficially resists shear but in the much larger deeper zone consists of collagen fibre arrangement principally designed to resist compressive stresses. Articular cartilage can also be thought of as a viscoelastic material in that it demonstrates both creep and stress relaxation behaviour. It is imperative to obtain an understanding of what these behaviours are but also understand the specific mechanisms which underlie them in articular cartilage.

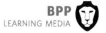

Biomechanically, we need to consider two phases in articular cartilage – a porous permeable solid phase and an interstitial fluid phase. What attracts the fluid in is the Donan Osmotic swelling pressure generated by all of the negatively charged glycosaminoglycan molecules in the aggrecans. However, we know that cartilage does not swell and burst as there is an opposing force of compressive stiffness imposed by the collagen-proteoglycan matrix which limits hydration to 40%. A useful analogy is to think of a balloon in a string bag.

We can now consider what happens during our creep and stress relaxation experiments. In creep, we impose a constant stress and witness deformation which gradually tails off until a steady state is achieved. What is happening is that as the cartilage is loaded fluid escapes from the porous structure causing deformation. However, as this fluid leaks out at the surface, the solid matrix is compacted which leads to a reduction in the size of the pores. This increases the frictional drag of the escaping fluid which limits this egress until an equilibrium state is reached. What also occurs as the compacted solid matrix exerts a greater hold on the remaining interstitial fluid is that the stiffness increases. Simply, if you push cartilage, it pushes back. In stress relaxation experiments deformation is kept constant and stress is shown to go down. This is explained by the time dependent internal redistribution of fluid to the compacted surface matrix reducing the stress here over time.

Ref:
Nordin M, Frankel V (2001) (3rd ed.) *Basic biomechanics of the musculoskeletal system*. Lippincott Williams & Wilkins, Philadelphia.

65.  **E**
Lubrication is the 'introduction of fluid between two surfaces in relative motion to reduce friction and wear'. In engineering terms there are two types of lubrication – boundary and fluid film. Several subtypes exist which the reader should be aware of as well as theorised mechanisms which are as yet unproven in vivo.

The determinants of what lubrication mechanism prevails are:
(a)  Load – magnitude, direction
(b)  Bearing surfaces – roughness, geometry, wettability
(c)  Velocity of bearing surfaces
(d)  Viscosity of lubricant

Fluid film:

In this form of lubrication, a thin film of fluid separates the surfaces. Consequently friction is determined solely by the viscous properties of the fluid. For this to occur you need to be able to generate a fluid film that is at least three times as thick as the surface roughness of the bearing surfaces. Advocates of modern large diameter hard bearings argue that such lubrication mechanisms are possible with the advent of improved sphericity, clearance, surface hardness and finish.

(a)  Hydrodynamic – load is supported by pressure in the fluid generated by relative motion between the entraining surfaces. This requires a high speed, high viscosity and low load.
(b)  Squeeze film – bearing surfaces approach each other without relative motion and fluid is trapped in between which eventually leaks out.

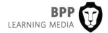

(c) Elastohydrodynamic – theorised in articular cartilage that loading causes deformation and increase in surface area and congruency which allows the trapped fluid film to persist for longer.

(d) Microelastohydrodynamic – further theorised that on loading tiny pools of lubricant between microasperities are also recruited as these peaks are flattened out.

Boundary lubrication:

This was put forward based on the finding of hyaluronidase treatment of synovial fluid reducing the viscosity to that of water with no change in lubrication characteristics supporting the argument that other mechanisms of lubrication must exist. If the fluid film does eventually disperse, then perhaps there is an adsorbed boundary lubricant coating each of the surfaces preventing contact. Therefore, friction would be independent of the physical characteristics of the bearing surfaces or lubricant viscosity and would solely depend on the chemical properties of the lubricant. Several candidate molecules have been put forward e.g. lubricin.

Mixed lubrication:

These are essentially hypothetical mechanisms thought to occur in articular cartilage mixing aspects of both boundary and fluid film models.

Boosted:

As bearing surfaces approach synovial fluid is pushed into the porous permeable matrix leaving behind a concentrated gel of lubricating molecules.

Weeping – Loading leads to fluid shifts through the porous matrix leading to escape of fluid at the cartilage periphery thereby renewing the fluid film.

Ref:
Nordin M, and Frankel V (2001) (3rd ed.) *Basic biomechanics of the musculoskeletal system.* Lippincott Williams & Wilkins, Philadelphia.

**66.** **B**

Troponin and Tropomyosin are regulatory molecules which are attached to actin thin filaments and regulate their interaction with thick myosin filaments. Tropomyosin sits on top of the actin molecules and prevent cross bridges from binding to the actin. The Troponin molecule is able to effect a conformational change in the Tropomyosin molecule to allow cross bridge attachment.

Troponin is composed of three subunits – Trop I (inhibitory), Trop C (binds to calcium) and Trop T (binds to tropomyosin). During muscle contraction the influx of calcium into the cell causes calcium to bind to the Troponin C. This displaces the troponin I which is normally sitting in a position which inhibits attachment to tropomyosin allowing the Trop T subunit to bind to and induce conformational change in the Tropomyosin molecule. This change allows actin and myosin to interact. This process is brought to an end when all of the calcium is actively transported back into the sarcoplasmic reticulum leading to troponin and tropomyosin resuming their inhibitory roles.

Ref:
Koeppen B, Stanton B (2008) (6th ed.) *Berne and Levy Physiology.* Mosby, Philadelphia.

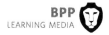

67.  **B**
A good way of remembering this is mentioned in the Stanmore Basic Sciences Guide and that is to think of a type 1 fibre as a 'slow red ox.'

Type I and II fibres can be considered almost polar opposites in terms of all of their features. One should envisage marathon runners when thinking of type I fibres and short distance sprinters for type II fibres.

Type I fibres   Slow contraction, low strength
      Small motor unit size
      High aerobic capacity, low anaerobic capacity
      Fatigue resistant

Type II fibres   Fast contraction, high strength
      Large motor unit size
      Low aerobic capacity, high anaerobic capacity
      Easily fatigued

Ref:
Koeppen, B and Stanton, B. (6th ed.) (2008) *Berne and Levy Physiology*, Mosby, Philadelphia.

68.  **C**
Other factors to increase stiffness are increasing the number of wires, reducing the ring diameter and placing the central rings closer to the fracture site.

Ref:
Buckwalter J, Einhorn T, Simon, S (2000) (2nd ed.) *Orthopaedic Basic Science: Biology and Biomechanics of the Musculoskeletal System*. American Academy of Orthopaedic Surgeons.

69.  **A**
At heel strike, the hip is usually flexed 25–30 degrees and the ground reaction force (GRF) is anterior to the joint producing a flexion moment. The hip extensors fire to counteract this moment whereas the flexors are silent.

From foot flat to heel rise, hip flexion decreases to about 15 degrees of extension. The GRF moves from anterior to posterior. Activity in the hip extensors gradually declines to counteract the diminishing flexion moment. As an extension moment develops there is negligible flexor activity to counteract this.

From heel rise there is slight further extension (20 degrees) until opposite contact is achieved and then the hip starts to flex as we move toward toe off. At this point the hip is still extended by 10 degrees. The GRF remains posterior to the joint and the flexors kick in with peak activity just after toe off.

In the swing phase, the hip flexes from 10 degrees extension to 30 degrees flexion. As the limb is freely in the air there is no GRF. Hip flexor activity peaks shortly after toe off during the initial swing to initiate motion. Thereafter the extensors take effect during terminal swing to decelerate the leg before heel strike.

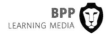
BPP
LEARNING MEDIA

Ref:

Whittle M (2001) (3rd ed.) *Gait analysis: an introduction.* Elsevier, Oxford.

**70. D**

The anterior Smith-Petersen approach has a superficial and deep internervous plane. The superficial plane is between sartorius and tensor fascia lata. The deep plane is between rectus femoris and abductor medius. The internervous plane is between the femoral and superior gluteal nerves.

Ref:

Hoppenfeld S, Deboer P (2003) *Surgical Exposures in Orthopaedics: The Anatomic Approach.* Lippincott Williams & Wilkins, Philadelphia.

**71. C**

OI has a prevalence 1 in 20000 children. Collagen type I is defective and the genes implicated include: Collagen 1A1 on chromosome 7q or mutation 1A2 on chromosome 17q.

Medical treatment includes bisphosphonates and vitamin D. Surgical treatment involves plaster, nailing, Sofield technique, scoliosis treatment.

Ref:
1. DiMeglio LA, Peacock M. Two-year clinical trial of oral alendronate versus intravenous pamidronate in children with osteogenesis imperfecta. *J Bone Miner Res* 2006; 21: 132–140.
2. Chevrel G, Schott AM, Fontanges E *et al.* Effects of oral alendronate on BMD in adult patients with osteogenesis imperfecta: a 3-year randomised placebo-controlled trial. *J Bone Miner Res* 2006; 21: 300–306.
3. Sillence DO, Senn A, Danks DM. Genetic heterogeneity in osteogenesis imperfecta. *J Med Genet* 1979; 16: 101–116.

**72. A**

The Risser classifiction is the degree of ossification of the iliac apophyses. '0' indicates no iliac apophyses ossified and hence a growing child. The likelihood of progression of scoliosis is related to growth.

Ref:

Herring JA (2002) *Tachdjian's Pediatric Orthopaedics.* Saunders, Philadelphia.

**73. D**

In children, supracondylar fractures typically remains extra-articular and involves the thin bone between coronoid fossa and olecranon fossa of the distal humerus;

Gartland classification:

2 types: extension type (95%) and flexion type.

Gartland classification for the extension fractures: This recognises that anterior cortex fails first with resultant posterior displacement of distal fragment

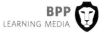

- Type I: non-displaced fracture
- Type II: displaced with intact posterior cottex
- Type III: displaced with no cortical contact

Ref:
Omid R, Choi PD, Skaggs DL. Supracondylar Humeral Fractures in Children. *J Bone Joint Surg [Am]* 2008; 90: 1121–1132.

**74.  E**

Several staging classifications are used to determine the severity of disease and prognosis in Perthes disease. These include the Catterall, Salter-Thomson, and Herring systems.

The Catterall classification is based on radiographic appearances and specifies four groups during the period of greatest bone loss.

Catterall staging is as follows:

- Stage I – Histologic and clinical diagnosis without radiographic findings
- Stage II – Sclerosis with or without cystic changes with preservation of the contour and surface of the femoral head
- Stage III – Loss of structural integrity of the femoral head
- Stage IV – Loss of structural integrity of the acetabulum in addition

The Salter-Thomson classification simplifies the Catterall classifications by reducing the groups to two. The first, called group A, includes Catterall groups I and II; for patients in this group, less than 50% of the head is involved. The second, called group B, includes Catterall groups III and IV; for patients in this group, more than 50% of the head is involved. For both classifications, if less than 50% of the femoral head is involved, the prognosis is better, whereas if more than 50% is involved, the prognosis is potentially poor.

The Herring classification addresses the integrity of the lateral pillar of the head. In lateral pillar group A, there is no loss of height in the lateral one third of the head, and there is little density change. In lateral pillar group B, there is a lucency and less than 50% loss of lateral height. Sometimes, the head is beginning to extrude from the socket. In lateral pillar group C, there is more than 50% loss of lateral height.

Ref:
Van Campenhout A, Moens P, Fabry G. Serial bone scintigraphy in Legg-Calve-Perthe's disease: correlation with the Catterall and Herring classification. *J Pediatr Orthop B* 2006; 15: 6–10.

**75.  E**
Achondroplasia patients have a normal trunk and short limbs – rhizomelic (Disproportionate) dwarfism.

**76.  A**
Ref:
Miller MD (ed.) (2008) *Review of Orthopaedics*. Saunders Elsevier, Philadelphia.

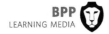

77. **B**

DDH is commonly seen in females (85%). SCFE is more common in African American children. The femoral head ossifies at about 3 months and radiographs become an impotant mode of investigation at this age. Forefoot adductus is a component of clubfoot. Kohler's disease is associated with osteonecrosis of the navicular.

Ref:
Miller MD (ed.) (2008) *Review of Orthopaedics*. Saunders Elsevier, Philadelphia.

78. **C**

Gilbert and Tassin were the first to indicate the importance of monitoring the return of biceps function as an indicator of brachial plexus recovery, which was subsequently confirmed by other studies. If normal biceps function fails to return by 3 months of age, the outcome at 2 years of age is abnormal.

Ref:
1.  Gilbert A, Tassin JL. Surgical repair of the brachial plexus in obstetric paralysis. *Chirurgie* 1984; 110: 70–75.
2.  Hardy AE. Birth injuries of the brachial plexus: Incidence and prognosis. *J Bone Joint Surg [Br]* 1981; 63: 98–101.
3.  Michelow BJ, Clarke HM, Curtis CG *et al*. The natural history of obstetrical brachial plexus palsy. *Plast Reconstr Surg* 1994; 93: 675–681.

79. **C**

During development, the tibio-femoral alignment changes during early years. At birth, the tibio-femoral alignment is 10–15 degrees of varus, which remodels to neutral at about 24 months of age and then becomes 10 degrees of valgus at the age of 3 years. Over the next 4 years, the tibio-femoral alignment gradually progresses to normal alignment of 7 degrees of valgus.

Ref:
Salenius P, Vankka E. The development of the tibio-femoral angle in children. *J Bone Joint Surg [Am]* 1975; 57: 259–261.

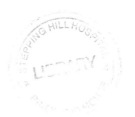

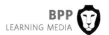

# More titles in the Progressing your Medical Career Series

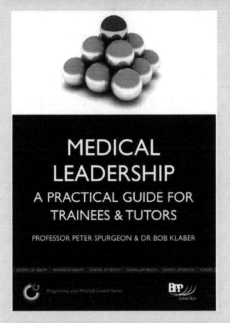

*Are you a doctor or medical student who wishes to acquire and develop your leadership and management skills? Do you recognise the role and influence of strong leadership and management in modern medicine?*

Clinical leadership is something in which all doctors should have an important role in terms of driving forward high quality care for their patients. In this up-to-date guide Peter Spurgeon and Robert Klaber take you through the latest leadership and management thinking, and how this links in with the Medical Leadership Competency Framework. As well as influencing undergraduate curricula and some of the concepts underpinning revalidation, this framework forms the basis of the leadership component of the curricula for all medical specialties, so a practical knowledge of it is essential for all doctors in training.

Using case studies and practical exercises to provide a strong work-based emphasis, this practical guide will enable you to build on your existing experiences to develop your leadership and management skills, and to develop strategies and approaches to improving care for your patients.

This book addresses:

- Why strong leadership and management are crucial to delivering high quality care

- The theory and evidence behind the Medical Leadership Competency Framework

- The practical aspects of leadership learning in a wide range of clinical environments (eg handover, EM, ward etc)

- How Consultants and trainers can best facilitate leadership learning for their trainees and students within the clinical work-place

Whether you are a medical student just starting out on your career, or an established doctor wishing to develop yourself as a clinical leader, this practical, easy-to-use guide will give you the techniques and knowledge you require to excel.

£19.99
November 2011
Paperback
978-1-445379-57-9

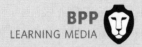

www.bpp.com/health

# More titles in the Progressing your Medical Career Series

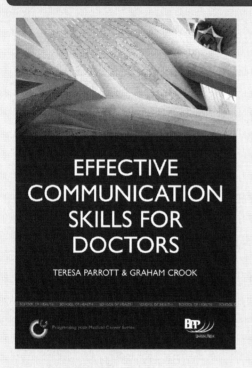

EFFECTIVE
COMMUNICATION
SKILLS FOR
DOCTORS

TERESA PARROTT & GRAHAM CROOK

£19.99
September 2011
Paperback
978-1-445379-56-2

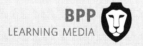

BPP
LEARNING MEDIA

*Would you like to know how to improve your communication skills? Are you looking for a clearly written book which explores all aspects of effective medical communication?*

There is an urgent need to improve doctors' communication skills. Research has shown that poor communication can contribute to patient dissatisfaction, lack of compliance and increased medico-legal problems. Improved communication skills will impact positively on all of these areas.

The last fifteen years have seen unprecedented changes in medicine and the role of doctors. Effective communication skills are vital to these new roles. But communication is not just related to personality. Skills can be learned which can make your communication more effective, and help you to improve your relationships with patients, their families and fellow doctors.

This book shows how to learn those skills and outlines why we all need to communicate more effectively. Healthcare is increasingly a partnership. Change is happening at all levels, from government directives to patient expectations. Communication is a bridge between the wisdom of the past and the vision of the future.

Readers of this book can also gain free access to an online module which upon successful completion can download a certificate for their portfolio of learning/Revalidation/CPD records.

This easy-to-read guide will help medical students and doctors at all stages of their careers improve their communication within a hospital environment.

www.bpp.com/health

# More titles in the Progressing your Medical Career Series

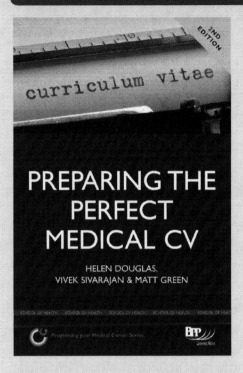

£19.99
October 2011
Paperback
978-1-445381-62-6

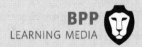

*Are you unsure of how to structure your Medical CV? Would you like to know how to ensure you stand out from the crowd?*

With competition for medical posts at an all time high it is vital that your Medical CV stands out over your fellow applicants. This comprehensive, unique and easy-to-read guide has been written with this in mind to help prospective medical students, current medical students and doctors of all grades prepare a Medical CV of the highest quality. Whether you are applying to medical school, currently completing your medical degree or a doctor progressing through your career (foundation doctor, specialty trainee in general practice, surgery or medicine, GP career grade or Consultant) this guide includes specific guidance for applicants at every level.

This time-saving and detailed guide:

- Explains what selection panels are looking for when reviewing applications at all levels.

- Discusses how to structure your Medical CV to ensure you stand out for the right reasons.

- Explores what information to include (and not to include) in your CV.

- Covers what to consider when maintaining a portfolio at every step of your career, including, for revalidation and relicensing purposes.

- Provides examples of high quality CVs to illustrate the above.

This unique guide will show you how to prepare your CV for every step of your medical career from pre-Medical School right through to Consultant level and should be a constant companion to ensure you secure your first choice post every time.

www.bpp.com/health

# More titles in the Progressing your Medical Career Series

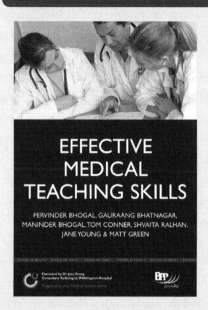

EFFECTIVE MEDICAL TEACHING SKILLS

PERVINDER BHOGAL, GAURAANG BHATNAGAR, MANINDER BHOGAL, TOM CONNER, SHVAITA RALHAN, JANE YOUNG & MATT GREEN

Foreword by Dr Jane Young
Consultant Radiologist, Whittington Hospital
Progressing your Medical Career Series

£19.99
October 2011
Paperback
978-1-445379-55-5

We *can all remember a teacher that inspired us, encouraged us and helped us to excel. But what is it that makes a good teacher and are these skills that can be learned and improved?*

As doctors and healthcare professionals we are all expected to teach, to a greater or lesser degree, and this carries a great deal of responsibility. We are helping to develop the next generation and it is essential to pass on the knowledge that we have gained during our experience to date.

This book aims to cover the fundamentals of medical education. It has been designed to be a guide for the budding teacher with practical advice, hints, tips and essential points of reflection designed to encourage the reader to think about what they are doing at each step.

By taking the time to read through this book and completing the exercises contained within it you should:

- Understand the needs of the learner

- Understand the skills required to be an effective teacher

- Understand the various different teaching scenarios, from lectures to problem based teaching, and how to use them effectively

- Understand the importance and sources of feedback

- Be aware of assessment techniques, appraisal and revalidation

This book aims to provide you with a foundation in medical education upon which you can build the skills and attributes to become a competent and skilled teacher.

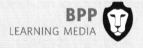

BPP LEARNING MEDIA

www.bpp.com/health

# More titles in the MediPass Series

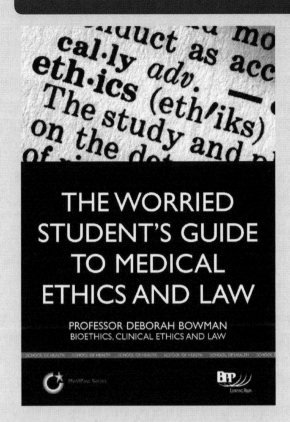

## THE WORRIED STUDENT'S GUIDE TO MEDICAL ETHICS AND LAW

PROFESSOR DEBORAH BOWMAN
BIOETHICS, CLINICAL ETHICS AND LAW

£19.99
October 2011
Paperback
978-1-445379-49-4

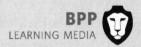
BPP
LEARNING MEDIA

*Are you confused about medical ethics and law? Are you looking for a definitive book that will explain clearly medical ethics and law?*

This book offers a unique guide to medical ethics and law for applicants to medical school, current medical students at all stages of their training, those attending postgraduate ethics courses and clinicians involved in teaching. It will also prove a useful guide for any healthcare professional with an interest in medical ethics and law. This book provides comprehensive coverage of the core curriculum (as recently revised) and clear demonstration of how to pass examinations, both written and practical. The title also considers the ethical dilemmas that students can encounter during their training.

This easy-to-use guide sets out to provide:

- Comprehensive coverage of the recently revised core curriculum

- Consideration of the realities of medical student experiences and dilemmas with reference to recently published and new GMC guidance for medical students

- Practical guidance on applying ethics in the clinical years, how to approach all types of examinations and improve confidence regarding the moral aspects of medicine

- A single, portable volume that covers all stages of the medical student experience

In addition to the core curriculum, this book uniquely explains the special privileges and responsibilities of being a healthcare professional and explores how professional behaviour guidance from the General Medical Council applies to students and medical professionals. The book is a single, accessible volume that will be invaluable to all those who want to thrive, not merely survive, studying and applying medical ethics day to day, whatever their stage of training.

www.bpp.com/health

# More titles in the Essential Clinical Handbook Series

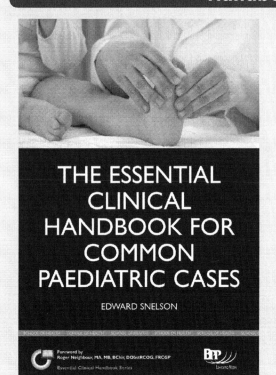

THE ESSENTIAL CLINICAL HANDBOOK FOR COMMON PAEDIATRIC CASES

EDWARD SNELSON

Foreword by
Roger Neighbour, MA, MB, BChir, DObstRCOG, FRCGP

Essential Clinical Handbook Series

BPP

£24.99
September 2011
Paperback
978-1-445379-60-9

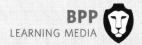

BPP
LEARNING MEDIA

*Not sure what to do when faced with a crying baby and demanding parent on the ward? Would you like a definitive guide on how to manage commonly encountered paediatric cases?*

This clear and concise clinical handbook has been written to help healthcare professionals approach the initial assessment and management of paediatric cases commonly encountered by Junior Doctors, GPs, GP Specialty Trainees and allied healthcare professionals. The children who make paediatrics so fun, can also make it more than a little daunting for even the most confident person. This insightful guide has been written based on the author's extensive experience within both a General Practice and hospital setting.

Intended as a practical guide to common paediatric problems it will increase confidence and satisfaction in managing these conditions. Each chapter provides a clear structure for investigating potential paediatric illnesses including clinical and non-clinical advice covering: background, how to assess, pitfalls to avoid, FAQs and what to tell parents. This helpful guide provides :

- A problem/symptom based approach to common paediatric conditions

- An essential guide for any doctor assessing children on the front line

- Provides easy-to-follow and step-by-step guidance on how to approach different paediatric conditions

- Useful both as a textbook and a quick reference guide when needed on the ward

This engaging and easy-to-use guide will provide you with the knowledge, skills and confidence required to effectively diagnose and manage commonly encountered paediatric cases both within a primary and secondary care setting.

www.bpp.com/health

# More titles in the Essential Clinical Handbook Series

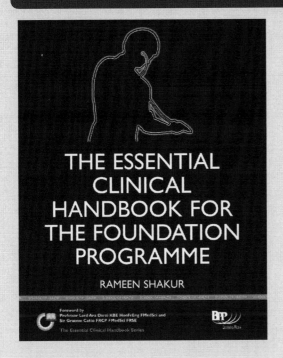

THE ESSENTIAL
CLINICAL
HANDBOOK FOR
THE FOUNDATION
PROGRAMME

RAMEEN SHAKUR

Foreword by
Professor Lord Ara Darzi KBE HonFrEng FMedSci and
Sir Graeme Catto FRCP FMedSci FRSE

The Essential Clinical Handbook Series

£24.99
October 2011
Paperback
978-1-445381-63-3

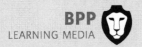

BPP
LEARNING MEDIA

*Unsure of what clinical competencies you must gain to successfully complete the Foundation Programme? Unclear on how to ensure your ePortfolio is complete to enable your progression to ST training?*

This up-to-date clinical handbook is aimed at current foundation doctors and clinical medical students and provides a comprehensive companion to help you in the day-to-day management of patients on the ward. Together with this it is the first handbook to also outline clearly how to gain the core clinical competencies required for successful completion of the Foundation Programme. Written by doctors for doctors this comprehensive handbook explains how to successfully manage all of the common cases you will face during the Foundation Programme and:

- Introduces the Foundation Programme and what is expected of a new doctor especially with the introduction of Modernising Medical Careers

- Illustrates clearly the best way to manage, step-by-step, over 150 commonly encountered clinical diseases, including NICE guidelines to ensure a gold standard of clinical care is achieved.

- Describes how to successfully gain the core clinical competencies within Medicine and Surgery including an extensive list of differentials and conditions explained

- Explores the various radiology images you will encounter and how to interpret them

- Tells you how to succeed in the assessment methods used including DOP's, Mini-CEX's and CBD's.

- Has step by step diagrammatic guide to doing common clinical procedures competently and safely.

- Outlines how to ensure your ePortfolio is maintained properly to ensure successful completion of the Foundation Programme.

- Provides tips and advice on how to start preparing now to ensure you are fully prepared and have the competitive edge for your CMT/ST application.

The introduction of the e-Portfolio as part of the Foundation Programme has paved the way for foundation doctors to take charge of their own learning and portfolio. Through following the expert guidance laid down in this handbook you will give yourself the best possible chance of progressing successfully through to CMT/ST training.

www.bpp.com/health

BPP
LEARNING MEDIA